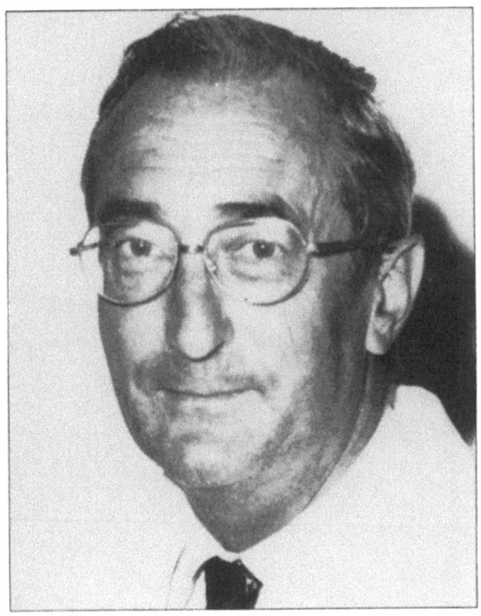

Professor W. Gepts
Scholar in the Pathology of the Diabetic Pancreas

to whom this Book is dedicated
at the Occasion of his Retirement from Academic Life

P. J. Lefèbvre   D. G. Pipeleers (Eds.)

The Pathology of the Endocrine Pancreas in Diabetes

With 72 Figures

Springer-Verlag Berlin Heidelberg New York
London Paris Tokyo

Professor Dr. Pierre J. Lefèbvre
Division of Diabetes, Nutrition and Metabolic Disorders
Department of Medicine
Centre Hospitalier Universitaire du Sart-Tilman
B-4000 Liège 1, Belgium

Professor Dr. Daniel G. Pipeleers
Dept. of Metabolism and Endocrinology
Vrije Universiteit Brussel
Laarbeeklaan 103
B-1090 Brussels, Belgium

Library of Congress Cataloging-in-Publication Data
The Pathology of the endocrine pancreas in diabetes P.J. Lefèbvre, D.G. Pipeleers (eds.)

ISBN-13: 978-3-642-72693-4 e-ISBN-13: 978-3-642-72691-0
DOI: 10.1007/978-3-642-72691-0

1. Diabetes-Pathophysiology. 2. Islands of Langerhans-Pathophysiology. I. Lefèbvre, P.J. (Pierre J.). II. Pipeleers, D.G. (Daniel G.), [DNLM: 1. Diabetes Mellitus-complications. 2. Islands of Langerhans-physiopathology. WK 835 P2975] RC660.P325 1988 616.4'6207-dc19 DNLM/DLC for Library of Congress

Softcover reprint of the hardcover 1s edition 1988

2127/3145-543210

Preface

Diabetes mellitus represents one of the most frequent and serious clinical syndromes in contemporary medicine. Since the end of the nineteenth century, the endocrine pancreas has been implicated in the pathogenesis of this disease. Several pathologists of the twentieth century detected various lesions and morphologic alterations in the pancreatic islets of diabetic patients, but the pathophysiologic basis of their findings remained long obscure. The systematic microscopic work of WILLY GEPTS clarified the views and related the variety in histopathology to differences in origin, duration and clinical expression of the disease. Over the past two decades, the concept of a multifactorial origin of diabetes has become widely accepted. Various agents and mechanisms have been identified which can lead to a quantitative or qualitative deficit in pancreatic B-cells. The purpose of this book is to bring an update on the many pathways which may induce an absolute or relative insufficiency in insulin release and hence a diabetic state. Rather than bringing a complete account on all research relevant to the understanding of the pathology of the diabetic pancreas, the authors of the various chapters of this volume have focussed on selected processes which can impair B-cell function, survival or regeneration. In combining contributions on in vitro research with chapters reviewing in vivo observations we may fail to promote uniform concepts concerning the origin of diabetes, but we hope to provide a broader and more provocative basis for the understanding and further exploration of the diverse pathology of the diabetic pancreas.

March 1988 Pierre Lefèbvre, Danny Pipeleers

Table of Contents

List of Contributors

ANDERSSON, A.
Department of Medical Cell Biology, Biomedical Centre, University of Uppsala, Box 571, 751 23 Uppsala, Sweden

ASKENSTEN, U.
Department of Tumor Pathology, Karolinska Institute, Karolinska Hospital, 104 01 Stockholm 60, Sweden

BÆKKESKOV, S.
Hagedorn Research Laboratory, Niels Steensensvej 6, 2820 Gentofte, Denmark

BONNER-WEIR, S.
Department of Medicine, New England Deaconess Hospital, Boston, MA 02115, USA

BOTTAZZO, G.F.
Department of Immunology, The Middlesex Hospital Medical School, 40–50 Tottenham Street, London W1P 9PG, United Kingdom

CERASI, E.
Department of Endocrinology and Metabolism, Hadassah University Hospital, P.O. Box 12000, 91 120 Jerusalem, Israel

DE VROEDE, M.
Department of Metabolism and Endocrinology, Vrije Universiteit Brussel, Laarbeeklaan 103, 1090 Brussels, Belgium

FALKMER, S.
Department of Tumor Pathology, Karolinska Institute, Karolinska Hospital, 104 01 Stockholm, Sweden

FOULIS, A.K.
Department of Pathology, Royal Infirmary, Glasgow, United Kingdom

HELLERSTRÖM, C.
Department of Medical Cell Biology, Biomedical Centre, University of Uppsala, Box 571, 751 23 Uppsala, Sweden

HELLMAN, B.
Department of Medical Cell Biology, Biomedical Centre, University of Uppsala, Box 571, 751 23 Uppsala, Sweden

IN'T VELD, P.A.
Department of Pathology, Vrije Universiteit Brussel, Laarbeeklaan 103, 1090 Brussels, Belgium

LACY, P.E.
Department of Pathology, Washington University School of Medicine, 660 South Euclid Avenue, St. Louis, MO 63110, USA

LEAHY, J.L.
Research Division, Joslin Diabetes Center, 1 Joslin Place, Boston, MA 02115, USA

LEFÈBVRE, P.J.
Division of Diabetes, Nutrition and Metabolic Disorders, Department of Medicine, Centre Hospitalier Universitaire du Sart-Tilman, 4000 Liège, Belgium

LEITER, E.H.
The Jackson Laboratory, Bar Harbor, ME 04609, USA

LERNMARK, Å.
Department of Medicine, University of Washington, Seattle, WA 98195, USA

LIKE, A.A.
Department of Pathology, University of Massachusetts Medical School, 55 Lake Avenue North, Worcester, MA 01605, USA

MALAISSE, W.J.
Laboratory of Experimental Medicine, Université Libre de Bruxelles, Boulevard de Waterloo 115, 1000 Brussels, Belgium

MANDRUP-POULSEN, T.
Steno Memorial Hospital, Niels Steensensvej 2, 2820 Gentofte, Denmark

MARKHOLST, H.
Hagedorn Research Laboratory, Niels Steensensvej 6, 2820 Gentofte, Denmark

MØLVIG, J.
Steno Memorial Hospital, Niels Steensensvej 2, 2820 Gentofte, Denmark

NERUP, J.
Steno Memorial Hospital, Niels Steensensvej 2, 2820 Gentofte, Denmark

PIPELEERS, D.G.
Department of Metabolism and Endocrinology, Vrije Universiteit Brussel, Laarbeeklaan 103, 1090 Brussels, Belgium

RAHIER, J.
Department of Pathology, University of Louvain School of Medicine, Hospital St. Luc, Avenue Hippocrate 10, 1200 Brussels, Belgium

SOMERS, G.
Department of Metabolism and Endocrinology, Vrije Universiteit Brussel, Laarbeeklaan 103, 1090 Brussels, Belgium

SPINAS, G.
Steno Memorial Hospital, Niels Steensensvej 2, 2820 Gentofte, Denmark

SWENNE, J.
Department of Medical Cell Biology, Biomedical Centre, University of Uppsala, Box 571, 751 23 Uppsala, Sweden

VAN DE WINKEL, M.
Department of Metabolism and Endocrinology, Vrije Universiteit Brussel, Laarbeeklaan 103, 1090 Brussels, Belgium

WEIR, G.C.
Department of Medicine, Brigham and Women's Hospital, Boston, MA 02115, USA

WERINGER, E.J.
University of Massachusetts, Medical School, 55 Lake Avenue North, Worcester, MA 01655, USA

WILSON, G.L.
Department of Anatomy, University of South Alabama College of Medicine, Mobile, AL 36688, USA

Clinical Forms of Diabetes Mellitus

P. J. Lefèbvre

Introduction

Heterogeneity in the presentation of diabetes mellitus has been recognized for many years. It was long considered, for instance, that the form of diabetes occurring in children, adolescents, and young adults was basically different from that appearing in older adults and elderly patients. As a consequence, *juvenile-onset type diabetes* and *maturity-onset type diabetes* were long opposed. This classification, based primarily on age at onset, was progressively abandoned when it was realized that some children aged 15 or less had all the typical characteristics of "maturity-onset type diabetes" and, in contrast, that some patients aged 75 or more had the features of "juvenile-onset type diabetes." Similarly, it was long implicitly considered that overt diabetes was preceded for some months or years by an intermediate state during which fasting blood glucose was normal but postprandial blood glucose higher than normal, particularly when an oral glucose load was used as a provocative test. For many years, patients exhibiting an abnormal oral glucose tolerance test were labeled as having "chemical diabetes". However, long-term studies performed in such individuals eventually revealed that, in a large percentage of them, overt diabetes failed to appear even after 25 or 30 years of consistently abnormal blood glucose levels on serial oral glucose tolerance testing. Labeling someone for 30 years a "chemical diabetic" when he or she will never become an "overt" or "true" diabetic is probably not scientifically sound, and certainly not psychologically and socioeconomically acceptable. Recently, the growth of knowledge regarding the etiology and pathogenesis of diabetes has stimulated national and international authorities to revise the criteria for the classification and diagnosis of diabetes mellitus and related disorders. Before reviewing the clinical forms of diabetes mellitus, I shall take a brief look at the recent efforts to improve the classification of diabetes and related disorders.

Classification of Diabetes Mellitus

Recent Attempts at Improvement by National and International Organizations

The major impetus for a revision of the criteria for classification and diagnosis of diabetes mellitus and related disorders came from the National Institutes of Health of the United States, which convened in 1978 an International Workgroup "to develop a nomenclature and classification system for diabetes mellitus." The conclusions of this workgroup were reported by the National Diabetes Data Group [41] and widely publicized. This classification and the revised criteria for the diagnosis of diabetes mellitus were reviewed by numerous organizations, including the American Diabetes Association, the British Diabetic Association, the Australian Diabetes Society, and the European Association for the Study of Diabetes. The Expert Committee on Diabetes of the World Health Organization accepted the major recommendations of the National Diabetes Data Group [65]. This classification comprises basically the following groups:

1. "Insulin-dependent" diabetes mellitus (IDDM) or type 1 diabetes mellitus
2. "Non-insulin-dependent" diabetes mellitus (NIDDM) or type 2 diabetes mellitus, viewed as a heterogeneous entity, in which at least two subclasses are to be considered depending on whether or not obesity is present (obese NIDDM and nonobese NIDDM)
3. A third group comprising a great variety of conditions and syndromes associated with diabetes mellitus, including pancreatic diseases, hormonal syndromes, use of numerous drugs or chemical agents, insulin receptor abnormalities, genetic syndromes, and various other conditions

In addition, the National Diabetes Data Group [41] recommended (a) that the term "gestational diabetes" should be restricted to women in whom glucose intolerance or diabetes develops or is discovered during pregnancy; (b) that the term "impaired glucose tolerance" should be used to qualify those individuals with plasma glucose levels intermediate between those considered normal and those considered diabetic, particularly during the course of an oral glucose tolerance test; and (c) that the terms "latent diabetes" and "prediabetes" should be abandoned. In a second report, the World Health Organization [66] recommended the adoption of a new entity, "malnutrition-related diabetes", which may well represent a subclass of "tropical diabetes" [1].

The New Classification from the Viewpoint of the Clinician

The new classification of diabetes mellitus and related disorders initially aimed to be used *"as a uniform framework to conduct clinical and epidemiological research"* and, from the beginning, it was explicitly stated that *"the classification is not an attempt to define guidelines for therapy of patients"* [41]. It has since become clear that the new classification and the revised criteria for diagnosis are used not only in clinical and epidemiological research, but also by numerous physicians in their daily practice. As a result, occasional problems are encountered in identifying a given patient as having type 1 (IDDM) or type 2 (NIDDM) diabetes mellitus or in considering a given patient as "normal," having "impaired glucose tolerance," or being "diabetic" [35]. In view of the extraordinary, and probably unexpected, impact that this new classification by the statisticians and epidemiologists has had on the routine clinical approach to the diabetic patient, it will be used throughout the present chapter.

Type 1 or Insulin-Dependent Diabetes Mellitus

Nomenclature

There is a general consensus to abandon the former terminology (juvenile diabetes, juvenile-onset diabetes, juvenile-onset type diabetes, ketosis-prone diabetes) and to use the term "type 1" to identify the particular form of diabetes mellitus occurring mainly but not only in young patients and characterized by a progressive loss of B-cell function due to the development of an autoimmune disease affecting the islets of Langerhans in genetically susceptible individuals. The National Diabetes Data Group [41], the World Health Organization [65, 66], and the leading journals in the field of diabetes have recommended regarding the terms "type 1 diabetes" and "insulin-dependent diabetes (mellitus)" as synonymous. This position has recently been challenged by TURNER et al. [61], who consider that it leads to some confusion.

Pathogenesis

EISENBARTH [15] has recently proposed dividing the development of type 1 diabetes into six stages, beginning with genetic susceptibility and ending with complete B-cell destruction.

The *first stage* is *genetic susceptibility*. That heredity is involved in the susceptibility to type 1 diabetes has long been suspected. The numerous studies on animal models of type 1 diabetes, reviewed in Chap. 15 by Like, have shown that at least one gene in the major histocompatibility region contributes to susceptibility to diabetes and that, at least in the nonobese diabetic (NOD) mouse and in the Bio-breeding diabetic rat (BB rat), the inheritance of diabetes is multigenic, involving one or more genes outside the major histocompatibility complex. In man, the susceptibility to type 1 diabetes is also linked to the major histocompatibility complex: among Caucasians, 90%-95% of type 1 diabetics express one or both of the histocompatibility alleles DR3 and DR4. It has been estimated that the relative risk of acquiring type 1 diabetes is 4-5 for individuals expressing DR3, 6-7 for those expressing DR4, and at least 15-20 for those expressing both DR3 and DR4. Concordance for type 1 diabetes in identical twins is about 50% [4], and as shown by JOHNSTON et al. [29], this rate is increased if the twins express both DR3 and DR4.

EISENBARTH's *second stage* is a hypothetical *triggering event* occurring in some genetically susceptible subjects. The role played by certain viruses will be reviewed in Chap. 6. Clinically suspected are Coxsackie viruses, measles virus, and congenital rubella infection. Other environmental factors such as drugs or even dietary changes have been implicated.

The *third stage* is *active autoimmunity*, a subject reviewed authoritatively in this book by pioneers and leaders in the field, namely BOTTAZZO, LERNMARK, and NERUP. The now classical islet-cell antibodies (ICAs) are the best known markers of the autoimmune process. They are found in 70%-95% of individuals at the time of diagnosis of type 1 diabetes [7], but their presence may *precede* the development of diabetes by more than 9 years [50, 53]. As reviewed by NERUP (see chapter 5), there is now evidence that the major damage to B-cells is due to T-lymphocytes, while the damaging role of ICAs, suggested by the observations of SVENNINGSEN et al. [55] is probably of lesser importance.

The *fourth stage* identified by EISENBARTH is a *progressive loss of glucose-stimulated insulin secretion*. For the clinician, the crucial marker here is a loss of first-phase insulin secretion (the peak insulin response 1-3 min after an intravenous glucose injection). It precedes the development of fasting hyperglycemia [51, 52] and probably reflects the reduction in B-cell mass.

The *fifth stage* is *overt diabetes*, which is considered to occur when 90% or more of the B-cell mass has been destroyed. Persistence of residual insulin secretion can be assessed by plasma C-peptide monitoring. Persistence of insulin secretion for months or years is frequent, and recent studies have indicated that it can be maintained in some patients by immunotherapy, administering cyclosporin A from the time of clinical diagnosis of diabetes [19, 54].

The *sixth and last stage* in the pathogenesis of type 1 diabetes corresponds to *complete disappearance of the B-cells in the islets of Langerhans*, evidenced by the absence of C-peptide in the blood, both in basal conditions and after meal-induced stimulation. Insulin lack is complete, and at this stage insulin deprivation leads to diabetic ketoacidosis, coma, and death: the patient has become totally insulin-dependent.

Some Clinical Aspects of Type 1 Diabetes Mellitus

Pre-Type 1 Diabetes

Some recent studies [11, 50, 53] have suggested that genetically susceptible individuals (subjects expressing DR3, DR4, or both, siblings of a diabetic sharing one or more haplotypes) in whom markers of anti-islet immunity (ICAs, spontaneous anti-insulin antibodies) are present and who have a defective insulin response to intravenous glucose are at high risk of developing type 1 diabetes. However, more precise evaluation of the risk would need larger and longer prospective studies. These are probably a prerequisite before considering any kind of immunotherapy in these subjects.

Remissions in Type 1 Diabetes

Clinicians have long known that after a few weeks of insulin therapy, the daily insulin needs progressively decline in many patients, leading in some of them to complete interruption of exogenous insulin while maintaining good metabolic control. Such "honeymoons" are less frequent in children and adolescents than in young adults. They are partly explained by reversal of the insulin resistance known to be present at the early clinical stage of type 1 diabetes [67]. Studies by MIROUZE and coworkers [39] have suggested that remission can be induced by early aggressive metabolic control by the artificial pancreas, by open-loop insulin infusion, or by intensive conventional insulin therapy. The possibility of spontaneous remission should always be considered when therapeutic intervention such as immunotherapy is considered in type 1 diabetes. In the recently published cyclosporin A trial performed in France [19], 18.6% of the patients in the placebo group were in complete remission at the 6th month vs 25.4% of the cyclosporin-treated patients (difference not significant). At 9 months of follow-up, however, 24.1% of the original cyclosporin group and only 5.8% of the original placebo group were in complete remission ($p < 0.01$).

Type 1 Diabetes Associated with Other Autoimmune Diseases

According to CUDWORTH [10] and BOTTAZZO et al. [6], 5%-10% of all type 1 diabetics present with autoimmune disorders affecting other organs: Graves' disease, primary myxedema, HASHIMOTO's thyroiditis, adrenal insufficiency, hypoparathyroidism, autoimmune hypogonadism, autoimmune hypophysitis, vitiligo, BIERMER's anemia, myasthenia gravis, etc. In these patients, diabetes becomes manifest somewhat later than in the classical type 1 diabetes, females are more affected than males, ICAs tend to persist longer in the plasma, and the haplotype DR3 is more frequently found. CUDWORTH [10] proposed creating a subclass 1B for these patients (as opposed to the most commonly found classical type 1 diabetes, which he proposed should be called subclass 1A).

"Brittle" Diabetes

In some patients with insulin-dependent diabetes, extreme fluctuations in metabolic control occur in spite of the best possible attempts at treatment. This situation was described by WOODYATT [64] as "brittle" diabetes. PICKUP [46] has recently proposed that the key element of brittle diabetes is *metabolic instability sufficient to cause disruption to the life-style or endanger the life of a patient.* This definition has the advantage that it makes no assumptions about the cause of brittleness and, in particular, "does not exclude inadvertent treatment errors by the physician or non-compliance and malefaction on the part of the patient" [46].

Type 2 or Non-Insulin-Dependent Diabetes Mellitus

Nomenclature

Type 2 or non-insulin-dependent diabetes mellitus affects 80% or more of all diabetic patients. The former terms used to identify these patients included adult-onset diabetes, maturity-onset diabetes, ketosis-resistant diabetes, and stable diabetes. Differentiation into two subclasses according to the presence or absence of obesity has been proposed [41]. Some confusion has emerged from the fact that even if these patients are usually not prone to ketosis and do not need insulin for the prevention of ketosis, they may require insulin for correction of symptomatic or persistent fasting hyperglycemia, if this cannot be achieved by means of diet or oral agents. When this is the case, the type 2 diabetic patient should be qualified as *insulin-requiring* (in opposition to the patient with type 1 diabetes in whom insulin is needed to prevent ketosis and to maintain life, and who is therefore *insulin-dependent*).

Pathogenesis

Heredity

There is a strong hereditary component in type 2 diabetes, but in contrast to type 1, there is no evidence of a link of type 2 diabetes mellitus with the genes of the major histocompatibility region (such as the class II genes of the HLA system).

Epidemiological studies have shown that the prevalence of type 2 diabetes is at least 2%-3% in places like the USA and Europe, with in addition a 1%-2% prevalence of undiagnosed cases, while it can reach 30%-35% in certain populations, for instance the Pima Indians in Arizona or the people living on some Pacific islands, such as Nauru [68]. Familial studies reported by KÖBBERLING and TILLIL [34] have shown that the risk for type 2 diabetes in brothers and sisters of a type 2 patient is 29%. The hereditary component is prominent in the so-called maturity-onset diabetes of young people (see below). The concordance rate of type 2 diabetes in identical twins is almost 100% [36]. Recent studies suggest that type 2 diabetes might be associated with specific alleles in the polymorphic region flanking the human insulin gene on the short arm of chromosome 11 [43]. Confirmation of the putative link between type 2 diabetes and a polymorphic locus near the insulin gene must await more extensive family studies [36]. Other recent studies have suggested that type 2 diabetes is associated with specific alleles in the region flanking the insulin receptor gene on the short arm of chromosome 19 [59].

Pathology

The islets of Langerhans of type 2 diabetes patients do not show the inflammatory lesions and progressive loss of B-cell mass that characterize type 1 diabetes. The mean features of the pancreas of patients with type 2 diabetes are reviewed in this book (see chapter 2 by RAHIER).

Impairment of Insulin Secretion

As reviewed by DE FRONZO and FERRANNINI [12], there is a whole spectrum of insulin secretion abnormalities in patients with type 2 diabetes, depending upon the duration and magnitude of the metabolic disorder, the presence or not of obesity, and the nature of the stimulus of insulin release. These factors are considered in detail in chapter 11 by CERASI.

Insulin Resistance

One of the key characteristics of type 2 diabetes is the existence of some degree of resistance to the action of insulin. The insulin resistance can be easily demonstrated by the "euglycemic-hyperinsulinemic glucose-clamp technique" [13]. The amount of glucose which has to be infused to maintain blood glucose at a predetermined level, despite infusion of insulin to achieve stable hyperinsulinemic plasma levels, is considerably less in patients with type 2 diabetes than in control subjects. Numerous studies have shown that insulin resistance concerns both the liver and the peripheral tissues. As recently summarized by TRUGLIA et al. [60], it seems that (1) insulin binding defects do not play a prominent role in the peripheral target tissues, and the status of receptors in human hepatic tissue is currently unknown; (2) a postbinding defect or defects leading to decreased insulin action appear(s) to be the primary lesion(s) in peripheral tissues; (3) increasing glucose intolerance is positively correlated with increasing resistance, so that the more severe the diabetes, the worse the cellular defect(s); (4) a relative insulin deficiency exists that becomes more pronounced as the hyperglycemia becomes greater; (5) although obesity is likely to play a major role in the development of impaired glucose tolerance and to contribute significantly to the insulin resistance of mild diabetes, its relative contribution diminishes as hyperglycemia increases. A major role in determining the severity of hyperglycemia in type 2 diabetes is played by the elevated rate of basal hepatic glucose output. For instance, in the study reported by REVERS et al. [47], in a group of untreated patients with type 2 diabetes, the mean rate of hepatic glucose production was twice that seen in control subjects (157 ± 6 vs 74 ± 4 mg/m^2/min) and a high degree of correlation ($r = 0.80$) was found between the basal rate of hepatic glucose output and the fasting glucose levels in individual subjects. A 2-week course of aggressive insulin therapy was subsequently shown to normalize this parameter [23].

The precise biochemical abnormality leading to insulin resistance in type 2 diabetes is not yet known. Using solubilized insulin receptors from circulating monocytes [25] or erythrocytes [24], two groups have reported defects in the protein kinase activity of the β-subunit of the insulin receptor in patients with severe insulin resistance. Whether or not similar abnormalities are responsible for the insulin resistance of the more common forms of type 2 diabetes remains to be ascertained by further studies.

Relationship Between Insulin Resistance and Insulin Secretion

In many diabetic patients with type 2 diabetes mellitus, plasma insulin levels, though normal in absolute terms, do not correspond with the level of hyperglycemia: *relative* insulin deficiency coexists with insulin resistance. As recently analyzed by FERRANNINI [18], the causal connection between the two defects is ambivalent:

> The B-cell may have been exhausted by the strain imposed, through hyperglycemia, by a primarily resistant periphery. Alternatively, an intrinsic secretory inadequacy of the endocrine pancreas may create gradually the milieu for the development of insulin resistance. This latter, in turn, will further stress the pancreas, thus triggering a full vicious circle. The case may be, in fact, different in different patients but the end-result is the same: tissues are refractory to insulin, free glucose builds up in the body, and the B-cell is unable to cope with the problem.

In a recent study, O'RAHILLY et al. [42] have evaluated glucose tolerance, B-cell function and insulin sensitivity in 154 first-degree relatives of 55 patients with type 2 diabetes. Reduced B-cell function was found with all degrees of glucose intolerance, whereas only the more severely hyperglycemic relatives had impaired insulin sensitivity. These data suggest that the primary defect in familial type 2 diabetes is B-cell dysfunction.

Some Clinical Aspects of Type 2 Diabetes Mellitus

Type 2 Diabetes and Obesity

Obesity is frequently associated with type 2 diabetes. Obesity by itself is a well-known factor in insulin resistance. Loss of weight reduces insulin resistance and improves diabetes control. The classical studies by VAGUE [62], confirmed by those carried out by KISSEBAH et al. [33] have shown a particularly strong statistical association between android (upper body) obesity and type 2 diabetes. Android obesity seems to play a role in the appearance of diabetes by unmasking the genetic predisposition to limited insulin secretory capacity through insulin resistance, which is one of its major characteristics. However, when diabetes is already present, possible worsening is not dependent upon the type of fat mass distribution [63].

Type 2 Diabetes of the Young

Initially described by TATTERSAL [57] and TATTERSAL and FAJANS [58] as "maturity-onset type diabetes of young people" (MODY)[1], this type of diabetes has a strong hereditary component and often affects many individuals in three or more generations. Two studies have shown that this type of diabetes is apparently not linked to the insulin gene [5, 44]. Microvascular complications are rare in MODY-type diabetes and, when present, nearly always mild [17].

Insulin-Requiring Type 2 Diabetes

As already mentioned, type 2 diabetic patients may require insulin for correction of symptomatic, or persistent, fasting hyperglycemia if this cannot be achieved by diet or oral agents. Objective estimation of the B-cell secretory capacity by determination of plasma insulin or C-peptide levels may help in determining those patients who have become insulin-requiring. However, a recent study has shown the importance of therapeutic traditions in the choice of treatment for type 2 diabetes. A typical model case of insulin-requiring patient was submitted to 400 physicians in each of three places, Northern Ireland, Norway, and Sweden. Analysis of the received forms indicated that insulin was suggested by 71% of the Norwegian doctors, but only 44% and 49% of those in Northern Ireland and Sweden respectively [9].

---

[1] Some authors prefer the term "Mason-type diabetes," Mason being the name of the family in which the syndrome was first described by TATTERSALL [57].

Tropical or Malnutrition-Related Diabetes

The 1980 World Health Organization classification of diabetes mellitus was revised in 1985 to include a new type of diabetes i.e., malnutrition-related diabetes mellitus (MRDM). Two subclasses have been identified: protein-deficient pancreatic diabetes mellitus (PDDM) and fibrocalculous pancreatic diabetes mellitus (FCPDM). This topic has been reviewed recently by BAJAJ [2], BAJAJ et al. [3], and ABU-BAKARE et al. [1]. There is a striking clinical and epidemiological association of PDDM and childhood undernutrition, such as kwashiorkor. This type of diabetes is usually not ketosis-prone. The pathognomonic feature of FCPDM is widespread formation of calculi in the main pancreatic duct and its branches. Epidemiological observations [37] have suggested an association between FCPDM and consumption of cassava (tapioca). Cyanogenic glycosides present in cassava have been implicated in the pathogenesis of FCPDM; it is likely that their deleterious effects are potentiated by concurrent low intake of proteins [2]. Another characteristic of MRDM is its frequent association with exocrine pancreatic deficiency [1].

Diabetes Associated with Other Conditions or Syndromes

In the "new classification" [41], one subclass of diabetes "forms part of certain other conditions or syndromes that often may have clinical features not associated with the diabetic state."

Pancreatic Disease

Occasionally, neonatal conditions are associated with diabetes; these include congenital absence of the pancreatic islets and the "transient diabetes of the newborn" found in infants who are small for gestational age and in the syndrome of functional immaturity of insulin secretion. Other causes of pancreatic disease include pancreatectomy, pancreatic trauma, chronic pancreatitis, tumors of the pancreas, and inherited disorders such as cystic fibrosis, hereditary relapsing pancreatitis, and hemochromatosis.

Hormonal Disorders

Diabetes or glucose intolerance can be associated with numerous endocrine disorders, including acromegaly, Cushing's syndrome, pheochromocytoma, glucagonoma, somatostatinoma, Conn's syndrome, and Laron's dwarfism.

Drugs and Chemical Agents

The list of drugs and chemical agents that can favor diabetes or glucose intolerance [41] include the following:

Diuretics and antihypertensive agents: chlorthalidone, clonidine, diazoxide, furosemide, metalazone, thiazides, etc.

Hormonally active agents: Adrenocorticotropin and derived compounds, glucagon, glucocorticoids (natural and synthetic), various oral contraceptives, somatotropin, thyroid hormones (at toxic doses), etc.

Psychoactive agents: chlorprothixene, haloperidol, lithium carbonate, phenothiazines, tricyclic antidepressants, marijuana, etc.

Catecholamines and other neurologically active agents: diphenylhydantoin, epinephrine, isoproterenol, levodopa, norepinephrine, etc.

Analgesic, antipyretic and anti-inflammatory agents: indomethacin, acetaminophen (overdose amounts), aspirin (overdose amounts), morphine.

Antineoplastic agents: alloxan, L-asparaginase, streptozotocin, megestrol acetate.

Miscellaneous compounds: isoniazid, nicotinic acid, rodenticides like Vacor, etc.

Insulin Receptor Abnormalities and Acanthosis Nigricans

KAHN et al. [30] were the first to describe two particular syndromes of insulin resistance associated with the skin condition known as *acanthosis nigricans.* Type A usually occurs in young females with signs of accelerated growth and/or virilization; the diabetes is due to a marked reduction in the number of insulin receptors. Type B is observed in older females with signs of other autoimmune diseases; the diabetes or decreased glucose tolerance is due to circulating anti-insulin receptor antibodies [20].

Genetic Syndromes

Inborn Errors of Metabolism

Diabetes Due to Secretion of a Structurally Abnormal Insulin. Recently several patients with an unusual diabetes associated with hyperinsulinemia have been described. In the original patient, the syndrome was shown to be due to an abnormal insulin in which leucine was substituted for phenylalanine in position B^{25} [56]. In another family, the mutation led to a substitution of phenylalanine B^{24} by serine [26]. In a last family, leucine substituted valine at position 3 of the insulin A-chain

[40]. Hyperinsulinemia is a feature of all patients with mutant insulins described to date [8]. Probably due to diminished clearance of the structurally abnormal insulin, these patients usually have a low C-peptide: insulin molar ratio in their peripheral plasma [27].
Others. Other inborn errors of metabolism potentially associated with diabetes or glucose intolerance include type 1 glycogen-storage disease, acute intermittent porphyria, hyperlipidemia, and hyperglycerolemia.

Insulin-Resistant Syndromes

Diabetes with insulin resistance has been described in ataxia-telangiectasia, myotonic dystrophy, MENDENHALL's syndrome, and various lipoatrophic syndromes.

Hereditary Neuromuscular Disorders

Diabetes or glucose intolerance has been described in association with numerous hereditary neuromuscular disorders, including optic atrophy, diabetes indipidus and nerve deafness, various muscular dystrophies, late-onset proximal myopathy, HUNTINGTON's chorea, MACHADO's disease, HERMAN's syndrome, FRIEDREICH's ataxia, ALSTROM's syndrome, LAURENCE-MOON-BIEDL syndrome, pseudo-Refsum's syndrome, and the syndrome associating retinopathy, hypogonadism, mental retardation, and nerve deafness.

Other Genetic Syndromes

Other genetic syndromes with which diabetes can be associated include the progeroid syndromes, PRADER-WILLI syndrome, achondroplasia, "steroid-induced ocular hypertension," epiphyseal dysplasia, and the cytogenetic syndromes of DOWN, TURNER, and KLINEFELTER.

Gestational Diabetes

The term "gestational diabetes" should be restricted to women in whom the onset or recognition of diabetes (or impaired glucose tolerance, see below) occurs *during* pregnancy. Diabetic women who *become* pregnant are not included in this class [41]. As recently reviewed by FREINKEL et al. [22], gestational diabetes mellitus (GDM) is encountered in about 2%-3% of all pregnancies. Perinatal complications are increased in these pregnancies, and probably more than half of the mothers will progress to frank diabetes mellitus under nongravid conditions [38]. The survey by FREINKEL et al. [22] emphasizes the phenotypic and genotypic heterogeneity of GDM; this condition may include slowly evolving type 1 diabetes, type 2 diabetes, and asymptomatic diabetes which antedated the pregnancy. Clinical recognition of GDM is important because therapy can prevent much of the associated perinatal morbidity and mortality. Furthermore, it has recently been recognized that the intrauterine environment may modify genetic expression in developing cells in the progeny and thereby increase the vulnerability to obesity or diabetes mellitus during later life [21, 45].

Impaired Glucose Tolerance

In the new criteria for "classification and diagnosis of diabetes mellitus and other categories of glucose intolerance" [41], the terms "impaired glucose tolerance" and "glucose intolerance" or "intolerance to glucose" are used indiscriminately. I have suggested [35] avoiding the designations "glucose intolerance" or "intolerance to glucose" because of the possible analogy with well-defined diseases due to precise inborn-errors of metabolism, such as "fructose intolerance" (deficiency of fructokinase or fructose 1-phosphate aldolase) or "galactose intolerance" (deficiency of galactose 1-phosphate uridyltransferase or galactokinase). In all likelihood such precise enzymatic defects do not underlie glucose intolerance, which is probably as heterogenous in nature as the established forms of diabetes mellitus. We have therefore suggested the use of "impaired glucose tolerance" only. Impaired glucose tolerance corresponds to a condition in which fasting plasma glucose concentration is less than that required for a diagnosis of diabetes (i.e., less than 140 mg/dl) and the plasma glucose during a 75-g oral glucose tolerance test is intermediate between normal and diabetic. "Impaired glucose tolerance" should replace terms such as "asymptomatic diabetes" and "latent diabetes" that implied the patient was at a stage of development of diabetes mellitus, which is far from being the rule [14]. In epidemiological studies, diabetes mellitus developed in 13.2% of patients within 5 years in the Whitehall survey [28], 15% over 10 years in the Bedford survey [32], 45.2% over 10 years in the study reported by Sartor et al. [48] and 38.5% over 7 years in a Japanese survey [49]. In addition, several studies of patients with impaired glucose tolerance have indicated increased prevalences of arterial disease, electrocardiographic abnormalities, and death from or increased susceptibility to atherosclerotic disease associated with other risk factors, including hypertension, hyperlipidemia, and adiposity [31].

Conclusions

Affecting at least 5% of the population in the Western World [16], diabetes mellitus is of major concern for the clinician. The "new classification" of diabetes mellitus initially aimed to be used "as a uniform framework to conduct clinical and epidemiological research," and from the beginning it was explicitly stated that "the classification is not an attempt to define guidelines for therapy of patients". The progress made over the last 8 years has largely confirmed the solid foundation of the new classification and criteria for diagnosis of diabetes mellitus. Type 1 diabetes mellitus has emerged as a disease characterized by a progressive loss of B-cell function due to the development of an autoimmune process affecting the islets of Langerhans in genetically susceptible individuals. Type 2 diabetes mellitus is a heterogeneous syndrome in which defects in insulin secretion and action are implicated and all factors increasing insulin resistance, such as obesity or sedentariness, lead to further metabolic deterioration. Malnutrition-related diabetes has been recently identified as a clinical entity of major concern in several parts of the world. Diabetes mellitus can also occur as a consequence of a mutation in the gene controlling the synthesis of insulin: although exceptional, such cases are of fundamental interest. Finally, diabetes mellitus can be associated with a myriad of pancreatic and nonpancreatic diseases, with the ingestion of numerous drugs and chemical agents, and with a growing number of genetic syndromes.

Acknowledgement. I acknowledge the expert secretarial help of E. VAESSEN-PETIT.

References

1. Abu Bakare A, Gill GV, Taylor R, Alberti KGMM (1986) Tropical or malnutrition-related diabetes: a real syndrome? Lancet I: 1135-1138
2. Bajaj JS (1986) Malnutrition-related fibrocalculous pancreatic diabetes. In: Serrano-Rios M, Lefèbvre PJ (eds) Diabetes 1985. Elsevier, Amsterdam, pp 1055-1060
3. Bajaj JS, Khardori R, Subba Rao G, Subba Rao J (1986) Malnutrition-related protein-deficient pancreatic diabetes. In: Serrano-Rios M, Lefèbvre PJ (eds) Diabetes 1985. Elsevier, Amsterdam, pp 1061-1066
4. Barnett AH, Eff C, Leslie RDG, Pyke DA (1981) Diabetes in identical twins: a study of 200 pairs. Diabetologia 20: 87-93
5. Bell JI, Wainscoat JS, Old JM, Chlouverakis C, Keen H, Turner RC, Weatherall DJ (1983) Maturity-onset diabetes of the young is not linked to the insulin gene. Br Med J 286: 590-592
6. Bottazzo GF, Doniach D, Dean BM, Cudworth AG (1981) Progrès récents sur les aspects autoimmuns du diabète. Journ Ann Diabetol Hôtel Dieu 21: 101-118
7. Bottazzo GF, Mann JI, Thorogood M, Baum JD, Doniach D (1979) Autoimmunity in juvenile diabetics and their families. Br Med J 2: 165-168
8. Chan SJ, Nanjo K, Miyano M, Lu Y-L, Welsh M, Nielsen D, Haneda M, Kwok SCM, Tager HS, Rubenstein AH, Steiner DF (1986) Abnormalities of insulin gene structure and expression: a minireview. In: Serrano-Rios M, Lefèbvre PJ (eds) Diabetes 1985. Elsevier, Amsterdam, pp 486-494
9. Criffiths K, McDevitt DG, Andrew M, Baksaas I, Helgeland A, Jervell J, Lunde PKM, Øydvin K, Agenäs I, Bergman U, Rosenqvist U, Sjöqvist F, Wessling A, Wiholm BE (1986) Therapeutic traditions in Northern Ireland, Norway and Sweden: I. diabetes. Eur J Clin Pharmacol 30: 513-519
10. Cudworth AG (1978) Type-1 diabetes mellitus. Diabetologia 14: 281-291
11. Dean BM, Becker F, McNally JM, Tarn AC, Schwartz G, Gale EAM, Bottazzo GF (1986) Insulin autoantibodies in the prediabetic period: correlation with islet-cell antibodies and development of diabetes. Diabetologia 29: 339-342
12. De Fronzo RA, Ferrannini E (1982) The pathogenesis of non insulin-dependent diabetes. An update. Medicine 61: 125-140
13. De Fronzo RA, Tobin JD, Andres R (1979) Glucose-clamp technique: a method for quantifying insulin secretion and resistance. Am J Physiol 237: E214-218
14. Diabetes Survey Working Party (1976) Ten year follow-up report on Birmingham diabetes survey. Br Med J 2: 35-37
15. Eisenbarth GS (1986) Type I diabetes mellitus: a chronic autoimmune disease. N Engl J Med 314: 1360-1368
16. Ekoe JM (1986) The diabetes mellitus syndrome: some epidemiological perspectives in the world. In: Serrano-Rios M, Lefèbvre PJ (eds) Diabetes 1985. Elsevier, Amsterdam, pp 43-49

17. Fajans SS, Clouthier MC, Crowther RL (1978) Clinical and aetiological heterogeneity of idiopathic diabetes mellitus. Diabetes 27: 1112-1125
18. Ferrannini E (1986) Insulin resistance, insulin deficiency and the pathogenesis of diabetes mellitus. Clin Physiol 6: 311-317
19. Feutren G, Assan R, Karsenty G, Du Rostu H, Sirmai J, Papoz L, Vialettes B, Vexiau P, Rodier M, Lallemand A, Bach J-F (1986) Cyclosporin increases the rate and lenght of remission in insulin-dependent diabetes of recent onset. Results of a multicenter double-blind trial. Lancet II: 119-124
20. Flier JS, Kahn CR, Roth J, Bar RS (1975) Antibodies that impair insulin receptor binding in an unusual diabetic syndrome with severe insulin resistance. Science 190: 63-65
21. Freinkel N, Metzger BE, Phelps RL, Dooley SL, Ogata ES, Radvahy RM, Belton A (1985) Gestational diabetes mellitus: heterogeneity of maternal age, weight, insulin secretion, HLA antigens, and islet-cell antibodies, and the impact of maternal metabolism on pancreatic B-cell and somatic development in the offspring. Diabetes 34 [Suppl 2]: 1-7
22. Freinkel N, Metzger BE, Phelps RL, Simpson JL, Martin AO, Radvany R, Ober C, Dooley SL, Depp RO, Belton A (1986) Gestational diabetes mellitus: a syndrome with phenotypic and genotypic heterogeneity. Horm Metab Res 18: 427-430
23. Garvey WT, Olefsky JM, Griffin J, Hamman F, Kolterman OG (1985) The effect of insulin tréatment on insulin secretion and insulin action in Type II diabetes mellitus. Diabetes 34: 222-234
24. Grigorescu F, Flier JS, Kahn CR (1984) Defect in insulin receptor phosphorylation in erythrocytes and fibroblasts associated with severe insulin resistance. J Biol Chem 259: 15003-15006
25. Grunberger G, Comi RJ, Taylor SI, Gorden P (1984) Tyrosine kinase activity of the insulin receptor of patients with type A extreme insulin resistance: studies with circulating mononuclear cells and cultured lymphocytes. J Clin Endocrinol Metab 59: 1152-1158
26. Haneda M, Chan SJ, Kwok SCM, Rubenstein AH, Steiner DF (1983) Studies on mutant human insulin genes: identification and sequence analysis of a gene encoding [Ser ^{B24}] insulin. Proc Natl Acad Sci USA 80: 6366-6370
27. Haneda M, Polonsky KS, Bergenstal RM, Jaspan JB, Shollson SE, Blix PM, Cham SJ, Kwok SCM, Wishner WB, Zeidler A, Olefsky JM, Freidenberg G, Tager HS, Steiner DF, Rubenstein AH (1984) Familial hyperinsulinemia due to a structurally abnormal insulin: definition of an emerging new clinical syndrome. N Engl J Med 310: 1288-1294
28. Jarrett RJ, Keen H, Fuller JH, McCartney M (1979) Worsening to diabetes in men with impaired glucose tolerance ("borderline diabetes"). Diabetologia 16: 25-30
29. Johnston C, Pyke DA, Cudworth AG, Wolf E (1983) HLA-DR typing in identical twins with insulin-dependent diabetes: difference between concordant and discordant pairs. Br Med J 286: 253-255
30. Kahn CR, Flier JS, Bar RS, Archer JA, Gorden P, Martin MM, Roth J (1976) The syndromes of insulin resistance and acanthosis nigricans. Insulin-receptor disorders in man. N Engl J Med 294: 739-745
31. Keen HJ, Jarrett RJ, Fuller JH (1974) Tolbutamide and arterial disease in borderline diabetics. In: Malaisse WJ, Pirart J (eds) Proceeding of the VIII congress IDF, Brussels, 15-20/7/1973. Excerpta Medica, Amsterdam, pp 588-602
32. Keen H, Jarrett RJ, McCartney P (1982) The ten-year follow-up of the Bedford survey (1962-1972): glucose tolerance and diabetes. Diabetologia 22: 73-78
33. Kissebah AH, Vydelingun N, Murray R, Evans DJ, Hartz AJ, Kalhoff RK, Adams PW (1982) Relation of body fat distribution to metabolic complications of obesity. J Clin Endocr Metab 54: 254-260
34. Köbberling J, Tillil H (1982) Empirical risk figures for first degree relatives of non-insulin dependent diabetics. In: Köbberling J, Tattersall R (eds) The genetics of diabetes mellitus. Academic, London, pp 201
35. Lefèbvre P (1982) Diabetes and the new criteria seen by the clinician. In: Eschwege E (ed) Advances in diabetes epidemiology. Elsevier, Amsterdam, pp 3-6
36. Leslie RDG, Pyke DA (1985) Genetics of diabetes. In: Alberti KGMM, Krall L (eds) The diabetes annual I. Elsevier, Amsterdam, pp 53-66
37. McMillan DA, Geevarghese PH (1979) Dietary cyanide and tropical malnutrition diabetes. Diabetes Care 2: 202-208

38. Metzger BE, Bybee DE, Freinkel N, Phelps RL, Radvany RM, Vaisrub N (1985) Gestational diabetes mellitus: correlations between the phenotypic and genotypic characteristics of the mother and abnormal glucose tolerance during the first year postpartum. Diabetes 34 [Suppl 2]: 111-115
39. Mirouze J, Selam J-L, Pham TC, Mendoza E, Orsetti A (1978) Sustained insulin-induced remissions of juvenile diabetes by mean of an external artificial pancreas. Diabetologia 14: 223-227
40. Nanjo K, Sanke T, Miyano M, Okai K, Sowa R, Kondo M, Nishimura S, Iwo K, Miyamura K, Given BD, Chan SJ, Tager HS, Steiner DF, Rubenstein AH (1986) Diabetes due to secretion of a structurally abnormal insulin (Insulin Wakayama). Clinical and functional characteristics of [Leu ^{A3}] insulin. J Clin Invest 77: 514-519
41. National Diabetes Data Group (1979) Classification and diagnosis of diabetes mellitus and other categories of glucose intolerance. Diabetes 28: 1039-1057
42. O'Rahilly SP, Rudenski AS, Burnett MA, Nugent S, Hosker JP, Darling P, Turner RC (1986) Beta-cell dysfunction, rather than insulin insensitivity, is the primary defect in familial type-2 diabetes. Lancet II: 360-364
43. Owerbach D, Nerup J (1982) Restriction fragment lenght polymorphism of the insulin gene in diabetes mellitus. Diabetes 31: 275-277
44. Owerbach D, Thomsen B, Johansen K, Lamm LU, Nerup J (1983) DNA insertion sequences near the insulin gene are not associated with maturity-onset diabetes of young people. Diabetologia 25: 18-20
45. Pettitt DJ, Bennett PH, Knowler WC, Baird R, Aleck KA (1985) Gestational diabetes mellitus and impaired glucose tolerance during pregnancy. Long-term effects on obesity and glucose tolerance in the offspring. Diabetes 34 [Suppl 2]: 119-122
46. Pickup JC (ed) (1985) Brittle diabetes. Blackwell, Oxford
47. Revers RR, Finck R, Griffin J, Olefsky JM, Kolterman OG (1984) Influence of hyperglycemia on insulin's in vivo effects in type II diabetes. J Clin Invest 73: 664-672
48. Sartor G, Schersten B, Carlström S, Melander A, Norden A, Persson G (1980) Ten year follow-up of subjects with impaired glucose tolerance: prevention of diabetes by tolbutamide and diet regulation. Diabetes 29: 41-49
49. Sasaki A, Suzuki T, Horiuchi N (1982) Development of diabetes in Japanese subjects with impaired glucose tolerance: a seven year follow-up study. Diabetologia 22: 154-157
50. Srikanta S, Ganda OP, Eisenbarth GS, Soeldner JS (1983) Islet-cell antibodies and beta cell function in monozygotic triplets and twins initially discordant for type 1 diabetes mellitus. N Engl J Med 308: 322-325
51. Srikanta S, Ganda OP, Gleason RE, Jackson RA, Soeldner JS, Eisenbarth GS (1984) Pre-type 1 diabetes: linear loss of beta cell response to intravenous glucose. Diabetes 33: 717-720
52. Srikanta S, Ganda OP, Jackson RA, Brink SJ, Fleischnick E, Yunis E, Alper C, Soeldner JS, Eisenbarth GS (1984) Pre-type 1 (insulin-dependent) diabetes: common endocrinological course despite immunological and immunogenetic heterogeneity. Diabetologia 27: 146-148
53. Srikanta S, Ganda OP, Jackson RA, Gleason RE, Kaldany A, Garovoy MR, Milford ER, Carpenter CB, Soeldner JS (1983) Type-1 diabetes mellitus in monozygotic twins: chronic progressive Beta cell dysfunction. Ann Intern Med 99: 320-326
54. Stiller CR, Dupré J, Gent M, Jenner MR, Keown PA, Laupacis A, Martell R, Rodger NW, Von Graffenried B, Wolfe BM (1984) Effect of cyclosporine immunosuppression in insulin-dependent diabetes mellitus of recent onset. Science 223: 1362-1367
55. Svenningsen A, Dyrberg T, Gerling I, Mackay P, Rabinowitch A (1983) Inhibition of insulin release after passive transfer of immunoglobulin from insulin-dependent diabetic children to mice. J Clin Endocrinol Metab 57: 1301-1304
56. Tager HS, Thomas N, Assoian R, Rubenstein AH, Saekow M, Olefsky J, Kaiser ET (1980) Semisynthesis and biological activity of porcine [Leu B^{24}] and [Leu B^{25}] insulin. Proc Natl Acad Sci USA 77: 3181-3185
57. Tattersal RB (1974) Mild familial diabetes with dominant inheritance. Q J Med 43: 339
58. Tattersal RB, Fajans SS (1975) A difference between the inheritance of classical juvenile-onset and maturity-onset type diabetes of young people. Diabetes 24: 44-53
59. Trembath RC, O'Connor G, Galton DJ (1986) An insulin receptor gene polymorphism and Type 2 (non-insulin-dependent) diabetes mellitus. Diabetologia 29: 601 A

60. Truglia JA, Livingston JN, Lockwood DH (1985) Insulin resistance: receptor and post-binding defects in human obesity and non insulin-dependent diabetes mellitus. Am J Med 79 [Suppl 2B]: 13-22
61. Turner RC, Holman RR, Matthews DR, O'Rahilly SP, Rudenski AS, Braund WJ (1986) Diabetes nomenclature: classification or grading of severity. Diabe Med 3: 216-220
62. Vague J (1956) The degree of masculine differentiation of obesities: a factor determining predisposition to diabetes, atherosclerosis, gout and uric calculous disease. Am J Clin Nutr 4: 20-34
63. Vague P, Vallo De Castro J, Vague J (1985) Association between adipose tissue distribution and non insulin dependent (type II) diabetes mellitus. In: Vague J, Björntorp P, Guy-Grand B, Rébuffé S, Vague P (eds) Metabolic complications of human obesities. Elsevier, Amsterdam, pp 77-84
64. Woodyatt RT (1938) Diabetes mellitus. In: Cecil R (ed) A textbook of medicine. Saunders, Philadelphia, p 620
65. World Health Organization (1980) Expert committee on diabetes mellitus. WHO Techn Rep Ser 646, Geneva
66. World Health Organization (1985) Study group on diabetes mellitus. WHO Tech Rep Ser 746
67. Yki-Järvinen H, Koivisto V (1986) Natural course of insulin resistance in type 1 diabetes. N Engl J Med 315: 224-230
68. Zimmet P, King H (1985) Epidemiology of diabetes mellitus: recent developments. In: Alberti KGMM, Krall L (eds) The diabetes annual I. Elsevier, Amsterdam, pp 1-15

The Diabetic Pancreas: A Pathologist's View*

J. Rahier

Introduction

The morphology of the pancreas in human diabetes has long received much attention. In 1845, more than 40 years before Von MERING and MINKOWSKI [105] demonstrated that pancreatectomy results in the advent of diabetes, autopsy findings had led BOUCHARDAT to the concept that diabetes is a pancreatic disease [11]. From this time on, many studies have improved our knowledge of the normal and diabetic pancreas. The most decisive one was the discovery of the islets by LANGERHANS in 1869 [51], followed, 30 years later, by the recognition of their heterogeneous composition [16]. In the early 1920s islet abnormalities were detected in the pancreas of diabetic patients [12, 49, 67, 90]. In 1951, about 30 years after the discovery of insulin by BANTING and BEST [3], the development of a bioassay for this hormone permitted differentiation of different forms of diabetes [9].

The introduction of new methodologies and concepts and the developments in the field of immunology and genetics contributed significantly to our understanding of the pathogenesis of diabetes but also revealed its diversity and complexity. It is now clear that diabetes is not a single clinical or morphological entity but corresponds to a group of diseases, sharing hyperglycemia.

Though we are still far from understanding the pathogenesis of the disease, it is clear that the endocrine pancreas is not primarily involved in all types of diabetes and that some of them are the consequence of peripheral abnormalities possibly having a secondary repercussion on the endocrine pancreas itself. This distinction is of critical importance in understanding the pathogenesis of the disease.

The classification of the World Health Organisation [119], which distinguishes insulin-dependent diabetes mellitus (IDDM) from non-insulin-dependent diabetes mellitus (NIDDM), can be useful for clinical purposes. It is, however, less well adapted to work on the morphology or pathogenesis of diabetes. Indeed, the pathogenesis of the disease and the morphological characteristics of the islets are completely different when the insulin dependency develops in children, adults, or patients with a long history of hemochromatosis.

Despite the frequency and seriousness of the disease, relatively few pathologists have focused their interest on the diabetic pancreas. This may result from the fact that the diagnosis of diabetes is not based upon a histopathological investigation. So far the only material available for morphological studies comes from autopsy

* The author's research referred to in this paper was supported by grant number 3.4560.81 of the FRSM, Brussels.

of diabetic patients. Exceptionally, biopsies have been obtained after surgery for chronic pancreatitis or from pancreatic grafts. For these reasons, it is difficult to obtain this material in a perfect state of preservation, thus restricting the use of several techniques such as electron microscopy. It is also impossible to follow the evolution of the pancreatic lesions in longitudinal studies in man.

However, the development of immunocytochemical techniques has improved the abilities of the pathologist interested in the islets of LANGERHANS. The availability of sensitive and specific antisera enables clear identification of the different endocrine cell types, quantification of their number, and some evaluation of their hormonal content. The volume density (i.e., ratio of endocrine cells to nonendocrine cells) of the immunostained cells can be assessed by morphometry and the corresponding values of total cell mass can be calculated. The advent of (semi)automatic image analyzers made it feasible to investigate large series of pancreases. Application of these immunocytochemical techniques in electron microscopy further allows a closer analysis of the functional characteristics of these cells.

The present chapter will review the contribution of pathology to the understanding of the pathogenesis of diabetes.

The Normal Pancreas, or Pancreas of Normoglycemic Subjects

Macroscopy

The normal pancreas is a compact organ, white to yellow in color, with a lobular structure. The mean weight of the adult pancreas is 75 g. Wide variation in this figure (35-150 g) has often been reported, apparently compatible with the maintenance of normoglycemia [81, 97]. KLÖPPEL has recently shown that the pancreatic weight is markedly increased in nondiabetic obese patients [45].

The pancreas is formed by the fusion of two embryological buds, the ventral and dorsal primordia [86, 95, 112]. The ventral primordium, located in the adult at the inferior and posterior part of the head, represents about 10% of the total mass of the pancreas [76]. Its relative weight is not influenced by the age of the patient [81]. Most of the PP-cells are located in this region [58, 68, 76].

Microscopy

Mesenchymal Fraction

With the exception of conditions such as cystic fibrosis [34] or Schwachman syndrome [92], the mesenchymal fraction of the human pancreas has never been studied extensively. From several recent works [78, 79, 81, 82], it can be inferred that the mesenchymal fraction is particularly high in the fetus (60%). It is reduced to

25% at birth and further decreases in infants, children, and young healthy adults. A slight increase occurs later in life.

The exact function of the pancreatic mesenchymal tissue is unknown. In chronic pancreatitis, as in other pathological conditions, the expansion of fibrous tissue often correlates with insular neoformation [4]. Currently we do not know whether this endocrine proliferation is related to the increase of mesenchymal tissue itself, to exocrine destruction, or to vascular perturbations [4, 41]. It is, however, interesting to mention that certain mesenchymal factors interfere with the ontogeny of the pancreas [19, 54] and that adjunction of collagen to monolayer cultures of pancreatic endocrine tissue, induces the three-dimensional formation of typical islets [62].

Pancreatic fat infiltration also increases with age. For still unknown reasons it is always less important in the PP-rich lobe than in the rest of the gland [71].

Insular Tissue

Most of the endocrine cells of the pancreas are located within the islets of Langerhans. However, in human neonates, up to 20% of the endocrine cells are extrainsular, scattered in the exocrine tissue, in ducts, or in their immediate vicinity [79]. The role and functional peculiarities of these non-insular endocrine cells have never been investigated. The islets are distributed throughout the whole pancreas but seem to be more numerous in the tail of the gland [60]. In the lobules they are probably not distributed at random, at least in neonates, where the regular large islets are located centrally and the small clusters more peripherally [35]. Such distribution is, however, not evident in the adult pancreas.

The amount of fibrous tissue is relatively low in healthy young subjects. With age, large fibrous septa may appear without any demonstrated repercussion upon islet function. Amyloid deposits are often detected within the islets of maturity-onset diabetic patients. They have, however, also been demonstrated in up to 23% of normoglycemic subjects. Their frequency is clearly age-related [5, 42, 67, 91, 111, 113-117].

Several reports have demonstrated that the composition of the islets depends on their embryological origin [58, 59, 68, 76] and that the proportion of each cell type varies with age [70, 78, 79].

As shown in Fig. 1, the islets which are embryologically derived from the ventral primordium are rich in PP-cells while the relative proportion of B-, D-, and mostly A-cells is clearly lower than that observed in the rest of the gland. In contrast, PP-cells are extremely rare in the dorsal primordium [59, 76].

Despite numerous studies in this field [37, 52, 98-99], the functional implication of this different cellular distribution is still unknown.

Proportion of the Different Endocrine Cell Types

The relative proportion of the different endocrine cell types also varies with age (Fig. 1) [70, 78, 79]. In the PP-poor islets of the neonate, B-cells represent approximatively 45% of the total mass of pancreatic endocrine cells, A-cells 23%, D-cells

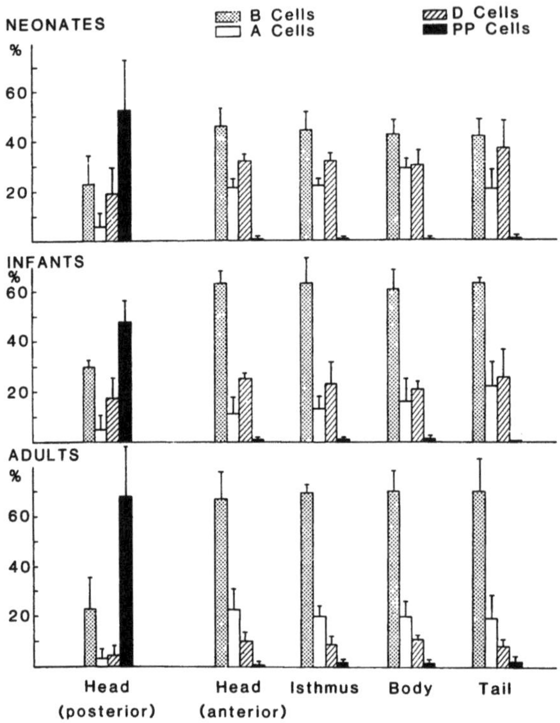

Fig. 1. Percentage of each endocrine cell type in the various regions of the pancreas of neonates, infants, and adults. [From 79]

32%, and PP-cells less than 1%. In adults, these proportions are respectively 66%, 20%, 10%, and 2%. The proportion of B-cells is thus lower in the normal neonate than in adults, whereas that of D-cells is much higher at birth than in adults. It tends to decrease in the early months of extrauterine life. The presence of a large number of somatostatin cells at birth may suggest that this hormone plays a particular and still undiscovered role during fetal or early extrauterine life. This hypothesis is reinforced by the demonstration of high levels of circulating somatostatin in the fetus [87]. Other organs, such as the thyroid, also contain a high proportion of somatostatin cells at birth [2]. In the lobe, which is rich in PP-cells, the most important modification with age is an increase in the proportion of PP-cells to the detriment of B-, A-, and D-cells [79].

Total Mass of Endocrine Tissue

The total mass of pancreatic endocrine tissue has been estimated at 300 mg in neonates, where it represents 10% of the pancreatic weight. In infants, it corresponds to 450 mg and represents 7% of the pancreatic weight [79], and in the adult it has been estimated at 1500 mg, i.e., 2% of the pancreatic weight [23, 79, 82]. So, when expressed in reference to the total pancreatic weight or to the body weight, the amount of endocrine tissue is the highest in neonates; it is lower in infants and lowest in adults. The reasons for such high proportion of endocrine tissue at birth are not clearly established. They may be related to the role of these hormones in growth and differentiation. The lower B-cell mass reported in hypotrophic neonates [103] is in agreement with this suggestion.

Individual Variations

In a given age group, the proportion of endocrine cell types is remarkably stable while the total mass of endocrine tissue varies over a wide range [79]. Normal glucoregulation can thus be maintained despite considerable variability of the endocrine cell mass. This also indicates that the maintenance of an adequate relative proportion of endocrine cells could be more critical for the maintenance of normoglycemia than their absolute mass. The variation of this proportion with age may also suggest that the hormonal interrelations could vary according to an age-related process.

The Normal Endocrine Pancreas: Its Definition on a Morphological Basis

In order to clearly determine the specific morphological abnormalities of the diabetic pancreas we should take into account all the factors which may influence the analysis. Some of them, such as the age of the patient and the origin of the specimen (from ventral or dorsal lobes) are easy to control. On the other hand, the clinical evolution of the patient and the drugs or nutrients administered before death could modify the hormonal content of the endocrine cells and interfere with their immunocytochemical quantification, but this is more difficult to control.

Large individual variations are observed in certain parameters, such as pancreatic weight and endocrine mass, and have to be taken into account.

Technical problems may also interfere with the definition of the normal endocrine pancreas: differences in the sensitivity of immunocytochemical detection resulting from the type of technique and from the quality of the antisera may influence the figures obtained in quantitative studies. This makes it sometimes difficult to compare data from different laboratories.

Finally, it is far from established that an endocrine pancreas should be considered as normal from the morphological point of view when the patient is normoglycemic and devoid of any disorders known to affect the endocrine pancreas (CUSHING's syndrome, hyperthyroidism, acromegaly, etc.). It is indeed conceivable that an adequate release of insulin (in amount and time) may be obtained with a reduced B-cell mass, as long as these cells are functionally normal. Thus, partial pancreatectomy does not result in the advent of diabetes. Also hyperinsulinism often persists after a 70% pancreatic resection in infants with persistent hypoglycemia where hyperfunction of B-cells has been implicated [83]. On the other hand, it is also possible that an abnormally low functional capacity of B-cells is compensated, at least temporarily, by an increase in their total number.

This means that what we consider to be a normal pancreas would better be called a "pancreas compatible with normal function". This would include cases where an adaptative reaction may have taken place. This concept, although liable to render the problem more complex, may also clarify certain cases and be closer to reality.

Type 1 Diabetes

The clinical distinction between juvenile-onset (type 1) and maturity-onset (type 2) diabetes was recognized a long time ago (see chapter by P. Lefèbvre in this volume). Surprisingly, this distinction was not always made in the morphological studies of the human diabetic pancreas. This may be due to the fact that cases of recent-onset insulin-dependent diabetes were more numerous in former studies. Furthermore, the recognition of four endocrine islet cell types and the knowledge that the composition of the islets varies according to the region from which they originate make it difficult to compare the data from recent studies with those from former works.

Macroscopy

In 1944, VARTIAINEN [104] mentioned the existence of a pancreatic atrophy in some cases of diabetes. MACLEAN and OGILVIE underlined the wide variability in the weight of the diabetic pancreas. As soon as a distinction was made between type 1 and type 2 diabetes, a relatively constant pancreatic atrophy was noted in type 1, amounting to 50% of the normal weight. This atrophy has even been documented after a clinical duration of only 1 year [82]. In pancreases from patients who died at the clinical onset of the disease, however, weight and macroscopic appearance are normal [44].

No correlations can be established between the weight of the pancreas, the age at onset of the disease, or its duration [82]. The reduction of pancreatic weight in chronic type 1 diabetic patients does not result from a diffuse or homogeneous atrophy: the lobe derived from the embryological ventral primordium is entirely preserved, and the atrophy is strictly limited to the PP-poor lobe derived from the dorsal primordium [81]. As a consequence, the relative weight of the PP-rich lobe (ratio PP-rich lobe/whole gland) will increase from 10% in healthy individuals to 20% and more in chronic juvenile-onset diabetics.

This atrophy is probably the morphological consequence of the disappearance of insulin, which is known to exert a trophic effect on the exocrine pancreas [1, 72, 94] as recently confirmed by experimental data [47].

Histological Appearance of the Islets

Type 1 Diabetes of Recent Onset

LECOMPTE [53], GEPTS [24], DONIACH and MORGAN [17], and JUNKER et al. [38] analyzed the morphology of the diabetic pancreas in the initial period of the disease. Their observations are invaluable, since the more recent advances in early diagnosis and treatment have made this type of material very rare. At the early stage of the disease, there are two types of islets. Some islets are small, shrunken, with a ribbon-like pattern and an irregular outline; in these, no immunoreactive B-cells can be detected. The second type is considered as hypertrophic, because its diameter exceeds 400 μm. This change probably results from a compensation for the atrophy of most of the other islets. While the old histochemical techniques such as aldehyde fuchsin were unable to demonstrate the presence of insulin in the hypertrophic islets, the more sensitive immunocytochemical methods revealed an abundance of B-cells, often partly degranulated [26]. In addition to degranulation, there are other signs of hyperactivity, such as the presence of numerous large and vesicular nuclei and an increase in the cytoplasmic RNA content, corresponding to the *Körnchen* of WEICHSELBAUM [24, 111].

Despite the occasional presence of hypertrophic and possibly regenerative islets, and although B-cells can still be detected in 14 out of the 16 recent-onset juvenile diabetics studied by Gepts, it is clear that, at the time of clinical onset, the B-cell mass is already markedly reduced (Fig. 2a) and atrophic islets are already present [24]. The recent study of a patient who died at the time of clinical onset confirms these data. Indeed, immunohistochemical quantitative methods allowed KLÖPPEL to demonstrate a reduction of the B-cell mass to one-fifth of the mean control values [44]. It is noteworthy that in this case, atrophic islets were already present.

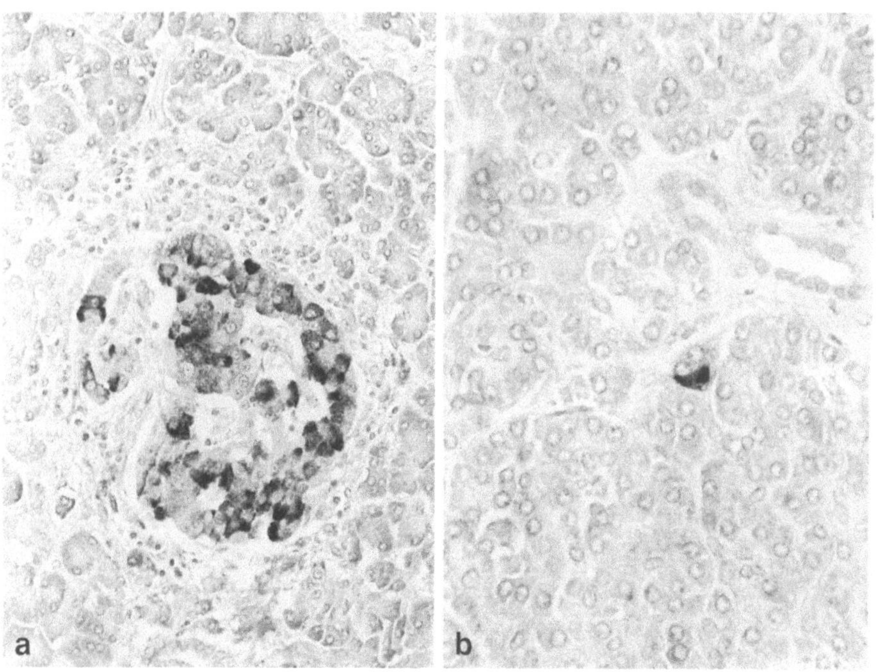

Fig. 2 a, b. Islet in type 1 diabetes. The number of immunostained B-cells is already decreased at the clinical onset (a - 190 ×). After a long duration of the disease, few B-cells can still be seen, scattered through the exocrine tissue. Immunostaining for insulin (b - 410 ×)

Variations in the size and number of islets have also been mentioned, but the relatively high variability of these parameters, even in controls, makes it difficult to draw a conclusion in the absence of quantitative studies. Insular fibrosis is also frequently mentioned in type 1 diabetes, but is more usual, although not constant, in chronic cases.

Insulitis, as initially described by VON MEYENBURG in 1940 [106], is characterized by lymphocytic infiltration of the islets. This lesion was described long ago by OPIE [67], SCHMIDT [90], and CECIL [12]. However, it was only later on that WARREN and ROOT [109], LECOMPTE [53], and GEPTS [24] recognized that this lesion is characteristic of recent-onset juvenile diabetic patients.

The lymphocytic infiltration does not involve all the islets at the same time and appears to be limited to those still containing B-cells. It is a fugacious lesion which occurs mainly in young diabetics less than 15 years old. This could explain the differences in the reported frequency of insulitis. Its exact significance has long been a matter of debate and this topic is treated in detail in another chapter of this volume (FOULIS and BOTTAZZO). It is, however, interesting to mention that in polyendocrine autoimmune disease, a similar lesion of insulitis can be observed without any insulin-requiring condition (Fig. 3; RAHIER, unpublished data). A similar case was presented by J. NERUP at the Franqui Foundation Colloquium, Brussels, in 1973.

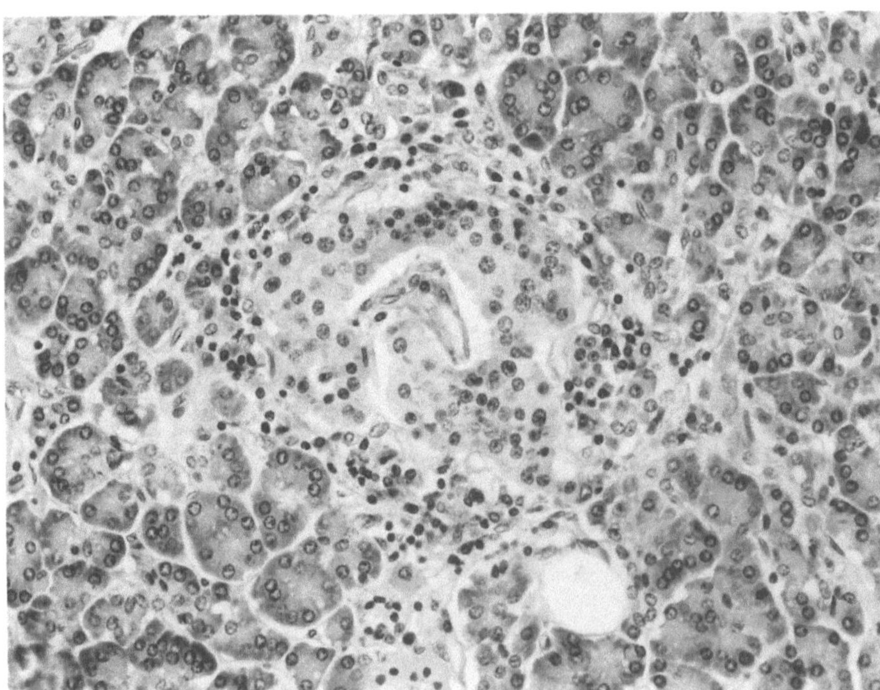

Fig. 3. Insulitis. Peri-insular lymphocytic infiltration in a patient with polyendocrine autoimmune disease. Hematoxylin eosin saffran (340 ×)

Type 1 Diabetes with Chronic Duration

After a long evolution of the disease, the insular structures become more difficult to visualize. Their form is irregular and their limits not easy to circumscribe. Thus, they share several features with the islets of the PP-rich region, where the proportion of B-cells is reduced with aging.

It has long been thought that in chronic type 1 diabetes the islets of Langerhans were entirely atrophic. The use of immunocytochemical methods has, however, demonstrated the presence of endocrine cells containing glucagon, somatostatin, and PP [26]. This is confirmed by electron-microscopic analysis (Fig. 4).

It has been suggested [69] that a hyperplasia of D-cells occurs in type 1 diabetic patients, just as in rats with streptozotocin-diabetes. However, quantitative immunohistochemical studies have shown that the increased volume density of D-cells in type 1 diabetics was only apparent, and secondary to an atrophy of the exocrine parenchyma [82]. Hyperplasia of PP-cells was also suggested [25] but further studies demonstrated that this apparent hyperplasia was secondary to a relative increase in volume of the PP-rich lobe [81]. Although rarely a few immunoreactive B-cells can be demonstrated in the pancreas of certain patients (Fig. 2b). Previous works [23, 24, 55, 56] have indicated a marked decrease in the mass of pancreatic

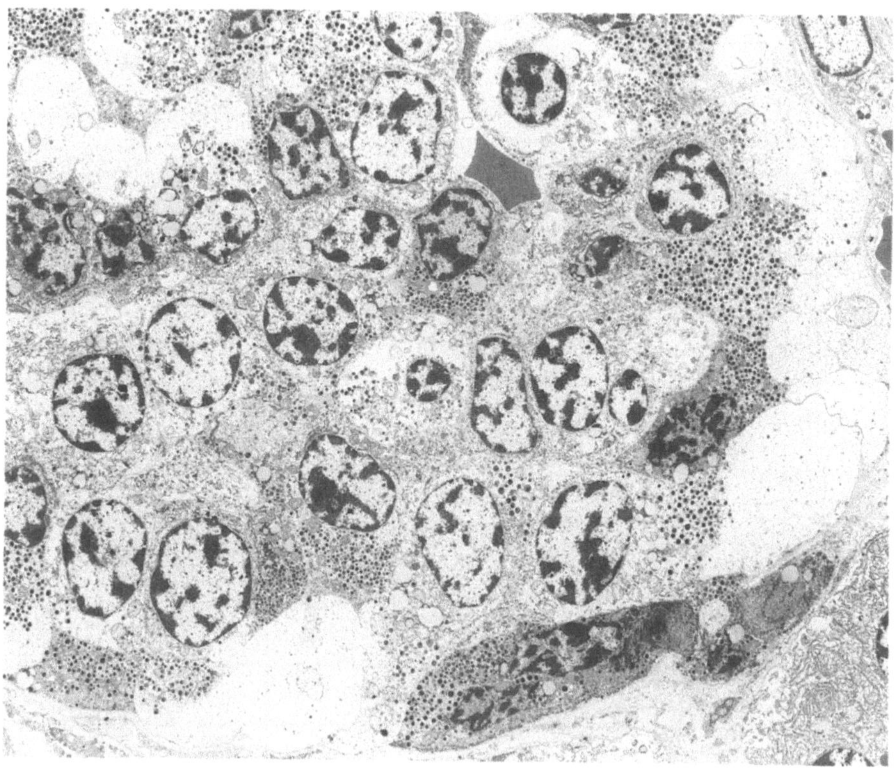

Fig. 4. Islet in type 1 diabetes after 20 years of disease. The "pseudoatrophic" islets still contain numerous well-granulated non-B-cells (2340 ×)

endocrine tissue. Quantitative immunocytochemical studies have demonstrated, moreover, that this reduction essentially affects the PP-poor lobe [82]. On the other hand, the proportion of B-cells in the PP-rich lobe is low, so that their disappearance does not affect substantially the amount of endocrine tissue in this lobe.

Although the volume density of A- and D-cells is increased, their total mass is slightly decreased (Fig. 5). This apparent discrepancy is again due to the atrophy of the exocrine pancreas. As a result of the near total disappearance of B-cells, the relative proportions of the different endocrine cell types are modified. However, the ratio of D to A does not change, suggesting that the disappearance of B-cells has no preferential influence on either of these two cell types. It can, from this, not

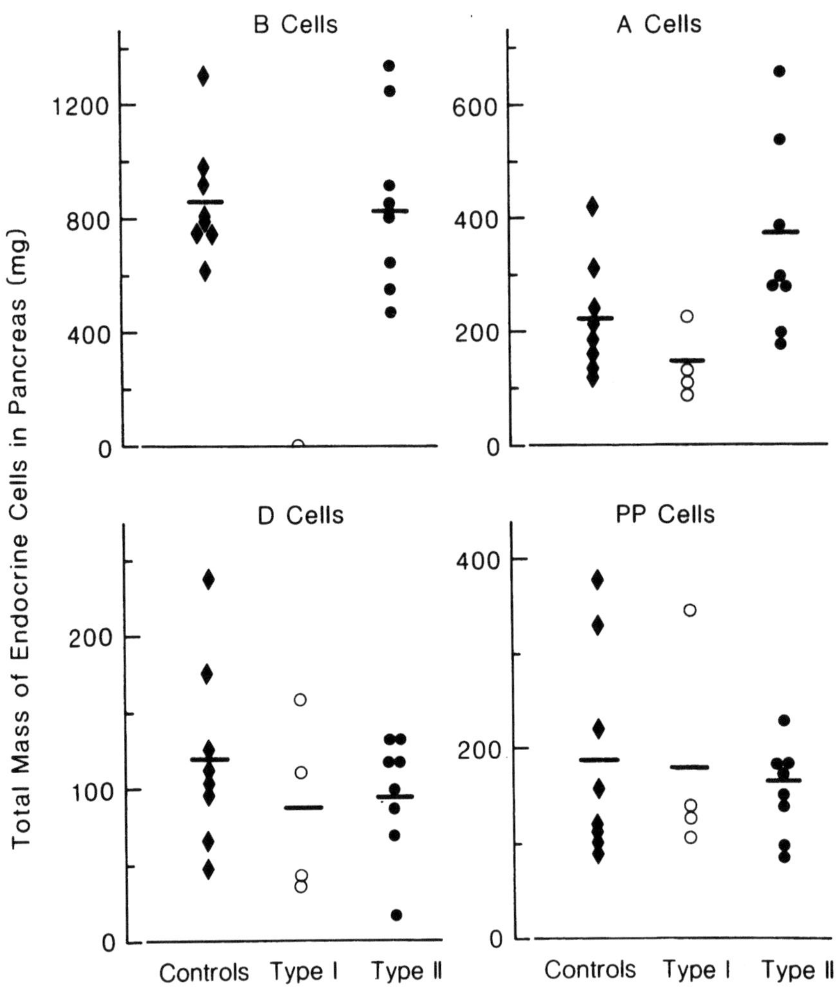

Fig. 5. Estimated total mass of each endocrine cell type in the pancreas of control and diabetic subjects [From 82]

be inferred that the interrelationship between A- and D-cells is insensitive to the architectural modification resulting from the loss of B-cells: it is for example noteworthy to mention that the proportion of D-cells which are scattered throughout the exocrine pancreas increases three- to fourfold in chronic type 1 diabetic patients [82].

Physiopathological Implications

Atrophy of the Pancreas

The atrophy of the pancreas in chronic type 1 diabetic patients may be easily explained: interactions have indeed been reported between endocrine and exocrine pancreas. The islets of Langerhans are scattered through the exocrine parenchyma, in the same way as the endocrine cells in the digestive tract. Peri-insular exocrine cells form a halo [76] where the nuclei are larger than those of the other exocrine cells [33]. Moreover, their zymogen content is higher than that of acinar cells located at distance from the islets [48], and biochemical analysis of the peri- and teloinsular acinar tissue has confirmed the existence of important differences between these two regions [57]. This may be the morphological and biological consequence of a local effect of pancreatic hormones on acinar tissue. Nevertheless, it is still unclear whether this effect is mediated by a portal system or by a paracrine mode of secretion. The role of insulin on exocrine tissue has been demonstrated in both clinical and experimental studies: it is well known that insulin stimulates pancreatic amylase excretion [1, 72, 94] and that the serum levels of amylase are lower in diabetic subjects than in healthy individuals [20]. Moreover, it has been demonstrated that the amount of messenger RNA coding for amylase synthesis is modulated by insulin [47]. The reduction in pancreas weight may thus reflect the disappearance of insulin secretion and consequently, the loss of its trophic effect on the parenchyma. However, in spite of the insulin treatment, the acinar cell nuclei from the PP-poor lobe, become, in diabetic patients, smaller than those of the PP-rich region [80]. This indicates that local insulin, more than circulating insulin, is responsible for a trophic effect.

The reason why the PP-rich region is protected from atrophy is obscure, since insulin cells also disappear from this lobe. It could be explained by a trophic local effect of PP on acinar tissue. Several arguments support this hypothesis. First, while in nondiabetic patients the nuclear volume (a marker for cellular functional activity) of exocrine cells is similar in both lobes, in juvenile-onset diabetic patients the nuclei of acinar cells are significantly larger in the PP-rich than in the PP-poor region [80]. Secondly, PP has been shown to increase the DNA synthesis of pancreatic exocrine cells in vitro [31]. Lastly, PP-cells present long cytoplasmic processes towards exocrine cells, suggesting a local interaction of PP [77].

Except for the weight reduction and, sometimes, a slightly darker colour, the general aspect of the gland is little affected. An increase in the fibrous component, although sometimes reported, is far from constant.

The Disappearance of B-Cells

Microscopically, the endocrine pancreas of chronic type 1 diabetic patients is characterized by a nearly complete loss of B-cells. This essential alteration is per se sufficient to explain the insulin-dependent state of these patients and their hyperglycemia.

However, the hyperglucagonemia reported in these patients [100, 102] may also be suspected to increase the glycemia. Though their absolute mass is slightly lowered, glucagon cells are still numerous in the islets of these patients. On the basis of the concept that insulin inhibits glucagon release [60], it can be postulated that the hyperglucagonemia results from the disappearance of insulin cells.

Insulitis

The cause of the B-cell destruction is still a matter of discussion and it remains unclear whether the mechanism involved is the same in all patients.

A possible pathogenic role has been attributed to the insulitis [24] but underlying mechanisms have not been defined. Since pancreases are usually analyzed after death of the patient, it is impossible to state precisely the frequency, the mode of appearance, and the evolution of the insulitis process.

The islet inflammatory infiltration could be secondary to B-cell necrosis due to viral infection or a toxic agent [75]. It may also correspond to a peculiar immunological reaction, indicative of or responsible for B-cell destruction. Currently, the hypothesis of *virus mediated B-cell destruction* is the one most often proposed to explain the disappearance of B-cells. Several indirect arguments, such as the seasonal occurrence of type 1 diabetes [8], the age distribution at clinical diagnosis, and the frequency of viral infection preceding onset are in agreement with this concept. Moreover, the isolation of Coxsackie-B4-like virus from the pancreas of a child dying from acute diabetes has recently been presented as a direct argument in favor of this hypothesis [120]. It must be pointed out that even in this case of acute clinical onset, atrophic shrunken islets devoid of B-cells were already present (GEPTS, personal communication). The demonstration of atrophic islets at the time of clinical onset, together with the occurrence of islet cell antibodies [29] long before the appearance of clinical symptoms, suggests that some B-cells have been destroyed before the last episode of viral infection and clinical onset.

Lymphocytic insular infiltration may constitute the morphological substrate of *immunological abnormalities.* A role for cell-mediated autoimmunity has been suggested by the results of many experimental and clinical studies and is discussed elsewhere in this volume. It is, however, interesting to remember the recurrence of diabetes in pancreatic grafts from HLA-identical twins or siblings [93]. The availability of repeated pancreatic biopsies makes this study most instructive. The appearance of well-documented insulitis, correlating with a progressive insulin deficiency, in the absence of islet cell antibodies or viral infection, reinforces the hypothesis of a specific and pathogenic role of cell-mediated autoimmunity whose morphological expression is characterized by insulitis.

The existence of a *genetic factor* predisposing to the disease has been inferred from a frequent association with HLA-B8, B15, DR3, and DR4 [14, 63]. Recent data suggest that an aberrant expression of class II antigens in conjunction with viral infection may participate in the autoimmune processes leading to B-cell destruction [10, 30].

How the combination of genetic susceptibility, autoimmunity, and virus infection can provoke diabetes is still questionable. The occurrence of repeated viral infections with each episode responsible for some degree of B-cell destruction, could lead to a progressive B-cell loss. Viral infections may also impair the function of B-cells without destroying them. Clinical diabetes would then develop in patients whose mass of functional B-cells, already reduced by autoimmune processes, is further reduced below a critical level. Transient functional recovery of the altered B-cells would explain the honeymoon period.

Type 2 Diabetes

Macroscopy

The gross appearance of the pancreas is little affected in type 2 diabetes. In our series the mean weight of the pancreas was only slightly reduced but in control series important variations were observed [82]. The relative weight of the lobe rich in PP-cells was, however, significantly increased, reaching 15% of the whole gland versus 10% in healthy individuals. KLÖPPEL has recently shown that the weight of the pancreas is higher in obese than in nonobese patients, whether they are diabetic or not [45].

The proportion of mesenchymal tissue is quite variable in type 2 diabetic patients. Fat infiltration or increased fibrotic tissue may be observed but are far from constant and are not specific for the disease.

Histological Appearance of the Islets

General Features: Hyalinosis

In some diabetic patients, the general appearance of the islets remains normal. In others, fibrosis of the islets has been reported [110]. This lesion, which may impair exchanges between blood and B-cells could explain a both delayed and insufficient insulin response. However, it is nonspecific, as it is also observed in the pancreas of nondiabetic subjects.

One of the most characteristic abnormalities is the hyalinosis of the islets, which was already described, at the beginning of this century, by OPIE [67] and WEICHSELBAUM and STRANGEL [111]. SEIFERT [91] estimates its frequency at about 50% in type 2 diabetes. It is not pathognomonic for the disease, since it is also encountered in healthy individuals. Several studies have shown that not only the incidence but also the proportion of altered islets and the degree of hyalinization increase with age [113]. Using electron microscopy, LACY has shown this hyalin material to be formed by fibrils which share the ultrastructural characteristics of amyloid. Indeed, it can easily be detected by polarization light examination after Congo red staining. The substance is completely different from the basement membrane material and is clearly distinct from the thickening of the basement membrane in small vessels. The location of the deposits between capillaries and B-cells suggests that this amyloid substance is a denaturated product of B-cell secretion. A recent immunohistochemical study has demonstrated that it possesses common antigenic determinants with the B-chain of insulin [117]. It is possible that, as in insulinoma, the amyloid deposits are related to a hyperproduction of insulin and to its evacuation outside B-cells in a denaturated form.

Although several previous studies have indicated a reduction in the number of islets, no precise quantitative immunocytochemical study is available to confirm or contradict these data. In contrast to the islets of type 1 diabetic patients, previously considered as atrophic, the islets of type 2 diabetic patients are not decreased in size. Moreover, OGILVIE has noticed that their size increases in obesity [64], a condition which is often associated with type 2 diabetes.

Mass of Insular Cells

The first quantitative studies concerning the mass of insular cells in diabetic patients stem from MACLEAN and OGILVIE [55] and GEPTS [23]. Both studies, performed on a large number of patients, conclude that there is a reduction of the endocrine cell mass in diabetics. However, an important overlap was noticed between normal and diabetic subjects, probably due to the lack of a clear-cut distinction between type 1 and type 2 diabetic subjects. The present development of quantitative immunohistochemical techniques and the availability of sensitive and specific sera raised to the various pancreatic hormones has led to reconsider this issue.

Despite adequate sampling methods and reproducible techniques for the detection and quantification of endocrine cells, conflicting results have been reported on the mass of B- and A-cells in type 2 diabetes. In the two patients studied by STEFAN et al. [96], the mass of insulin and pancreatic polypeptide cells was within the limits of the 13 nondiabetic values in the PP-rich lobe, whereas the mass of glucagon cells was increased in this lobe. In the PP-poor region, no difference was detected in the masses of endocrine tissue, except for the mass of B-cells in one case, which was lower than the lowest nondiabetic value. From our own study [82] performed on eight control and eight type 2 diabetic subjects, it becomes evident that a high variability exists in the diabetic subjects as far as the mass of B- or A-cells is concerned (Figs. 5, 6). In our series, the mean value of the B-cell mass was virtually unchanged, two patients had a mass of insulin cells at the upper limits of the normal range, three corresponded to the mean control value, and the three others were lower than the lowest value observed in controls. It is noteworthy that the only two patients who had amyloid deposits exhibited a decrease of 40% in B-cell mass.

The latter observation is in agreement with a study on 12 type 2 diabetic patients with large amyloid deposits, in which WESTERMARK and WILANDER [116] also found a decrease in the mass of islet cells of about 40%.

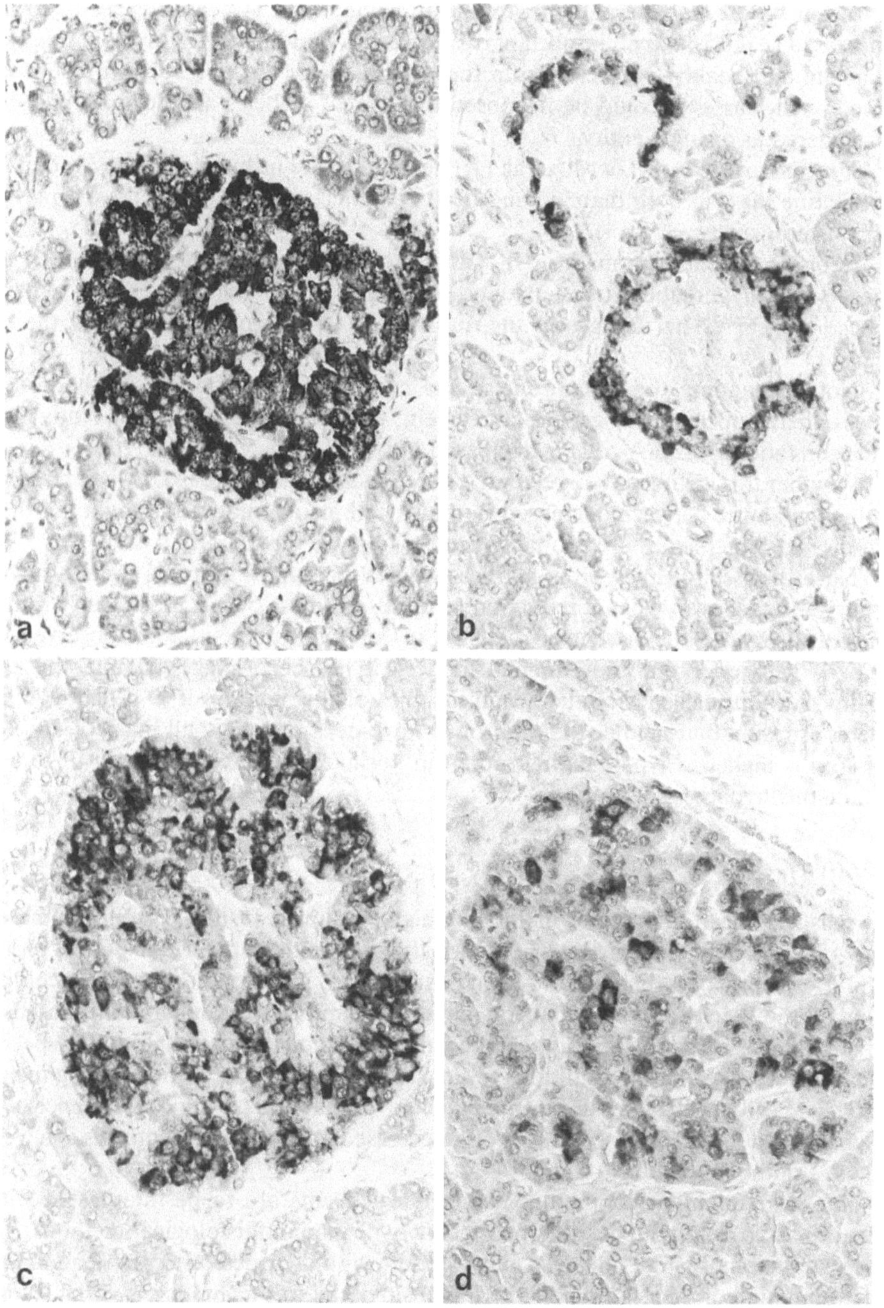

Fig. 6a-d. Different aspects of the insulin content in a normoglycemic subject (**a**) and in type 2 diabetes (**b, c, d**). The amount of insulin-containing cells is decreased in patients with large deposits of amyloid (**b**). Non-B-cells or fibrous septa sometimes dissociate the mass of B-cells (**c**). B-cells may be found scattered through the islet (**d**). These morphological peculiarities are, however, not specific for type 2 diabetes (220 ×)

In our type 2 diabetic patients, the mean value of the A-cell mass seems to be increased ($p = 0.5$), but an important overlap exists between the figures obtained in diabetic and healthy subjects. From the heterogeneity of the results, for both B- and A-cell masses it could be proposed that type 2 diabetes should no longer be considered as a single entity.

A recent article by Klöppel et al. [45] devoted to the influence of obesity on the endocrine mass in both diabetic and healthy subjects may explain, at least partly, this heterogeneity.

In obese patients, the mass of B-cells is increased whether they are diabetic or not. However, in diabetic obese patients, it remains, on average, lower than in non-obese diabetics. The changes in the mass of the A-cells parallel those of the B-cells.

Notwithstanding the discordant results concerning the changes in the A-cell mass, there appears to be general agreement, with the exception of one study [88], that the ratio of B- to A-cells is decreased in type 2 diabetes [45, 82, 96].

Whether this is linked to a decreased B-cell mass, to an increased A-cell mass or to an imbalance between decreased B- and A-cell mass remains unknown. Further studies on larger series are probably needed to solve this point.

Nevertheless, it is likely from all these studies that type 2 diabetes is not a single entity and that even when a reduction of the B-cell mass occurs, it is clearly insufficient to explain the advent of diabetes, in contrast to the situation observed in type 1 diabetes. From experimental models, it has been suggested that the impaired insulin release is related to an increase of the number of D-cells [69]. The demonstration that neither the ratio of D- to B-cells nor the total mass of D-cells (Fig. 5) is higher in type 2 diabetes than in normal individuals, allowed us to exclude this hypothesis [82].

Activity of B-Cells

B-cells have been reported to maintain a high amount of insulin granules in maturity-onset diabetic patients [5]. This contrasts with the degranulated aspect of residual B-cells in type 1 diabetes of recent onset. It can, however, hardly be concluded that all the B-cells of type 2 diabetic patients are still fully granulated and insensitive to glucose. In fact, immunocytochemical techniques performed under specifically selected technical conditions reveal striking differences in the labeling intensity from cell to cell, at least in some patients. Whether this is the consequence of a hypersecretion of certain B-cells or of a decrease in their insulin synthesis is nevertheless questionable.

All these quantitative immunocytochemical results are to be interpreted with caution. It is clear that, despite the sensitivity of immunohistological methods, the degranulation of endocrine cells may interfere with their detection and lead to underestimation of their number [83]. The sensitivity of this technique is variable and highly dependent upon many technical conditions and the reagents used. Moreover, we have to keep in mind that all the studies are performed on post-mortem material and that differences in clinical and therapeutic conditions may also interfere with the results.

Pathophysiological Implications

B-Cell Deficiency

As discussed above, the B-cell mass has been evaluated as either moderately decreased or within the range of normal values. In this context, the hyperglycemia of these patients is particularly surprising and it must be concluded that the function, more than the B-cell mass, is responsible for the disease. Several recent clinical studies have demonstrated the existence of functional abnormalities in B-cells. The shift of the dose-response curve for glucose-induced insulin release has led to the hypothesis of a decreased sensitivity to glucose [13]. A lack of the first-phase insulin response to intravenous glucose has been documented [73]. The rapid insulin release in response to arginin or isoproterenol still increases with the elevation of the ambient glucose level in type 2 diabetic patients [32], but remains as the other responses consistently lower than in controls, documenting again the impaired B-cell sensitivity to glucose. Finally, the recent demonstration of a decreased maximal insulin responsiveness to the potentiating effect of glucose also suggests the existence of an important functional defect in B-cells [108].

Possible Functional Implications of the Morphological Abnormalities

The morphological substrate of these secretory abnormalities, if any, remains a matter of debate. The sluggish insulin response could perhaps result from a decreased availability of glucose to the B-cells. The presence of amyloid deposits between B-cells and capillaries has been incriminated as a possible responsible factor. One must consider against this hypothesis, the lack of specificity of these deposits; however, they are most often far less abundant in nondiabetic than in diabetic patients. The observation that B-cells located in the vicinity of amyloid deposits are often markedly granulated gives some support to this concept [115]. The apparent lack of morphological signs of hyperactivity in B-cells, such as a decreased Golgi area [40, 114] has also been considered as supporting the hypothesis of a B-cell insensitivity to glucose [27]. On the other hand, morphometrical studies have demonstrated the existence of an increased rate of B-cell polyploidy in maturity-onset diabetic patients [74]. Whether this expresses a cellular hyperactivity or a pathological consequence of a prolonged exposure of B-cells to hyperglycemia (glucose stress) is still unclear [118]. The persistence of well-granulated B-cells has been interpreted as the consequence of an insulin release deficiency, secondary to a decrease in B-cell sensitivity to glucose. It is, however, not established that all B-cells are fully granulated. Indeed, as already stated above, under selected technical conditions, immunocytochemistry reveals variable levels of labeling from cell to cell in some maturity-onset diabetes patients.

In conclusion, despite the numerous morphological changes occurring in the maturity-onset diabetes pancreas their inconstancy and lack of specificity make it still difficult to ascertain which one if any, could be responsible for the disease.

Insulin Resistance

Although it has been previously questioned, it seems now clear that a B-cell deficiency, associated with peripheral insulin resistance and hepatic glucose hyperproduction, contributes to the hyperglycemia in type 2 diabetic patients [66, 108]. Insulin resistance may be due to a decrease in the number of receptors, possibly associated with a postreceptor defect, both leading to a lowering of glucose transport. States of mild insulin resistance are essentially attributable to a decrease in receptor number, whereas in patients with severe diabetes, the participation of a postreceptor defect becomes more prominent [46]. Adequate treatment partially reverses (50%–70%) this insulin resistance [89].

The increased hepatic production of glucose also intervenes in the occurrence of hyperglycemia and diabetes. It could be the consequence of hyperglucagonemia but may also result from the liver insulin resistance. The role of this glucose hyperproduction is primordial in determining fasting hyperglycemia whereas peripheral insulin resistance is mainly responsible for postprandial hyperglycemia. The relative importance of these factors is, however, still unknown. It remains also difficult to decide which of these is the primary event initiating the disease [65, 66].

A certain degree of insulin resistance is often associated with obesity. Overstimulation of B-cells produces hyperinsulinism and secondary downregulation of the receptors. For a certain time, the pancreas would be able to compensate with a B-cell hyperplasia [18, 39]. This would explain the higher mass of B-cells measured in obese patients [45, 64]. Exceeding the ability of the pancreas to compensate would result in the development of diabetes. Formal morphological proof is not yet available to corroborate this interpretation.

Bihormonal Dysregulation

It has been said that diabetes is a disease implicating a bihormonal dysregulation, since the metabolic abnormalities can only be explained by the coexistence of both an absolute or relative insulin deficiency and a glucagon oversecretion [100, 102].

Most of the morphological studies agree in concluding that the A/B ratio is clearly increased in diabetes. Furthermore, the presence of islets where glucagon cells are by far more numerous than B-cells could also account for a glucagon hypersecretion if one takes into consideration that insulin regulates glucagon secretion [60, 61]. The precise contribution of these abnormalities to the development of diabetes is still unclear.

Conclusions

The specific contribution of pathology to the understanding of the pathogenesis of diabetes has been reviewed. Four major concepts emerge from this analysis.

1. It is difficult to establish the limits and criteria of "morphological normality" of the endocrine pancreas. This partly results from a lack of information concern-

ing the possible effects of various factors (such as aging, environmental factors, circumstances of death, and ethnic origin) upon the morphology of this tissue.
2. In type 1 diabetes, the disease is secondary to the disappearance of B-cells, but the pathogenesis of this event is still unclarified. From a morphological point of view, the early clinical stage of the disease is characterized by a lymphocytic infiltration of the islets, the latter being considered as the expression of an autoimmune process, in which a viral infection may possibly play a role.
3. In type 2 diabetes, the mass of B-cells may be increased, normal, or moderately decreased, and various morphological abnormalities are observed, though not systematically, in the islets of these patients. From these data, it can be inferred that:
   a) The diabetic symptomatology does not result from an overt decrease of the B-cell mass but rather from abnormal B-cell function and/or impaired peripheral responsiveness to insulin. It is still unknown which morphological abnormality (if any) is related to the disease.
   b) Maturity onset diabetes can no longer be considered as a single entity, and further studies are needed to explain the clinical and morphological heterogeneity observed in these patients.
4. Progress in the understanding of this disease is dependent on the development of new tools, allowing a more functional analysis of the various parameters available to the pathologist.

Acknowledgements. I thank J. M. Ketelslegers for critical reading of the manuscript and E. Vaes for secretarial assistance.

References

1. Adler G, Kern HF (1975) Regulation of exocrine pancreatic secretory process by insulin in vivo. Horm Metabol Res 7: 290-296
2. Alumets J, Hakanson R, Lundqvist G, Sundler F, Thorell J (1980) Ontogeny and ultrastructure of somatostatin and calcitonin cells in the thyroid gland of the rat. Cell Tissue Res 206: 193-201
3. Banting FG, Best CH (1922) The internal secretion of the pancreas. J Lab Clin Med 7: 251-266
4. Bartow SA, Mukai K, Rosai J (1981) Pseudoneoplastic proliferation of endocrine cells in pancreatic fibrosis. Cancer 47: 2627-2633
5. Bell ET (1953) The incidence and significance of degranulation of the B cells in diabetes mellitus. Diabetes 2: 125-129
6. Bell ET (1959) Hyalinization of the islets of Langerhans in nondiabetic individuals. Am J Pathol 35: 801-805
7. Berson S, Yalow R (1961) Plasma insulin in health and disease. Am J Med 31: 882
8. Bloom A, Haes TM, Gamble DR (1975) Register of newly diagnosed diabetic children. Br Med J 3: 580-583
9. Bornstein J, Lawrence RD (1951) Plasma insulin in human diabetes mellitus. Br Med J 1: 1541-1548
10. Bottazzo GF, Pujoll Borell R, Hanafusa T (1983) Role of aberrant HLA-DR expression and antigen presentation in induction of endocrine autoimmunity. Lancet 2: 1115-1119
11. Bouchardat A (1845) Quoted by Kraus EJ (1929)
12. Cecil RL (1909) A study of the pathological anatomy of the pancreas in 90 cases of diabetes mellitus. J Exp Med 2: 266

13. Cerasi E, Luft R, Efendic S (1972) Decreased sensitivity of the pancreatic beta cells to glucose in prediabetic and diabetic subjects. Diabetes 21: 224-234
14. Cudworth AG (1978) Type 1 diabetes mellitus. Diabetologia 14: 281-291
15. Defronzo RA, Ferrannini E, Koivisto V (1983) New concepts in the pathogenesis and treatment of noninsulin-dependent diabetes mellitus. Am J Med, Diabetes Symposium, 52-76
16. Diamare V (1889) Studi comparativi sulle isole di Langerhans del pancreas. Mem La Int Monat Anat Physiol 16: 155-208
17. Doniach I, Morgan AG (1973) Islets of Langerhans in juvenile diabetes mellitus. Clin Endocrinol 2: 233-248
18. Fajans SS (1983) Heterogeneity of diabetes mellitus. In: Mngola EN (ed) Diabetes 1982. Excerpta Medica, Amsterdam, pp 229-235
19. Filosa S, Pictet R, Rutter WJ (1975) Positive control of cyclic AMP on mesenchymal factor controlled DNA synthesis in embryonic pancreas. Nature 257: 702-704
20. Foo Y, Rosalki SB, Ramdial L, Mikhailidis D, Dandona P (1980) Serum isoamylase activities in diabetes mellitus. J Clin Pathol 33: 1102-1105
21. Foulis AK, Stewart JA (1984) The pancreas in recent-onset Type 1 (insulin-dependent) diabetes mellitus: insulin content of islets, insulitis and associated changes in the exocrine acinar tissue. Diabetologia 26: 456-461
22. Fujita T (1966) D-Zellen der Pankreasinseln beim Diabetes mellitus mit besonderer Berücksichtigung ihrer Argyrophilie. Z Zellforsch 69: 363-370
23. Gepts W (1958) Die histopathologischen Veränderungen der Langerhansschen Inseln und ihre Bedeutung in der Frage der Pathogenese des menschlichen Diabetes. Endokrinologie 36: 185-211
24. Gepts W (1965) Pathological anatomy of the pancreas in juvenile diabetes mellitus. Diabetes 14: 619-633
25. Gepts W, De Mey J, Marichal-Pipeleers M (1977) Hyperplasia of "pancreatic polypeptide" cells in the pancreas of juvenile diabetics. Diabetologia 13: 27-34
26. Gepts W, De Mey J (1978) Islet cell survival determined by morphology. An immunocytochemical study of the islet of Langerhans in juvenile diabetes mellitus. Diabetes 27 [Suppl 1]: 251-261
27. Gepts W, LeCompte PH (1981) The pancreatic islets in diabetes. Am J Med 70: 105-115
28. Gepts W (1982) Pathology of the pancreas in diabetes. In: Brodoff BN, Bleicher SJ (eds) Diabetes mellitus and obesity. Williams and Wilkins, Baltimore, pp 622-633
29. Gorsuch AN, Lister J, Dean BM, Spencer KM, McNally JM, Bottazzo GF (1981) Evidence for a long prediabetic period in type I (insulin-dependent) diabetes mellitus. Lancet 19/26: 1363-1366
30. Gorsuch AN, Spencer KM, Lister J, Wolf E, Bottazzo GF, Cudworth AG (1982) Can future type diabetes be predicted? A study in families of affected children. Diabetes 31: 862-867
31. Greenberg GR, Mitznegg P, Bloom SR (1977) Effect of pancreatic polypeptide on DNA-synthesis in the pancreas. Experienta 33: 1332-1333
32. Halter JB, Graf RJ, Porte D (1979) Potentiation of insulin secretory responses by plasma glucose levels in man: evidence that hyperglycemia in diabetes compensates for impaired glucose potentiation. J Clin Endocrinol Metab 48: 946-954
33. Hellman B, Wallgren A, Peterson B (1962) Cytological characteristics of the exocrine pancreatic cells with regard to their position in relation to the islets of Langerhans. Acta Endocrinol 39: 465-473
34. Imrie JR, Fagan DG, Sturgess JM (1979) Quantitative evaluation of the development of the exocrine pancreas in cystic fibrosis and control infants. Am J Pathol 95: 697-708
35. Jaffe R, Hashida Y, Yunis EJ (1980) Pancreatic pathology in hyperinsulinemic hypoglycemia of infancy. Lab Invest 42: 356-365
36. Jarotsky AJ (1899) Über die Veränderungen in der Größe und im Bau der Pankreaszellen bei einigen Arten der Inanition. Virchows Arch 155: 409-450
37. Jarousse C, Jeanrenaud B (1982) Functional differences of the endocrine pancreas due to specific blood supply. Diabetologia 23: 177
38. Junker K, Egeberg J, Kromann H (1977) An autopsy study of the islets of Langerhans in acute onset juvenile diabetes mellitus. Acta Pathol Microbiol Scand [Sect A] 85: 699-706
39. Karam JH (1982) Obesity and diabetes in humans. In: Brodoff BN, Bleicher SJ (eds) Diabetes mellitus and obesity. Williams and Wilkins, Baltimore, pp 294-400

40. Kawanishi H, Akazawa Y, Machii B (1966) Islets of Langerhans in normal and diabetic humans. Acta Pathol Jpn 16: 177-197
41. Klöppel G, Bommer G, Commandeur G, Heitz PU (1978) The endocrine pancreas in chronic pancreatitis. Virchows Arch [A] 377: 157-174
42. Klöppel G (1981) Endokrines Pankreas und Diabetes mellitus. In: Doerr W, Seifert G (eds) Spezielle pathologische Anatomie, vol 14. Springer, Berlin Heidelberg New York, pp 523-728
43. Klöppel G (1984) Islet histopathology in diabetes mellitus. In: Klöppel G, Heitz PU (eds) Pancreatic Pathology. Livingstone, Edinburgh
44. Klöppel G, Drenck CR, Oberholzer M, Heitz PU (1984) Morphometric evidence for a striking B-cell reduction at the clinical onset of type 1 diabetes. Virchows Arch 403: 441-452
45. Klöppel G, Löhr M, Habich K, Oberholzer M, Heitz PU (1985) Islet pathology and the pathogenesis of type 1 and type 2 diabetes mellitus revisited. Surv Synth Path Res 4: 110-125
46. Kolterman OG, Gray RS, Griffin J (1981) Receptor and post-receptor defects contribute to the insulin resistance in non-insulin dependent diabetes mellitus. J Clin Invest 68: 957-969
47. Korc M, Owerbach D, Quinto C, Rutter WJ (1981) Pancreatic islet-acinar cell interaction: Amylase messenger RNA levels are determined by insulin. Science 213: 351-353
48. Kramer MF, Tan HT (1968) The peri-insular acini of the pancreas of the rat. Z Zellforsch 86: 163-170
49. Kraus EJ (1929) Die pathologisch-anatomischen Veränderungen des Pankreas beim Diabetes mellitus. In: Henke F, Lubarsch O (eds) Handbuch der speziellen Pathologischen Anatomie und Histologie. Julius Springer, Berlin, vol 5, Part 2: 622-747
50. Lacy PE (1964) Pancreatic beta cell. In: Aetiology of diabetes mellitus and its complications. Ciba Foundation Colloquia on Endocrinology, Boston, Little, Brown and Company. Vol 15: 75-88
51. Langerhans P (1869) Beiträge zur mikroskopischen Anatomie der Bauchspeicheldrüse. Inaugural Dissertation, Friedrich Wilhelms Universität, Berlin
52. Leclercq-Meyer V, Marchand J, Malaisse WJ (1983) Insulin and glucagon release by the perfused ventral and dorsal parts of the rat pancreas. Diabetologia 25: 175
53. LeCompte PM (1958) "Insulitis" in early juvenile diabetes. Arch Path 66: 450-457
54. Levine S, Pictet R, Rutter WJ (1973) Control of cell proliferation and cytodifferentiation by a factor reacting with the cell surface. Nature New Biol 246: 49-52
55. Maclean N, Ogilvie RF (1955) Quantitative estimation of the pancreatic islet tissue in diabetic subjects. Diabetes 4: 367-376
56. Maclean N, Ogilvie RF (1959) Observations on the pancreatic islet tissue of young diabetic subjects. Diabetes 8: 83-91
57. Malaisse-Lagae F, Ravazolla M, Robberecht P, Vandermeers A, Malaisse WJ, Orci L (1975) Exocrine pancreas: evidence for topographic partition of secretory function. Science 190: 795-797
58. Malaisse-Lagae F, Stefan Y, Cox J, Perrelet A, Orci L (1979a) Identification of a lobe in the adult human pancreas rich in pancreatic polypeptide. Diabetologia 17: 361-366
59. Malaisse-Lagae F, Orci L, Perrelet A (1979b) Anatomic and hormonal markers for the ventral primordium in the human pancreas. N Engl J Med 300: 436
60. Maruyama H, Hisatomi A, Orci L, Grodsky GM, Unger RH (1984) Insulin within islets is a physiologic glucagon inhibitor. J Clin Invest 74: 2296-2299
61. Maruyama H, Tominaga M, Bolli G, Orci L, Unger RH (1985) The alpha cell response to glucose change during perfusion of anti-insulin serum in pancreas isolated from normal rats. Diabetologia 28: 836-840
62. Montesano R, Mouron P, Amherdt M, Orci L (1983) Collagen matrix promotes reorganization of pancreatic endocrine cell monolayers into islet-like organoids. J Cell Biol 97: 935-939
63. Nerup J, Platz P, Anderson O, Christy M, Egeberg J, Lyngsoe J (1976) HLA, autoimmunity and insulin dependent diabetes mellitus. In: Creutzfeld W, Köbberling J, Neel JV (eds) The genetics of diabetes mellitus. Springer, Berlin Heidelberg New York, pp 106-114
64. Ogilvie RF (1933) The islands of Langerhans in 19 cases of obesity. J Pathol Bacteriol 37: 473-481
65. Olefsky JM (1985) Diabetes mellitus. In: Wyngaarden JB, Smit LH (eds) Cecil textbook of medicine, 17th edn. Saunders, Philadelphia, pp 1320-1339

66. Olefsky JM (1985) Pathogenesis of insulin resistance and hyperglycemia in non-insulin-dependent diabetes mellitus. Am J Med 79: 1-7
67. Opie EL (1900) On the relation of diabetes mellitus to the lesions of the pancreas. Hyaline degeneration of the islets of Langerhans. J Exp Med 5: 397-428
68. Orci L, Baetens D, Ravazzola M, Stefan Y, Malaisse-Lagae F (1976a) Pancreatic polypeptide and glucagon: non-random distribution in pancreatic islets. Life Sci 19: 1811-1816
69. Orci L, Baetens D, Rufener C, Amherdt M, Ravazzola M, Studer P, Malaisse-Lagae F, Unger RH (1976b) Hypertrophy and hyperplasia of somatostatin containing D cells in diabetes. Proc Natl Acad Sci USA 73: 1338-1342
70. Orci L, Stefan Y, Malaisse-Lagae F, Perrelet A (1979a) Instability of pancreatic endocrine cell population throughout the life. Lancet I: 615
71. Orci L, Stefan Y, Malaisse-Lagae F, Perrelet A, Patel Y (1979b) Pancreatic fat. N Engl J Med 301: 1292
72. Palla JC, Abdeljlil AB, Desnuelle P (1968) Action de l'insuline sur la biosynthèse de l'amylase et de quelques autres enzymes du pancréas du rat. Biochim Biophys Acta 158: 25-35
73. Pfeifer MA, Halter JB, Porte D (1981) Insulin secretion in diabetes mellitus. Am J Med 70: 579-588
74. Pohl MN, Swartz FJ, Carstens PHB (1981) Polyploïdy in islets of normal and diabetic humans. Hum Pathol 12: 184-186
75. Prosser PR, Karam JH (1978) Diabetes mellitus following rodenticide ingestion in mass. JAMA 239: 1148-1150
76. Rahier J, Wallon J, Gepts W, Haot J (1979) Localization of pancreatic polypeptide cells in a limited lobe of the human neonate pancreas: Remnant of the ventral primordium? Cell Tissue Res 200: 359-366
77. Rahier J, Wallon J (1980) Long cytoplasmic processes in pancreatic polypeptide cells. Cell Tissue Res 209: 365-370
78. Rahier J, Wallon J, Henquin JC (1980) Abundance of somatostatin cells in the human neonatal pancreas. Diabetologia 18: 251-254
79. Rahier J, Wallon J, Henquin JC (1981) Cell populations in the endocrine pancreas of human neonates and infants. Diabetologia 20: 540-546
80. Rahier J, Wallon J, Haot J (1983a) A trophic role of pancreatic polypeptide on acinar cells in the human pancreas? Regul Pept [Suppl 2]: S73
81. Rahier J, Wallon J, Loozen S, Lefevre A, Gepts W, Haot J (1983b) The pancreatic polypeptide cells in the human pancreas: the effects of age and diabetes. J Clin Endocrinol Metab 56: 441-444
82. Rahier J, Goebbels RM, Henquin JC (1983c) Cellular composition of the human diabetic pancreas. Diabetologia 24: 366-371
83. Rahier J, Fält K, Müntefering G, Becker K, Gepts W, Falkmer S (1984) The basic structural lesion of persistent neonatal hypoglycemia with hyperinsulinism: deficiency of pancreatic D cells or hyperactivity of B cells. Diabetologia 26: 282-289
84. Reaven GM, Bernstein A, Davis B, Olefsky JM (1966) Nonketotic diabetes mellitus: insulin deficiency or insulin resistance? Am J Med 60: 80-88
85. Rizza RA, Mandarino LJ, Gerich JE (1981) Mechanism and significance of insulin resistance in non-insulin-dependent diabetes mellitus. Diabetes 30: 990-995
86. Romanoff AL (1960) The avian embryo. Structural and functional development. Macmillan, New York, p 527
87. Saito H, Saito S, Sano T, Hosoi E, Saito H (1983) Fetal and maternal plasma levels in immunoreactive somatostatin at delivery: evidence for its increase in the umbilical artery and its arterio-venous gradient in the feto-placental circulation. J Clin Endocrinol Metab 56: 567-571
88. Saito K, Yaginuma N, Takahashi T (1979) Differential volumetry of A, B and D cells in the pancreatic islets of diabetic and nondiabetic subjects. Tohoku J Exp Med 129: 273-283
89. Scarlett JA, Gray RS, Griffin J, Olefsky J, Kolterman OG (1982) Insulin treatment reverses the insulin resistance of Type II diabetes mellitus. Diabetes Care 5: 353-363
90. Schmidt MB (1902) Über die Beziehung der Langerhansschen Inseln des Pancreas zum Diabetes mellitus. Münch Med Wochenschr 49: 51-54

91. Seifert G (1959) Die pathologische Morphologie der Langerhansschen Inseln, besonders beim Diabetes mellitus des Menschen. Verh Dtsch Gesamt Pathol 18: 50-84
92. Shwachman H, Diamond LK, Oski FA (1964) The syndrome of pancreatic insufficiency and bone marrow dysfunction. J Pediatr 65: 645
93. Sibley RK, Sutherland DER, Goetz F, Michael AF (1985) Recurrent diabetes mellitus in the pancreas iso- and allograft. A light and electron microscopic and immunohistochemical analysis of four cases. Lab Invest 53: 132-144
94. Söling HD, Unger KO (1972) The role of insulin in the regulation of alpha-amylase synthesis in the rat pancreas. Eur J Clin Invest 2: 199-212
95. Spooner BS, Walther BT, Rutter WJ (1970) The development of the dorsal and ventral mammalian pancreas in vivo and in vitro. J Cell Biol 47: 235-246
96. Stefan Y, Orci L, Malaisse-Lagae F, Perrelet A, Patel Y, Unger RH (1982) Quantification of endocrine cell content in the pancreas of nondiabetic and diabetic humans. Diabetes 31: 694-700
97. Testut L, Latarjet A (1949) Traité d'anatomie humaine, vol 4, 9th edn. Douin, Paris, pp 712-713
98. Trimble ER, Renold AE (1981) Ventral and dorsal areas of rat pancreas: islet hormone content and secretion. Am J Physiol 240: E422-E427
99. Trimble ER, Halban PA, Wollheim CB, Renold AE (1982) Functional differences between rat islets of ventral and dorsal pancreatic origin. J Clin Invest 69: 405-413
100. Unger RH, Aguilar-Parada E, Muller WA, Eisentraut AM (1970) Studies of pancreatic alpha cell function in normal and diabetic subjects. J Clin Invest 49: 837-848
101. Unger RH, Grundy S (1985) Hyperglycemia as an inducer as well as a consequence of impaired islet cell function and insulin resistance: implications for the management of diabetes. Diabetologia 28: 119-121
102. Unger RH, Orci L (1975) Hypothesis: the essential role of glucagon in the pathogenesis of diabetes mellitus. Lancet 1: 14-16
103. Van Assche FA, Aerts L (1979) The fetal endocrine pancreas. Contrib Gynecol Obstet 5: 44-57
104. Vartiainen I (1944) Studien über den Diabetes mellitus in Finnland: die makroskopischen Organveränderungen der Diabetiker im Lichte des Obduktionsmaterials. Acta Med Scand 118: 538-589
105. von Mering S, Minkowski O (1889) Diabetes mellitus nach Pankreasexstirpation. Arch Exp Pathol Pharmakol 26: 371-387
106. von Meyenburg H (1940) Über "Insulitis" bei Diabetes. Schweiz Med Wochenschr 21: 554-557
107. Ward WK, Beard JC, Halter JB, Pfeifer MA, Porte D (1984) Pathophysiology of insulin secretion in non-insulin-dependent diabetes mellitus. Diabetes Care 7: 491-502
108. Ward WK, Bolgiano DC, McKnight B, Halter JB, Porte D (1984) Diminished B cell secretory capacity in patients with noninsulin-dependent diabetes mellitus. J Clin Invest 74: 1318-1328
109. Warren S, Root HF (1925) The pathology of diabetes, with special reference to pancreatic regeneration. Am J Pathol 1: 415-430
110. Warren SH, LeCompte PH (1952) The pathology of diabetes mellitus, 3rd edn. Kimpton, London, pp 53
111. Weichselbaum A, Stangl E (1901/02) Zur Kenntnis der feineren Veränderungen des Pankreas bei Diabetes mellitus. Wien Klin Wochenschr 14: 968
112. Wessells NK, Cohn IH (1967) Early pancreas organogenesis: morphogenesis, tissue interactions and mass effects. Dev Biol 15: 237-270
113. Westermark P (1972) Quantitative studies of amyloid in the islets of Langerhans. Upsal J Med Sci 77: 91-94
114. Westermark P (1973) Fine structure of islets of Langerhans in insular amyloïdosis. Virchows Arch 359: 1-18
115. Westermark P (1977) Amyloïd of human islets of Langerhans. Virchows Arch 373: 161
116. Westermark P, Wilander E (1978) The influence of amyloid deposits in the islets volume in maturity onset diabetes mellitus. Diabetologia 15: 417-421
117. Westermark P, Wilander E (1983) Islet amyloid in type 2 (non-insulin-dependent) diabetes is related to insulin. Diabetologia 24: 342-346

118. White JW, Swartz FJ, Swartz AF (1985) Excess glucose intake induces accelerated B cell polyploidisation in normal mice: a possible deleterious effect. J Nutr 115: 271–278
119. World Health Organisation expert committee on diabetes mellitus (1980) Second report. Technical report series. WHO, Geneva
120. Yoon JW, Austin M, Onodera R, Notkins AL (1979) Virus induced diabetes mellitus. Isolation of a virus from the pancreas of a child with diabetic ketoacidosis. N Engl J Med 300: 1173–1179

Insulitis in the Human Pancreas

A. K. Foulis and G. F. Bottazzo

The Establishment of the Concept of Insulitis

Most people interested in the pathogenesis of type 1 diabetes associate the term "insulitis" with one name - that of WILLY GEPTS. In what must be one of the most cited references in the diabetic literature, he showed that this lesion, comprising a predominantly chronic inflammatory cell infiltrate of the islets of LANGERHANS, was present in 15 of 22 patients who had died of "juvenile" diabetes within a year of presentation [13]. The lesion was not seen in diabetes of more prolonged duration.

While insulitis had been described in recent-onset diabetic in children since the beginning of this century, it had been regarded as a rare lesion until the work of LECOMPTE [17] who described it in four patients. There has continued to be debate concerning the frequency of insulitis in recent-onset type 1 diabetes. JUNKER et al. [16a] found it in six of 11 cases, but it was not seen in 13 patients studied by DONIACH and MORGAN [10a]. The patients in the latter study (who died before the advent of insulin therapy) may have been slightly atypical in that four had diabetes for more than 6 months and three were thought to have no residual B-cells in the sections of pancreas available for study. The question of the incidence of insulitis has been partially resolved by the finding of the lesion in 47 of 60 (78%) patients who had died of recent-onset type 1 diabetes [11]. In this study the frequency of insulitis was very similar to that found by GEPTS [13] and both authors suggested it was an underestimate, since in many of the cases in which insulitis was not found only limited pancreatic material was available for examination.

LECOMPTE [17] and GEPTS [13] noted that there was a marked reduction in the number of insulin-secreting B-cells in the pancreas of recent-onset type 1 diabetics. The latter also described the secretory hyperactivity in the residual B-cells which might explain why basal serum insulin levels are only marginally below normal in some patients at clinical presentation.

The Development of the Concept of Insulitis

With the advent of modern immunohistochemistry, GEPTS and DE MEY [14] showed that there were two principal types of islets present in recent-onset diabetes. The most common, previously thought to be atrophic, was devoid of B-cells but contained relatively normal numbers of the other pancreatic endocrine cells.

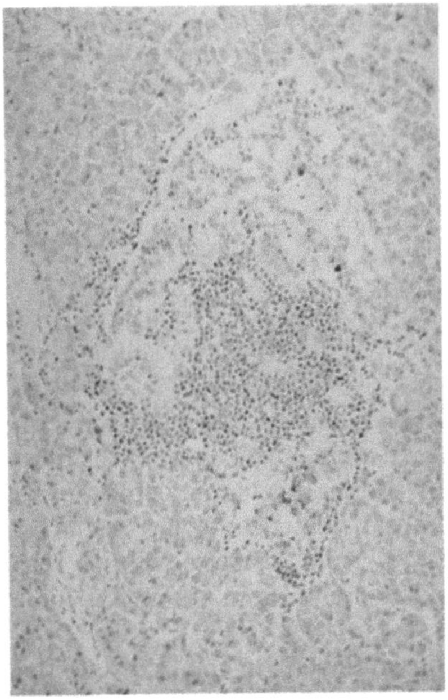

Fig. 1. Insulitis. There is a heavy lymphocytic infiltrate in this islet and only scattered B-cells remain. Indirect immunoperoxidase technique for insulin, ×80

The second population of islets contained residual B-cells and was found in 14 of the 16 recent-onset cases studied. Insulitis was present in 11 cases in this series, and in one pancreas it was noted that all the inflamed islets contained B-cells. This case provided the first real clue that insulitis represented an immune reaction specifically directed at B-cells. More histological evidence for this concept has recently been provided [11]. In a study of 50 cases in which insulitis was present, the lesion was seen in 889 of 3931 (23%) islets which contained B-cells but in only 93 of 7892 (1%) islets which were insulin-deficient. A spectrum of changes was noted suggesting progressive destruction of B-cells within an islet. In early insulitis, characteristically there was infiltration by small lymphocytes at the periphery of an insulin-containing islet in which the number of B-cells often appeared relatively normal. In the next stage there was a more diffuse inflammatory cell infiltrate within the islet accompanied by a marked drop in the number of B-cells (Fig. 1). Occasionally, islets in which no B-cells were detectable were also inflamed. This probably represented the end-stage of the destructive phase.

Since the clinical onset of diabetes is often quite abrupt, it had been assumed that the pathological process which destroyed the B-cells must be fairly acute. GEPTS [13] questioned this, suggesting on the basis of his histological findings that the disease must have a protracted course. The finding of islet cell antibodies years before clinical presentation of diabetes [15], the presence of residual B-cells in the pancreas years after diagnosis [14] and the presence of insulitis up to 6 years after the onset of diabetes [11] all support GEPTS' original suggestion that B-cells may be destroyed over a long period.

Given that the destructive process affecting B-cells is a chronic one, it is not surprising that there is evidence of regeneration of residual B-cells in the pancreas at clinical presentation. In many cases some insulin-containing islets are enlarged and contain an increased number of B-cells, some of which have polyploid nuclei. GEPTS maintained that a proportion of these islets had been formed in postnatal life from ductal elements, i.e. islet neoformation [14]. In support of this he photographed an islet surrounding a central duct [13]. One of us (AKF) has studied a large number of cases of recent-onset diabetes and has examined up to 40 serial sections through many insulin-containing islets so that they could be assessed in their entirety. No convincing evidence of islet neoformation from ducts was observed. An alternative view would therefore be that B-cell regeneration takes place in residual undamaged insulin-secreting islets and that there is no neoformation of whole islets.

In his description of the inflammatory cell content of insulitis, GEPTS noted that while there were no plasma cells, the predominant cell types were lymphocytes, "reticular" cells (? macrophages) and occasional polymorphs [13]. It is only recently that a more detailed characterisation of the inflammatory cells has been possible [6]. Pancreatic material from an autopsy was snap-frozen, which allowed the application of specific monoclonal antibodies to differentiate the inflammatory and endocrine cell types. The majority of lymphocytes around the islets in this case were activated T-lymphocytes, with a predominance of those belonging to the CD8 phenotype (? cytotoxic) subpopulation. While helper T-lymphocytes and natural killer cells were also present in small numbers, macrophages were not seen. Cells of the B-lymphocyte lineage were also present, with a predominance of immunocytes containing cytoplasmic IgG. In addition, IgG (but not IgM or IgA) deposition was detected both on the surface of some islet endocrine cells and within their cytoplasm. The complement component C9 was found to codistribute with the IgG on endocrine cells, suggesting the presence of complement fixation by immune complexes. The finding of IgG deposition both within and on endocrine cells was confirmed by examination of fixed sections in a larger series of patients with type 1 diabetes [27].

Insulitis and Autoimmunity

In 1965, 9 years prior to the discovery of islet cell cytoplasmic antibodies in type 1 diabetes [3], GEPTS suggested that insulitis "might have an immunological origin". Since then evidence has accumulated to support the concept that many cases of type 1 diabetes fulfill the criteria of an organ-specific autoimmune disease [4]. There is evidence for both cell-mediated [22] and humoral immunity. Islet cell cytoplasmic antibodies were found in up to 85% of newly diagnosed type 1 diabetics [18]. In addition, islet cell surface antibodies have been described, some of which lyse cultured rat B-cells in preference to A-cells, D-cells, and PP-cells [10]. Recently antibodies to insulin have been found in a proportion of newly diagnosed type 1 diabetics, even prior to treatment [23].

The Connection Between Class II MHC Genes and Autoimmunity to B-Cells

While the presence of insulitis and the various immunological phenomena described support the concept that many cases of type 1 diabetes are autoimmune in origin, there is another line of evidence which suggests that there is a very large genetic component to this disease linked to the major histocompatibility complex (MHC) genes. Initially the linkage was thought to be with class I MHC genes (HLA-A, B, C in man) but it has now been established that the major relationship is with class II MHC genes (HLA-DR, DP and DQ in man). Thus up to 98% of all type 1 diabetics were positive for either DR3 or DR4, and 51% possessed both these antigens [30]. The relative risk with DR3 was 5.0, with DR4, 6.8 and with both antigens, 14.3. By contrast, the relative risk with DR2 was 0.1, i.e. the presence of this antigen apparently protected against diabetes.

While class I MHC molecules are present on most nucleated cells in the body, cellular expression of class II MHC products is more restricted. They are found on B-lymphocytes, activated T-lymphocytes, antigen-presenting cells, capillary endothelial cells and certain epithelial cells. In the normal human pancreas, islet endocrine cells do not express class II MHC [2, 21]. Acini are normally also negative, but duct epithelium may be positive [12]. Capillary endothelial cells are consistently positive and comprise the positive cells seen in and around islets.

It is thought that the principal function of class II products is to facilitate antigen presentation. Helper T-lymphocytes, which will initiate an immune response, only recognise the antigen to which they are directed if it is "presented" to them by a cell expressing the same class II MHC as themselves. It has been proposed that the initial event in many organ-specific autoimmune diseases may be aberrant expression of class II MHC by the target cells [5]. If a cell did not normally express class II MHC on its surface, then any cell-specific autoantigens it may possess would never have been "presented" to potentially autoreactive helper T-lymphocytes. Thus, even though the latter may exist there would be no immune response. If, however, the cell were induced to express class II MHC, it may become a functional antigen-presenting cell and "present" its particular cell surface antigen to potentially autoreactive helper T-lymphocytes which would then initiate an autoimmune response. This hypothesis was prompted by observations in the thyroid. Normal cultured thyrocytes did not express class II MHC but became positive after addition of mitogens [24]. Most importantly, thyrocytes in thyroid autoimmune diseases expressed class II MHC spontaneously [16].

While this observation has been extended to other tissues affected by autoimmunity [8], the pancreas in type 1 diabetes offers a unique opportunity to test this hypothesis further. It is worth emphasizing that of the four hormone-producing cells in the pancreas, only the B-cells are destroyed. Thus, if the hypothesis were true, aberrant class II MHC expression would be confined to B-cells and would not be seen on A-cells, D-cells or PP-cells.

The abnormal presence of class II MHC expression on islets was initially tested in the case of a child who died of recent-onset diabetes and in whom frozen pancreas was available [6]. Class II MHC positive islet endocrine cells were identified but were not numerous. They were found particularly in islets showing little inflammation. By double immunofluorescence with a monoclonal antibody to human C-peptide, it was shown that all the class II MHC-positive endocrine cells were functional B-cells (Fig. 2). Other islets contained B-cells which did not express class II MHC. A-cells and D-cells never showed this expression.

With the advent of a monoclonal antibody which recognised a formalin-resistant epitope found on the non-polymorphic part of the alpha-chain of DR, DP and DQ [1] a similar study could be done on historical cases where formalin-fixed, paraffin-embedded pancreatic material was available [12]. The pancreases of 14 children who had died of type 1 diabetes were studied. Two cases in which no residual insulin-secreting B-cells were present displayed no evidence of class II MHC product expression on endocrine cells. Insulin-containing islets were pre-

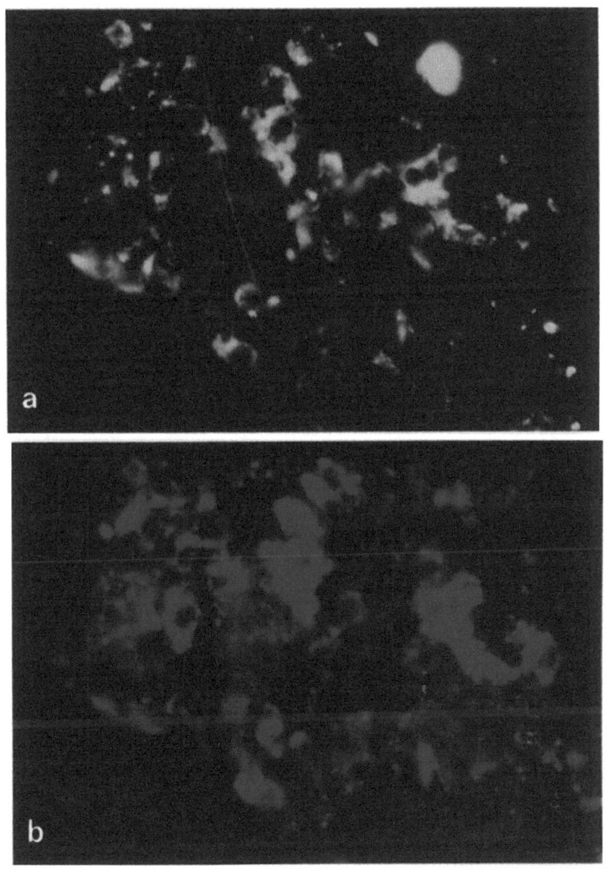

Fig. 2 a, b. Class II MHC in the pancreas in recent-onset diabetes. **a** HLA-DR molecule expression is seen in capillaries and some large cells. **b** The same field is stained in red for reactivity with a monoclonal antibody to C-peptide, indicating that HLA-DR-positive B-cells are present. Double-stained sections using a fluorescein conjugate to demonstrate HLA-DR and a rhodamine conjugate to demonstrate C-peptide were used. Indirect immunofluorescent techniques were used for both, ×200

sent in the remainder, and some class II MHC-positive endocrine cells were found in each of these cases. On adjacent serial sections from all 14 cases it was shown that endocrine cells expressing class II MHC were present in 171 of a total of 630 insulin-containing islets. However, class II MHC-positive endocrine cells were not seen in 2060 insulin-deficient islets. Sections double-stained for class II MHC and the respective pancreatic hormones confirmed that of the four hormone-producing cells in the pancreas, only the B-cells expressed class II MHC. This study also examined pancreases from 26 patients aged under 12 years who had died of diseases unrelated to the pancreas, 12 patients who had died of cystic fibrosis, seven patients with chronic pancreatitis and six patients with type II diabetes. Endocrine cells expressing class II MHC were not observed in any of these cases. Thus the presence of aberrant expression of class II MHC on pancreatic B-cells is as characteristic of type 1 diabetes as is the presence of insulitis.

Which Came First: Chicken or Egg?

The crucial question to be answered in the light of these studies is whether aberrant class II MHC expression precedes insulitis or is the consequence of insulitis. Since all pathological studies on type 1 diabetes have been done when at least 70% of the B-cells have been destroyed, presumably by insulitis, this may seem an impossible question to answer. It has been argued, however [12], that at clinical presentation there are three populations of islets - insulin-depleted islets (the majority), insulin-containing islets affected by insulitis and insulin-containing islets unaffected by any destructive process. The same three populations can be seen up to 6 years after diagnosis, although obviously the proportions are different from those seen at presentation, with markedly fewer insulin-containing islets. By extrapolation it can be assumed that the pancreas in the prediabetic phase, when islet cell antibodies are present, may have the same three islet populations, but with fewer insulin-depleted islets. If this argument is correct, then abnormalities detected in the pancreas at clinical presentation may be similar to abnormalities present at the onset of B-cell destruction. It has been noted that the majority of islets in which aberrant expression of class II MHC was found had no evidence of insulitis [4, 7, 12]. Both insulitis and aberrant class II MHC expression can be focal within an islet, and a single section of an islet may be misleading with regard to their presence or absence. In a recent study [31], 40 serial sections of pancreas were cut from three cases of recent-onset type 1 diabetes. The middle section was stained for insulin and the remainder for class II MHC. Using this method, "whole" islets could be examined for the presence of class II MHC and insulitis. One hundred and thirty insulin-containing islets were studied, 57 of which had insulitis. Thirteen of these 57 inflamed islets had no evidence of class II MHC expression on B-cells. Class II-positive endocrine cells were present in 88 of the insulin-containing islets, but in only 44 of these was insulitis present. Thus there was no convincing evidence for a direct relationship between insulitis and class II MHC expression on B-cells.

Gamma-interferon, a lymphokine produced by T-lymphocytes, has been shown to cause aberrant expression of class II MHC on thyrocytes in vitro [29]. Thus it has been argued that the class II expression on thyrocytes seen in thyroid autoimmune disease may be a consequence of adjacent inflammation and not the primary abnormality. However, the situation in the pancreas appears to be different. While gamma-interferon induced class II expression on cultured pancreatic exocrine cells in vitro, no such expression was seen on cultured pancreatic endocrine cells [9, 25]. Equally, alpha-interferon, beta-interferon, interleukin-2 and supernatants from activated lymphocytes derived from islet cell antibody-positive, prediabetic family members failed to induce class II expression on islet endocrine cells [25]. Recently it has been shown that pancreatic endocrine cells cultured in the presence of both tumor necrosis factor and gamma-interferon can be induced to express class II MHC [26]. However, this aberrant expression was seen on A-cells as well as B-cells. Thus, to date, no chemical mediators of inflammation liable to be released in the insulitis process have been shown capable of causing selective expression of class II MHC on B-cells in vitro similar to that seen in vivo. This is in keeping with the failure to observe class II MHC expression on islet endocrine cells in chronic inflammatory diseases of the pancreas such as cystic fibrosis and chronic pancreatitis [12].

In what is liable to be a unique study, SIBLEY et al. [28] reported the recurrence of diabetes in four patients who had received pancreatic organ grafts from their normal identical twins. The recipients had had diabetes for at least 17 years. Because these were isografts no suppressive immunotherapy was given in three of the patients. As soon as 6 weeks after transplant, insulin-depleted islets and insulitis were found in biopsy specimens of the grafted pancreases. Glucagon- and somatostatin-secreting cells maintained their normal numbers. Islet cell cytoplasmic antibodies were not present in any preoperative sera and reappeared in only one of the four recipients in the post-transplant period. CD8-positive (? cytotoxic) T-lymphocytes again predominated in the inflammatory infiltrate. Interestingly, aberrant class II MHC expression on islet cells, though sought, was not found. A possible interpretation of this finding is that while aberrant class II MHC expression on B-cells may be involved in the induction of autoimmunity (and may have been present on the recipients' own pancreases when they originally presented with diabetes), once a sufficient number of cytotoxic T-lymphocytes have been generated and tolerance overcome, B-cells can be destroyed and insulitis be present without induction of more aberrant class II MHC expression.

Thus the finding of aberrant class II MHC expression on B-cells in islets unaffected by insulitis in recent-onset diabetes, the absence of such expression on B-cells in pancreatic inflammatory diseases or when B-cells are cultured in the presence of gamma-interferon and other inflammatory mediators, and the lack of the phenomenon in the transplanted twin pancreases all suggest that within a given islet aberrant class II MHC expression on B-cells may precede insulitis.

Aberrant expression of class II MHC by B-cells may provide a rational explanation for the genetic link between the HLA-DR type of an individual and his/her risk of developing diabetes. Theoretically, DR3 and DR4 antigens could be more readily inducible on B-cells than others. Alternatively, their particular shape, charge or other property could make them act as "immune response genes", i.e.

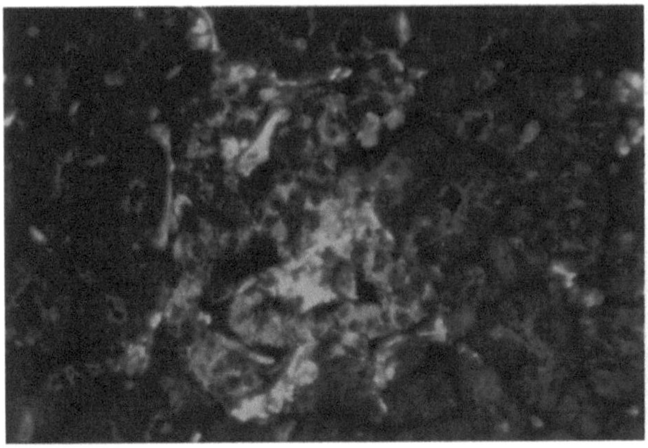

Fig. 3. Section of the same diabetic pancreas as shown in Fig. 2 stained by a double immunofluorescent technique with monoclonal antibodies to capillary endothelial cells (stained *orange*) and to human proinsulin (staines *green*). Note the hypertrophy of capillaries around and inside the islet which still contains functional B-cells ×150

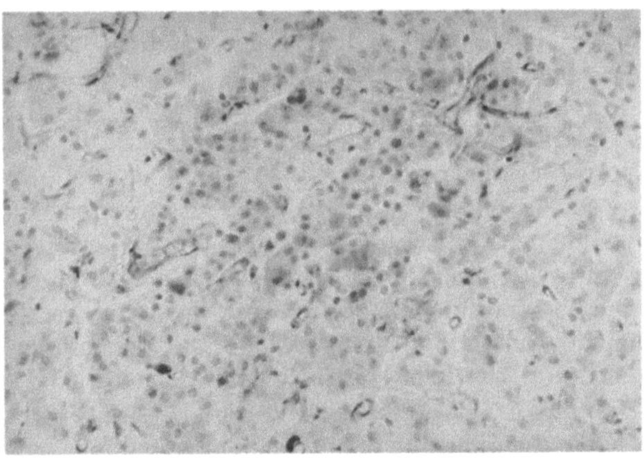

Fig. 4. Pancreas of a child who died 6 years after diagnosis of type 1 diabetes. Several endocrine cells (shown to be B-cells on double labelling) can be seen to express class II MHC aberrantly. There is swelling of capillary endothelial cells which also hyperexpress class II MHC. There is no evidence of insulitis in the islet. Indirect immunoperoxidase technique for class II MHC used monoclonal antibody TAL 1B5, ×100

once expressed they might be more capable of presenting particular autoantigens on B-cells than other class II products.

While it has been shown that thyrocytes expressing class II MHC (but not normal thyrocytes) can act as antigen-presenting cells by presenting either thyroid-specific autoantigens [20] or foreign antigen [19] to the appropriate cloned T-lymphocytes, such studies have not yet been done with pancreatic B-cells. Thus it has yet to be established that B-cells expressing class II MHC can effectively present autoantigen.

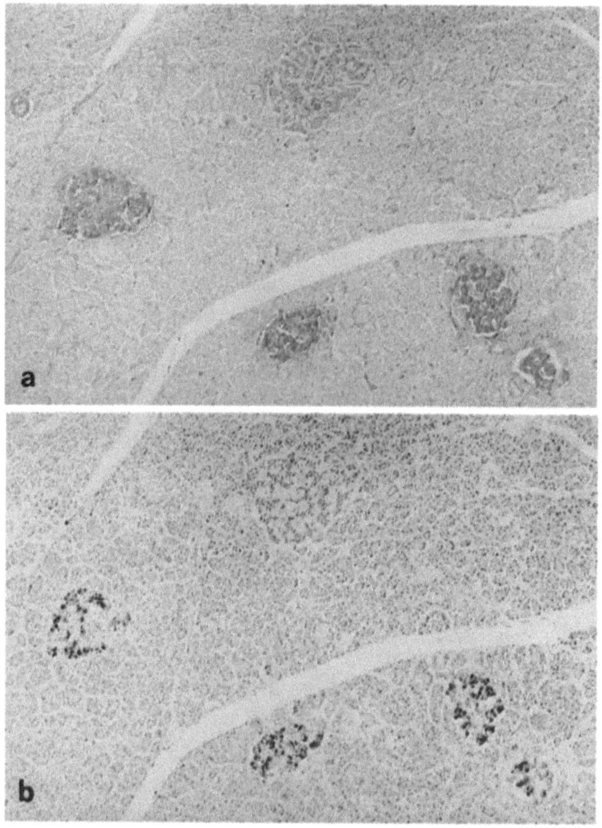

Fig. 5 a, b. Expression of Class I MHC in the pancreas of recent-onset type 1 diabetic patient. **a** All islets except the large islet at the top hyperexpress class I MHC. Indirect immunoperoxidase for class I MHC, ×30. **b** This large islet is devoid of B-cells. Indirect immunoperoxidase for insulin, ×30

Capillary endothelial cells in islets with aberrant class II MHC expression on B-cells are usually swollen and strongly class II-positive [6] (Figs. 3, 4). This is the case even when multiple serial sections show no evidence of insulitis in the islet [12]. This suggests an important role for the capillaries in facilitating the "homing" of potentially autoreactive lymphocytes. The enhanced class II expression by endothelial cells could be important in this process, by possibly enabling these cells to present antigens cross-reactive with B-cells or antigens which have leaked from target endocrine cells.

It was observed that there was hyperexpression of class I MHC products on endocrine cells in some islets in recent-onset type 1 diabetes [6]. This phenomenon has been investigated further [31]. Ninety-seven per cent of insulin-containing islets in pancreases from 19 patients with recent-onset type 1 diabetes hyperexpressed class I MHC. This hyperexpression appeared to affect all the endocrine cells in the islets equally. By contrast, only 1% of insulin-deficient islets hyperexpressed class I MHC (Fig. 5). Since the A-cells and D-cells only hyperexpressed class I MHC in affected islets when they were adjacent to B-cells, a possible explanation is that some B-cells secrete an immune modulator (? an interferon) which has a paracrine affect on neighbouring endocrine cells. Cytotoxic T-lymphocytes only recognise the antigen to which they are directed in the context of class I MHC molecules. Thus the hyperexpression of class I MHC found on insulin-containing islets may facilitate the presentation of B-cell-specific antigens to invading cytotoxic T-lymphocytes resulting in the eventual destruction of the B-cells.

The Future

If the pancreas of a patient who has had diabetes for many years is studied, B-cells will probably be completely absent. In his classic paper on recent-onset type 1 diabetes, Willy Gepts examined the preceding pathology and established the presence and incidence of insulitis. He went on to suggest that this lesion represented the destructive process which leads to B-cell loss. The present studies have tried to reach back even further into the events which result in diabetes. It now seems possible that aberrant expression of class II MHC on B-cells precedes insulitis and is the crucial step in the induction of autoimmunity. It is also possible that class I MHC hyperexpression on islet endocrine cells is an important homing mechanism for autoreactive cytotoxic T-lymphocytes. Further study of the pancreas of patients with recent-onset diabetes may allow detection of agents which could be responsible for these abnormalities in MHC expression. The following important message is thus emerging: pancreatic B-cells are not so passive as was originally thought [7]. While the pancreas at clinical presentation of the disease has given us clues as to the pathogenesis of B-cell destruction, a new era will dawn in this study if safe pancreatic biopsy can be done on predisposed individuals before the onset of their disease.

Willy Gepts highlighted the morphological presence of insulitis. We are currently undertaking research in an attempt to bring the whole process to life by suggesting functional abnormalities which precede the inflammation of islets and final destruction of B-cells. Will this approach succeed in demonstrating the initial abnormalities in the islets and offer new clues to prevent and cure the disease? We shall see.

Acknowledgements. Miss May Habbick has shown remarkable patience and goodwill in dealing with both the Scottish and Italian versions of this manuscript.

References

1. Adams TE, Bodmer G, Bodmer WF (1983) Production and characterisation of monoclonal antibodies recognising the alpha chain subunits of human Ia alloantigens. Immunology 50: 613-624
2. Alejandro R, Shienvold FL, Hajek SV, Ryan U, Miller J, Mintz DH (1982) Immunocytochemical localization of HLA-DR in human islets of Langerhans. Diabetes 31: [Suppl 4] 17-22
3. Bottazzo GF, Florin-Christensen A, Doniach D (1974) Islet cell antibodies in diabetes mellitus with autoimmune polyendocrine deficiences. Lancet 2: 1279-1282
4. Bottazzo GF (1984) Beta-cell damage in diabetic insulitis: are we approaching a solution? Diabetologia 26: 241-249

5. Bottazzo GF, Pujol-Borrell R, Hanafusa T, Feldmann M (1983) Role of aberrant HLA-DR expression and antigen presentation in induction of endocrine autoimmunity. Lancet 2: 1115-1118
6. Bottazzo GF, Dean BM, McNally JM, MacKay EH, Swift PGF, Gamble DR (1985) In situ characterization of autoimmune phenomena and expression of HLA molecules in the pancreas in diabetic insulitis. N Engl J Med 313: 353-360
7. Bottazzo GF (1986) Death of a beta cell: homicide or suicide? Diabetic Med 3: 119-130
8. Bottazzo GF, Todd I, Mirakian R, Belfiore A, Pujol-Borrell R (1986) Organ-specific autoimmunity: a 1986 overview. Immunol Rev 94: 137-169
9. Campbell IL, Bizilj K, Colman PG, Tuch BE, Harrison LC (1986) Interferon-gamma induces the expression of HLA-A, -B, -C but not HLA-DR on human pancreatic beta cells. J Clin Endocrinol Metab 62: 1101-1109
10. Dobersen MJ, Scharff JE (1982) Preferential lysis of pancreatic Beta cells by islet cell surface antibodies. Diabetes 31: 459-462
10a. Doniach I, Morgan AG (1973) Islet of Langerhans in juvenile Diabetes mellitus. Clin Endocrinol 2: 233-248
11. Foulis AK, Liddle CN, Farquharson MA, Richmond JA, Weir RS (1986) The histopathology of the pancreas in Type I (insulin-dependent) diabetes mellitus: a 25-year review of deaths in patients under 20 years of age in the United Kingdom. Diabetologia 29: 267-274
12. Foulis AK, Farquharson MA (1986) Aberrant expression of HLA-DR antigens by insulin containing beta cells in recent onset Type I (insulin-dependent) diabetes mellitus. Diabetes 35: 1215-1224
13. Gepts W (1965) Pathologic anatomy of the pancreas in juvenile diabetes mellitus. Diabetes 14: 619-633
14. Gepts W, De Mey J (1978) Islet cell survival determined by morphology - an immunocytochemical study of the islets of Langerhans in juvenile diabetes mellitus. Diabetes 27: [Suppl 1] 251-261
15. Gorsuch AN, Spencer KM, Lister J, McNally JM, Dean BM, Bottazzo GF, Cudworth AG (1981) Evidence for a long prediabetic period in Type I (insulin-dependent) diabetes mellitus. Lancet 2: 1363-1365
16. Hanafusa T, Pujol-Borrell R, Chiovato L, Russel RCG, Doniach D, Bottazzo GF (1983) Aberrant expression of HLA-DR antigen on thyrocytes in Graves' disease. Relevance for autoimmunity. Lancet 2: 1111-1115
16a. Junker K, Egeberg S, Kromann H Nerup J (1977) An autopsy study of the islet of Langerhans in acute-onset juvenile diabetes mellitus. Acta Pathol Microbiol Scand [A] 85: 699-706
17. LeCompte PM (1958) "Insulitis" in early juvenile diabetes. Arch Pathol 66: 450-457
18. Lendrum R, Walker G, Cudworth AG, Theophanides C, Pyke DA, Bloom A, Gamble DR (1976) Islet-cell antibodies in diabetes mellitus Lancet 2: 1273-1276
19. Londei M, Lamb JR, Bottazzo GF, Feldmann M (1984) Epithelial cells expressing aberrant MHC Class II determinants can present antigen to cloned human T cells. Nature 312: 639-641
20. Londei M, Bottazzo GF, Feldmann M (1985) Human T-cell clones from autoimmune thyroid glands: specific recognition of autologous thyroid cells. Science 228: 85-89
21. Natali PG, DeMartino CD, Quaranta V, Nicotra MR, Frezza F, Pellegrino MA, Ferrone S (1981) Expression of Ia-like antigens in normal human non-lymphoid tissues. Transplantation 31: 75-78
22. Nerup J, Andersen OO, Bendixen G, Egeberg J, Poulsen JE (1971) Anti-pancreatic cellular hypersensitivity in diabetes mellitus. Diabetes 20: 424-427
23. Palmer JP, Asplin CM, Clemons P, Lyen K, Tatpati O, Raghu PK, Paquette TL (1983) Insulin antibodies in insulin-dependent diabetics before insulin treatment. Science 222: 1337-1339
24. Pujol-Borrell R, Hanafusa T, Chiovato L. Bottazzo GF (1983) Lectin-induced expression of DR antigen on human cultured follicular thyroid cells. Nature 304: 71-73
25. Pujol-Borrell R, Todd I, Doshi M, Gray D, Feldmann M, Bottazzo GF (1986) Differential expression and regulation of MHC products in the endocrine and exocrine cells of the human pancreas. Clin Exp Immunol 65: 128-139
26. Pujol-Borrell R, Todd I, Doshi M, Bottazzo GF, Sutton R, Gray D, Adolf GR, Feldmann M

(1987) HLA Class II induction in human islet cells by Interferon-γ plus tumor necrosis factor or lymphotoxin. Nature 326: 304-306
27. Sai P, Kremer M, Nomballais MF, Aillet G (1984) Antibodies spontaneously bound to islet cells in Type I diabetes. Lancet 2: 233-234
28. Sibley RK, Sutherland DER, Goetz F, Michael AF (1985) Recurrent diabetes mellitus in the pancreas iso- and allograft. A light and electron microscopic and immunohistochemical analysis of four cases. Lab Invest 53: 132-144
29. Todd I, Pujol-Borrell R, Hammond LJ, Bottazzo GF, Feldmann M (1985) Interferon-γ induces HLA-DR expression by thyroid epithelium. Clin Exp Immunol 61: 265-273
30. Wolf E, Spencer KM, Cudworth AG (1983) The genetic susceptibility to Type 1 (insulin-dependent) diabetes: analysis of the HLA-DR association. Diabetologia 24: 224-230
31. Foulis AK, Farquharson MA, Hardman R (1987) Aberrant expression of class II major histocompatibility Complex molecules by B cells and hyperexpression of class I major histocompatibility complex molecules by insulin containing islets in Type I (insulin-dependent) diabetes mellitus. Diabetologia 30: 333-343

Circulating Signs of Autoimmune Islet Disease*

Å. Lernmark, H. Markholst and S. Bækkeskov

Introduction

Nearly 100 years ago, the pathogenesis of diabetes mellitus was linked to the pancreas [1]. Later, at the beginning of this century, some investigators reported islet lesions in diabetic individuals which included fibrosis, hyalinosis, hydropic degeneration, atrophy and inflammatory reactions [2]. However, the islets of LANGERHANS were yet to be linked to the production of insulin and the etiology and pathogenesis of diabetes remained unclear. Insulin was extracted from the pancreas in 1921 and proved to ameliorate most of the diabetic symptoms [3]. It soon became clear, however, that insulin was not a cure for diabetes. In 1965, Gepts [4] reported that the major morphologic alteration in the pancreas at the onset of IDDM was a disruption of the architecture of the islets of LANGERHANS and a loss of B-cells. The number of B-cells was reduced to less than 10% of normal values and in 68% of the pancreases examined, the islets were infiltrated by mononuclear cells. Islet inflammation, insulitis, was therefore suggested to be of pathogenetic importance [4-7]. Infiltration of the islets of LANGERHANS has also been associated with experimental diabetes induced by immunization with insulin [8-9], by multiple injections of low-dose streptozotocin [10], or following infection with diabetogenic viruses [11, 12].

Further support to the hypothesis that IDDM has an autoimmune pathogenesis was obtained from the demonstration of a hypersensitivity reaction to pancreatic antigens [13], islet cell antibodies [14, 15], and a close association with the HLA locus on chromosome 6 [16-18]. The pathogenesis of IDDM may therefore be linked to an abnormal immune response directed against the pancreatic B-cells, causing a specific loss of these cells and resulting in diabetes.

The possibility that the immune system was somehow involved in the process of B-cell destruction was not evident until the now classical 1965 paper by WILLY GEPTS [4]. However, GEPTS had already reported in 1963 that the B-cells are reduced in every case of juvenile-onset diabetes [19]. In acute-onset patients, the B-cells may still be present, but in numbers well below normal values. GEPTS also pointed out the necessity of quantitative studies [19], which were an important part of the 1965 study [4], but could not refrain from reporting in 1963 that in the pancreas of juvenile-onset diabetics there may be both peri- and intrainsular inflam-

* The work in the authors' laboratory has been supported by the foundation Nordisk Insulinlaboratorium, The National Institutes of Health (grants DK26190, DK33873), and the Juvenile Diabetes Foundation. Steinunn Bækkeskov is supported by a Juvenile Diabetes Foundation Career Development Award.

matory infiltrates, insular fibrosis, changes in the acinar tissue, and vascular lesions. The similarities with other organ-specific autoimmune disorders, such as HASHIMOTO'S, GRAVES', and ADDISON'S diseases were obvious and resulted in an intensive search for islet cell autoantibodies (ICA). If ICA were detected, it would be a major support to the hypothesis that insulin-dependent diabetes has an autoimmune pathogenesis.

Antibodies reactive with insulin were first described in sera from diabetic patients tested on pancreatic sections [20], but these antibodies were likely to be induced by a polyclonal reaction to the injected insulin rather than to ICA. Technical improvements such as better fluorescent reagents and the introduction of epi-illumination in the fluorescence microscope, as well as thorough methodological study on the reactivity of human serum and antibodies with the exocrine portion of the pancreas [21], were the prerequisites for the first description of the islet cell antibodies in 1974 (Table 1). Publishing a month apart, BOTTAZZO et al. [14] and MACCUISH et al. [22] described the presence of ICA in sera from patients with the simultaneous presence of insulin-dependent diabetes mellitus (IDDM) and polyendocrine disease.

In subsequent investigations, LENDRUM and coworkers [23, 24] showed that ICA were particularly prevalent at the time of clinical diagnosis in young IDDM patients and that the ICA disappeared with increasing length of insulin therapy. The typical patient with ICA would therefore tend to be a young individual who has recently developed diabetes rather than an older patient with organ-specific autoimmunity and late-onset insulin-dependent diabetes.

The ICA reaction was found to involve all islet cells [14, 22]. However, several studies show a specific reduction of the islet B-cells only at the time of clinical diagnosis of IDDM [4, 5, 7]. The obvious question to ask was whether IDDM patients had antibodies reactive with antigenic determinants which would be specif-

Table 1. Circulating signs of autoimmune islet disease

Preparation to detect islet antigen	Method of detection	Islet cell autoantibody	References
Frozen sections of human pancreas	Indirect immunofluorescence	Islet cell cytoplasmic (ICA, ICCA)	14, 22, 44
Human insulinoma cells	Indirect immunofluorescence	Human insulinoma cell	25, 26
Dispersed rat islet cells	Indirect immunofluorescence	Islet cell surface (ICSA)	15
Monolayers of rat islet cells	^{51}Cr-release	Islet cell cytotoxic (C'AMC)	28
Purified rat islet B cells	Indirect immunofluorescence	B-cell specific ICSA	29
Transformed (hamster) islet cells	^{51}Cr-release	Antibody-dependent cellular cytotoxicity (ADCC)	69, 72
Human islets	Immunoprecipitation	64 K protein	30, 32

ically expressed on the surface of the B-cells. Antibodies binding to the cell surface were initially described using human insulinoma cells [25]; however, it was uncertain whether these cells produced insulin, and the experiments could not be reproduced due to the loss of the cells [26]. Later, normal rat islets dispersed into single cells [27], which primarily would contain B-cells, were used to demonstrate islet cell surface antibodies (ICSA) in sera from patients with IDDM [15]. Monolayer rat islet cell cultures in a combined immunofluorescence and cytotoxicity test showed the ICSA to mediate complement-dependent cytotoxicity [28]. Novel methods to separate rat islet B-cells from the non-B-cell population allowed the detection of B-cell-specific ICSA [29].

Several methods are now available to detect ICA and ICSA [30, 31]. The tissue preparations may be of human origin, but due to the lack of material, nonhuman tissue preparations are most often used. A major lack in understanding the autoimmune phenomena in IDDM resides in the fact that we have yet to determine what the antibodies are able to recognize and bind to in the islet tissue. So far, only one antigen, a protein of M_r 64000 (64 K protein) has been detected [30, 32]. It was recently demonstrated that about one-third of newly diagnosed IDDM patients have insulin autoantibodies as well [33]. The multitude of islet cell autoantibodies appears confusing. In part this confusion is due to the fact that the antibodies are named according to the way they are detected and not by the antigen used to detect them. It is therefore important to briefly review current views on the initiation of an immune response in order to understand how circulating signs of an autoimmune islet disease may develop.

The Normal Immune Response

The pathway of cellular interactions involved when the immune system mounts a response against a foreign antigen is complex and not yet fully understood (Fig. 1). This pathway is assumed also to be involved in a reaction against "self antigens" or autoantigens. In brief, an antigen is taken up by antigen-presenting cells (APC), which are macrophages or macrophage-like cells. The APC processes the antigen by means of limited proteolysis. The fragments of the antigen are thought to be

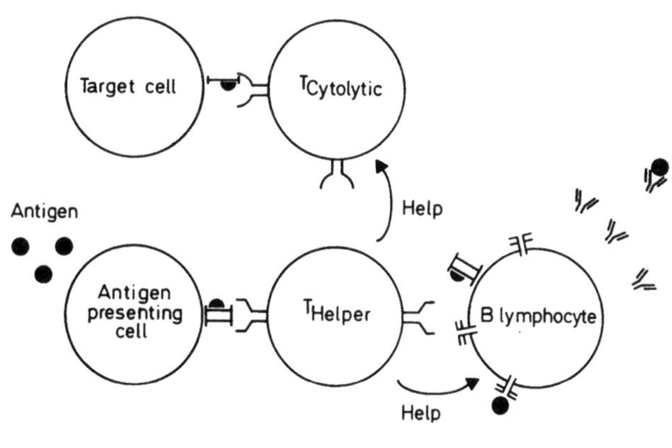

Fig. 1. Pathways of an immune response to an antigen. ⊢⊣ and ⊨⫤ represent class I and II MHC molecules respectively

presented as epitopes on the APC surface in conjunction with, or perhaps even bound to, a class II molecule. The latter is encoded in the major histocompatibility complex (MHC) or HLA on the short arm of the human chromosome 6.

A helper T-lymphocyte expressing a specific T-cell receptor is activated when the antigen (epitope) - class II complex is recognized. The activation of helper T-lymphocytes provides stimulus to self-proliferation and causes clonal expansion and differentiation of effector cells.

Effector cells are antigen-specific T-lymphocytes with either cytotoxic or suppressive properties and/or B-lymphocytes. Cytotoxic T-lymphocytes are able to recognize and kill target cells which express the particular epitope of a foreign antigen on their cell surface. However, the killing is restricted to target cells which share class I molecules (HLA-A, B, C region gene products) with the cytotoxic T-lymphocyte.

B-lymphocytes express membrane-bound antibody molecules, which also serve as antigen receptors. These bind circulating foreign antigen, but they will only proliferate and differentiate into plasma cells when they receive help from T-lymphocytes. B-lymphocytes have also been shown to process and present antigens. Plasma cells secrete large amounts of antibody that combine with circulating foreign antigen to form complexes. Recent evidence suggests that each clone of antigen-activated B-lymphocytes experience rapid somatic mutations at the rate of 10^{-3} per base pair per cell division, thus modifying the immunoglobin genes to provide an increasing degree of antigen specificity.

The binding of the antibody to an invading organism, results in an effective activation of the complement pathway. The end result is lysis of the organism. Similarly, an antibody may bind to the surface of a cell, thereby eliminating this cell by the same mechanism. Antibodies may also arm killer cells (leukocytes, macrophages) to seek a target antigen on a cell surface to mediate an antibody-dependent cellular cytotoxic reaction. Finally, an antibody may bind to a specific receptor, either to mimic the receptor ligand or to act as an antagonist.

The synthesis and release of an antibody seems to be controlled both by the availability of antigen and, in part, by a feedback mechanism. The latter phenomenon involves the formation of antibodies which recognize the antigen-binding portion of the original antibody. This portion of the antibody is referred to as the idiotype and the antibody formed against the idiotype is termed anti-idiotypic antibody.

The Autoimmune Response

It is assumed that the above-mentioned cellular interactions are involved in an immune response which develops against an autoantigen. A foreign antigen may induce antibodies which cross-react with an antigen or autoantigen of the host. A well-known example of this is the occasional occurence of hemolytic episodes during mycoplasmal pneumonia infections, in which antibodies known as cold agglutinins also react with the group I receptor of erythrocytes to cause complement-dependent hemolysis [34]. Infection with group A streptococci may cause rheumatic fever in an HLA-DR-associated manner to involve autoreactivity against cardiac valve receptors [35]. The *Yersinia enterocolitica* membrane possesses a saturable binding site for the thyroid-stimulating hormone (TSH) to mimic the thyroid cell TSH receptor, which may explain why epidemics of *Yersinia* are followed by an increased incidence of Graves' disease [36].

These pathways may be circumvented by factors which induce a polyclonal activation. Epstein-Barr virus (EBV), which causes infectious mononucleosis, may induce antibodies directed against various autoantigens present in diverse tissues and cells such as smooth muscle, nuclear proteins, lymphocytes, and erythrocytes [37]. Parasitic [38] and protozoan [39] infections have also been shown to cause unspecific B-lymphocyte stimulation. A phenomenon which still requires explanation is the by now classical association between certain HLA types and autoimmune diseases. The hypothesis is that genes encoded in the MHC confer susceptibility to certain autoimmune reactions; however, the mechanisms involved remain to be clarified.

If autoimmunity is important in the etiology and pathogenesis of diabetes, there is inadequate information concerning the initial steps of the process involved when the B-cell becomes the specific target of the immune system.

Detection of Antibodies

The structure and function of immunoglobulin (Ig) molecules allow their detection in a variety of ways (Fig. 2). The property of an antibody to bind to its antigen via the variable region (V) or the idiotype region is used in standard binding assays. The ability of the antibody to bind to a labeled antigen is often tested in competition binding experiments using unlabeled antigen. This approach allows the binding characteristics of an antibody to be fully described. The antibody may, for example, be given numbers expressing its association and dissociation constants, avidity, or antigenic specificity. The latter is only possible when structural

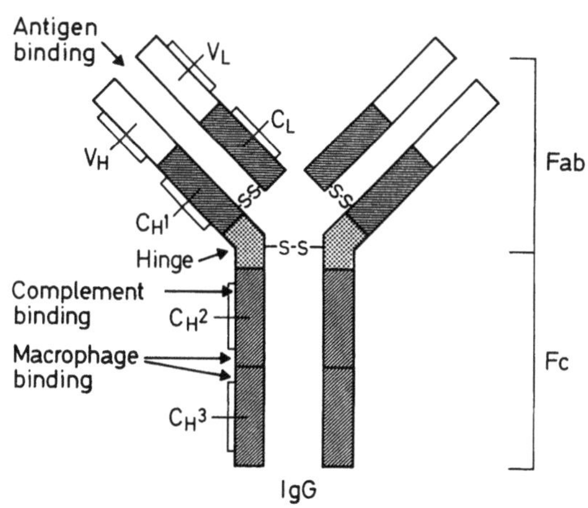

Fig. 2. A schematic representation of an IgG molecule indicating various parts often used to detect tissue-bound antibodies. The three constant regions *(C_H1 -C_H3)* of the heavy chain, the constant region of the light chain *(C_L)*, and the variable portions of the heavy *(V_H)* and light *(V_L)* chains along with disulphide bridges (-S-S) are also indicated

analogues of the antigen are available. In current studies on the humoral autoimmune response against the pancreatic islet cells this is not yet possible, since preparations of entire tissues or cells are used to determine the presence of bound antibodies.

The parts of an Ig molecule which show allotype (F_c + V) specificity (Fig. 2) are antigenic in other animals. Antisera against human IgM, IgG, or IgA, which are commercially available from a very large number of sources, are polyvalent and react with different parts of the corresponding Ig molecule. These reagents are most often available as fluorescent molecules after conjugation with fluorescein isothiocyanate, rhodamine, or Texas red. These second antibody reagents allow an effective although not always quantitative way to detect an Ig molecule bound to its antigen.

The isotype or F_c portion of an IgG molecule (Fig. 2) offers yet other means by which an antibody bound to its antigen can be detected. First, certain bacterial wall proteins such as protein A [40] or protein G [41] show specific binding to the F_c portion. Numerous investigations have shown the great utility of these reagents in detection of antigen-bound Ig.

Antibodies are also able to activate complement [42]. The complex formed between an antigen and an antibody results in a conformational change in the F_c portion which allows binding of C_1 and the initiation of the complement cascade to be used as a measure of the presence of an antibody. Finally, many cells express receptors for the F_c portion on their cell membranes. In this way such cells, which

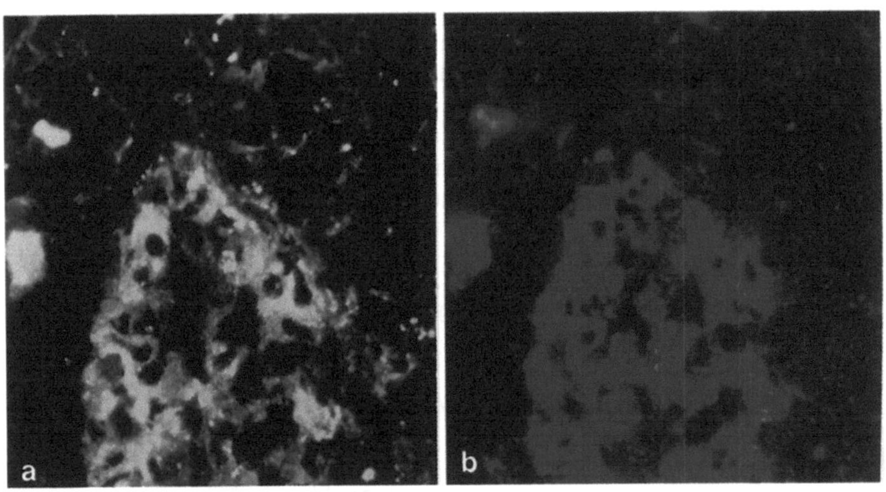

Fig. 3. Islet cell antibody (ICA) detected by indirect immunofluorescence on a section of frozen human pancreas. The *left* panel shows the indirect immunofluorescence reaction with a serum from a patient with newly diagnosed insulin-dependent diabetes mellitus. The presence of ICA is visualized by a second antibody reagent labeled with fluorescein-isothiocyanate. The *right* panel shows staining with a mouse monoclonal IgG specific for human proinsulin. The binding of this antibody is visualized with a Texas red-labeled second antibody. The procedure used in simultaneous staining for these antibodies was developed at the Hagedorn Research Laboratory by Dr. O. D. Madsen, who also kindly provided these photomicrographs

include macrophages or leukocytes, may become armed with an antibody and express antigen-specific cellular killing to mark the presence of an antibody against a specific antigen.

Islet Cell (Cytoplasmic) Antibodies (ICA): Methods of Detection

The indirect immunofluorescence test on sections of frozen human pancreas has become the routine approach to detect ICA [43-48]. Human blood group 0 pancreas, frozen as quickly as possible, is used and 1- to 3-μm sections are cut. The frozen sections are dried onto slides and incubated with serum. After careful rinsing, the sections are incubated with a second antibody reagent, which is fluorescent anti-human Ig serum or an IgG-binding reagent such as Protein A. The fluorescent reaction is viewed in a fluorescence microscope with epi-illumination (Fig. 3). Unless the serum samples are ICA-positive, islets of Langerhans will not be detected. Serum or plasma samples are usually tested without being diluted and are scored negative or positive. In the case of a particular series of sections not containing any islets, there is a risk of false-negative determinations.

Several modifications to detect ICA have been reported. One is to allow bound antibodies to fix complement, i.e., to bind C1 present in normal human serum and allow the complement-cascade reactions to occur. The complex is then visualized by fluorescently labeled antibody against human C3b [44]. These antibodies have been referred to as complement-fixing ICA or CF-ICA. Similarly, the F_c portion of bound Ig may be detected by fluorescent protein A (SpA) [45]. Protein A does not bind all IgG subclasses and this antibody may be referred to as SpA-ICA [45]. It should also be possible to develop very sensitive detection systems for ICA using enzyme-linked immunoassay systems. A first attempt with a peroxidase-labeled second antibody reagent to vizualize tissue-bound ICA (or PAP-ICA) was recently reported [46].

Circulating ICA in Autoimmune Diabetes

A synthesis of numerous studies indicates that ICA:

1. Are most prevalent among newly diagnosed IDDM patients.
2. Decrease both in prevalence and titer with increasing duration of IDDM.
3. In high titers are associated with a more rapid loss of endogenous C-peptide.
4. May be present up to several years before the clinical onset of IDDM.
5. May often be associated with a later development of IDDM in some patients with NIDDM.
6. May be evanescent in the nonaffected twin among monozygotic twins who remain discordant for IDDM.

7. May decrease in titer following cyclosporin A treatment in newly diagnosed IDDM patients and show a rebound when the treatment is discontinued.

These [see reviews in 42, 46-49] and other observations are taken as an evidence that the presence of ICA mark an ongoing or active immune process against islet cells. However, the qualitative approach to determine ICA is questionable and the first effort to standardize ICA measurements in a workshop was recently published [50].

The major problem in current ICA assays is the fact that the nature of the antigen(s) is not known. Proper displacement studies have therefore not been carried out. Assay reproducibility and precision have been improved in two-colour immunofluorescent assays [45, 51] to identify the islets by specific monoclonal antibodies (Fig. 3). However, once the antigen(s) is isolated, precise, reproducible, and high-capacity assays are likely to quickly outdate the current ICA assays.

Islet cell surface antibodies

Islet cell surface antibodies are defined by their ability to bind to antigens expressed on the cell membrane of an islet cell [15]. Islet B-cell-specific ICSA have been described [29]. It is not possible to use intact islets to detect ICSA, but islets dispersed into single-cell suspensions allow binding of the antibody to the very surface of the individual cells. Insulin-producing, cloned cell lines of rat [52] or hamster [53-55] origin, or alternatively, newborn rat islet cells [28] and human fetal islet cells [56], which are kept in monolayer cultures, may be used. The frequent occurrence of antibodies reactive with rodent determinants necessitates that all samples are first absorbed to cells or tissue of the same species as the insulin-producing cell which will be used to detect ICSA.

Antibodies bound to the cell surface are detected with the same type of second reagents as those described for ICA. Two major approaches have been used. One is indirect immunofluorescence [15, 28, 54], the other employs radioactive second antibodies [57] or ^{125}I-protein A [58].

The prevalence of ICSA reactive with rat, mouse, or hamster islet cells was reported to be 50%-70% [15, 28, 52], while the prevalence in the monolayer islet tumor cell assays was lower [54]. The ICSA tended to be evanescent among the IDDM patients. The frequencies of ICSA among studies vary markedly, probably because rodent target cells are used and sera have not always been preabsorbed to remove cross-reactive antibodies. Further studies are therefore needed to isolate and characterize the cell surface antigens detected by ICSA. As a circulating sign of islet autoimmune disease, the ICSA remain of particular interest, since it cannot be excluded that some ICSA may recognize islet cell surface molecules which are involved in the regulation of insulin release. At the time of clinical diagnosis, IDDM patients may have Ig which interfere with the islet B-cell function in vitro [59, 60]. Further studies will be needed to substantiate the hypothesis that ICSA have a direct effect on the in vivo B-cell function.

Cytotoxic Islet Cell Antibodies

It was observed early that human serum or plasma is cytotoxic to single-cell preparations of islet cells [61], the action being probably mediated by activation of the alternative complement pathway [62]. In retrospect, perhaps some of these cytotoxic effects were due to the presence of interleukin-1 [63]. Cytotoxic islet cell antibodies or, more correctly, complement-dependent antibody-mediated cytotoxicity (C'AMC) would be those ICSA which bind to the islet cell surface. The ICSA should withstand washing and, after addition of serum as a source of complement, they should bind the complement component C1. Thereby they initiate the complement cascade which results in cellular killing by making holes in the cell membrane and the eventual complete lysis of the cells. Animal sera are often used as the source of complement, and care must be taken to avoid preparations which themselves are toxic to the islet cells. The ability to fix complement varies among Ig subclasses [42] and may explain any discrepancies between ICSA and C'AMC determinations.

Several methods are available to estimate cell viability in a C'AMC test. The classical test is to use ^{51}Cr-labeling of the target cell and to measure release of the isotope as a measure of cytotoxicity. Other tests involve viability stains such as trypan blue or ethidium bromide. The isotope assays are quantitative, independent of observer bias, and can be the subject of intra- and interassay standardizations. It is difficult to test the role of C'AMC in the pathogenesis of IDDM due to the lack of human pancreatic islet cells.

The prevalence of C'AMC at the clinical onset of IDDM varies from 30% to 70% [28, 64–67]. In one prospective study [65], the C'AMC tended to remain longer than ICA with increasing duration of IDDM. The C'AMC was observed at an increased frequency among first-degree relatives compared to healthy controls [28, 66]. The possible association between appearance of C'AMC against islet B-cells and a later development of IDDM remain to be determined. The C'AMC assays utilizing insulin-producing islet cell lines [52, 66, 67] are attractive, since a large number of samples can be tested. At the same time, proper inter- and intra-assay control samples can be included in each assay. Whether the C'AMC activity detected in IDDM sera in vitro is at all related to the function of remaining islet B-cells remains a matter of controversy. Using a two-wavelength immunofluorescence system, Smets and Gepts [68] demonstrated that B-cell-specific ICSA in IDDM sera were able to bind complement at both 4 °C and 37 °C. In contrast, ICSA in IDDM sera able to bind both B-cells and non-B-cells were able to fix complement on all cell types at 4 °C but only on B-cells at 37 °C. It was therefore suggested that ICSA have a B-cell-specific cytotoxic effect in the presence of complement at physiological temperature. It will be important to substantiate these in vitro studies further by in situ experiments.

Antibody-Dependent Cellular Cytotoxicity

Macrophages or leukocytes are normally not cytotoxic to other cells. Primarily in vitro, but also in vivo, such cells may become cytotoxic and serve as effector cells if armed with an antibody against an islet cell. The effector cells express F_c receptors which will bind antibodies present in circulation or better when bound to a target cell. In this way an ICSA may form a bridge between the effector and target islet cell. The close proximity between the target and effector cell allows the latter to kill the former. The mechanism of killing is not known in detail, but probably involves monokines as well as a protein which has properties similar to the complement factors which mediates perforation of cell membranes.

In the antibody-dependent cellular cytotoxicity (ADCC) assay, the target cells are usually labeled with ^{51}Cr and the release of the radioactivity taken as a measure of viability. In general, it is assumed that the ^{51}Cr radioactivity which leaks out of a dying or dead cell is bound to large-molecular-weight compounds. Radioactivity appearing in the supernatant is therefore not taken up by other viable cells. However, since the effector cells in this assay are effective phagocytic cells, care must be taken to optimize effector/target (E/T) cell ratios, as well as the time of incubation, to minimize this possible artifact. It should also be noted that a labeled target cell, such as a transformed insulin-producing cell, may be killed by natural killer cells present in the effector cell population. The activity of such cells would yield the background activity observed without the addition of serum containing ICSA.

In ADCC assays carried out so far, the target islet cells have been of rodent origin [69-71], while the serum and the effector cells have been from man. ADCC has been observed among 30%-50% of newly diagnosed IDDM patients. Among healthy individuals 2%-4% were positive [68-70]. The most effective ADCC killing was observed when the effector cells were from the same individual whose serum was being tested [70].

It has yet to be determined in a prospective analysis whether islet cell ADCC precede the clinical onset of IDDM and to what extent positive reactions correlate with an alteration in islet B-cell function. Interleukin-1 (IL-1) and other monokines are cytotoxic to rat and human islet cells in vitro [63]. Since the insulitis also involves cells which are typical effectors in an ADDC assay, IL-1 production in sufficiently high concentrations would kill any islet cell in a nonspecific manner. However, the specific loss of the islet B-cells would be easily explained if macrophages are armed by B-cell-specific ICSA. In this way these killer cells would recognize the islet B-cells only, and by a direct and close interaction exert a lytic effect.

Are Autoantibodies Against B-Cell-Specific Proteins Circulating Signs of Islet Autoimmunity?

An explanation of the specific loss of the insulin-producing cells would be easy if antigen-specific effectors, either cytotoxic T-lymphocytes or antibodies, could furnish the immune system with a mechanism by which to detect only the pancreatic B-cells. What particular molecule of the B-cells, including those transplanted to spontaneously diabetic BB rats [73], is recognized by the immune system? The approach to detect islet autoantigens has been to label islet proteins by metabolic labeling in vitro and then immunoprecipitate the labeled proteins with sera from BB rats [74], or subjects with [30, 32] or later developing [75] IDDM. Antibody-antigen complexes formed are absorbed to Protein A-Sepharose, washed, and boiled in SDS to denature and solubilize the bound proteins. SDS gel electrophoresis of the solubilized material separates the proteins according to their electrophoretic mobility. It was detected that autoantibodies in diabetic sera specifically recognized a protein of about M_r 64000 [30, 32]. Among 14 subjects followed prospectively until the development of IDDM [75], antibodies against this 64 K protein was consistently detected in 11 (Fig. 4). M_r 64 K antibodies were detected before ICA in two patients. These studies suggest that 64 K antibodies are an early marker of B-cell autoimmunity and may be useful to predict a later onset of IDDM. IDDM sera were also able to bind a rat islet B-cell protein of similar molecular mass, while this protein could not be detected in nonislet tissues [76].

So far, this protein and insulin autoantibodies [33] are the only islet B-cell-specific antigens which might be involved in the pathogenesis of IDDM. Insulin autoantibodies have now been reported not only in newly diagnosed IDDM patients [32, 77], but also in individuals either susceptible to IDDM [78, 79] or later developing the disease [80]. However, unless the insulin molecule is somehow expressed at the cell surface, which has been suggested [81], it is difficult to understand how immune effectors would be able to use this antigen to kill B-cells. The pancreatic islet cells synthesize and express class I antigens [82, 83], and should therefore be easy targets for T-cytotoxic (CTL) killing, if the proper antigen is presented and seen by the CTL receptor. In this context, the nature of the 64 K protein remains obscure, except that it is a membrane-associated molecule and may be present in minor concentrations on the cell surface of human and rat islet cells [32]. Whether it is a receptor molecule of importance to specific properties of the B-cells such as glucose-stimulated insulin biosynthesis, storage, or release remains to be determined.

It is assumed that the formation of autoantibodies against the islet B-cells is preceded by antigen processing, presentation, and activation by a proper helper-T lymphocyte of the B-lymphocyte circuit. It is still unclear to what extent the B-cell itself may serve as an APC. Given an exogeneous challenge such as a viral infection, the B-cell might express class II antigens and perhaps itself present the autoantigens, such as the 64 K protein. Although some class II molecule-positive islet cells were reported in one subject [6], islet cells in diabetic BB rats failed to express class II molecules [84]. It is therefore equally plausible that the initial antigen presentation causing later B-cell intolerance is initiated away from the islets of LANGERHANS, and that the immune recognition of the B-cells occurs later on.

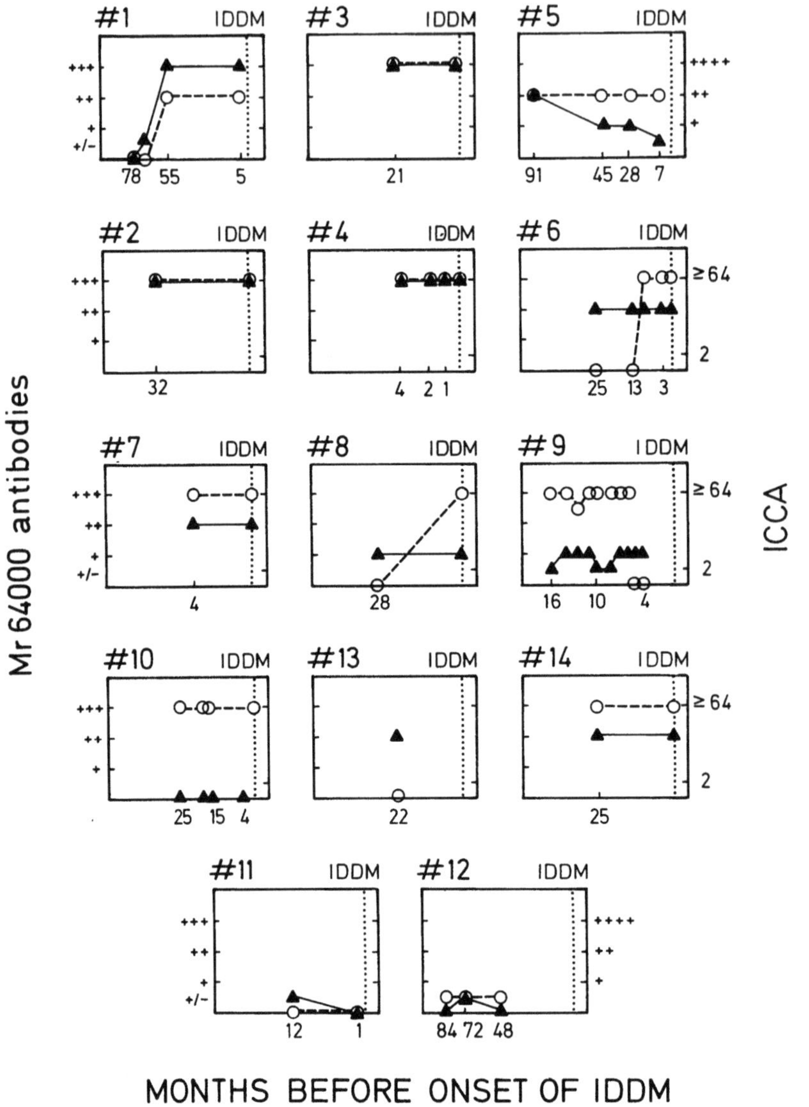

Fig. 4. Presence of islet cell antibodies (ICA) ○—○) and 64 K protein antibodies (▲—▲) in 14 individuals followed up for 4-91 months before the clinical onset of insulin-dependent diabetes mellitus (IDDM). The levels of ICA were estimated either by end-point titrations or arbitrarily. The levels of 64 K protein antibodies were estimated on the basis of the autoradiographic intensity of immunoprecipitated 64 K component on a 0-3+ scale. (Data from 75)

Organ-Specific Autoantibodies

Apart from antibodies directed against islet cells, many studies have shown the presence of a number of autoantibodies against various tissues such as thyroid, gastric mucosa, and adrenal. This break of tolerance, which seems to affect several endocrine tissues, is not understood. In addition, circulating immune complexes were detected in 25% newly diagnosed IDDM patients, as compared to 7% of controls [85, 86]. Whether these complexes reflect an increased autoimmunity or are of pathological significance remains to be clarified.

Discussion and Future Directions

A large number of assays to detect antibodies which react with islet cells and islet cell antigens have been described. The presence of ICA at high titer and frequency at the time of clinical diagnosis of IDDM may reflect an active immune process against the B-cells. In selected individuals followed for as long as 5–8 years before the clinical diagnosis in parallel with progressive B-cell failure, islet cell (cytoplasmic), insulin, and 64 K protein autoantibodies have also been demonstrated. It needs to be clarified, however, why patients with newly diagnosed IDDM have a multitude of autoantibodies also reactive with other endocrine organs or cell constituents. It is therefore central to the understanding of autoimmune IDDM to determine which B-cell-specific antigens are recognized by the immune system, by T-lymphocytes as well as by B-lymphocytes and antibodies secreted from the latter cells.

Foreign antigens such as a virus or bacterium induce a humoral immune response which follows immediately after the antigen has been in circulation for a short period of time. IgM antibodies against the antigen appear first, and a continued presence of the antigen will then lead to the disappearance of the IgM antibodies and their replacement by IgG antibodies. In time, the IgG antibodies alter in structure to display an increasing specificity toward the antigen. In autoimmune IDDM we are ignorant of any such processes. Are islet cell (auto)antigens ever detected in the blood? Do IgM islet cell (auto)antibodies exist, and if so, when do they switch to IgG? What is the time-span from antigen presentation to clinical diagnosis of IDDM? These and other questions would be possible to answer once one or several islet autoantigens become available. The prospects have never been better that the mechanisms of the B-cell-specific killing in IDDM, first demonstrated by WILLY GEPTS, will eventually be understood.

The spectacular achievements in purifying individual islet cell types [87, 88, 89] have already made it possible for PIPELEERS, GEPTS and their colleagues [29, 68, 89] to obtain evidence that the circulating signs of islet cell immune-mediated killing may be B-cell-specific surface antibodies.

Recent advances in molecular and cell biology should permit the cloning and complete sequence determination of the antigen(s) recognized by these autoantibodies. It will then be possible to study the mechanisms of processing and presentation of these (auto)antigens to determine their immunogenicity and antigenicity in systems which involve not only the use of patient sera and monoclonal antibodies, but also cloned T-lymphocytes trained to recognize relevant antigen epitopes in the context of HLA class II specificities. Since susceptibility for IDDM is associated with certain HLA specificities, such experiments should provide the necessary information about the pathways which control the humoral immune response to the B-cells. Finally, techniques of antigen-specific immune suppression will eventually be used to test whether the course of an autoimmune islet disease can be obstructed or prevented.

Acknowledgement. We thank Lone Hesselholdt for expert help in preparing this review.

References

1. von Mering J, Minkowski O (1889) Diabetes Mellitus nach Pankreasextirpation. Arch Exp Pathol Pharmacol 26: 371-387
2. Gepts W, Pipeleers D (1976) The endocrine pancreas. Functional morphology and histopathology. In: Luft R (ed) Insulin. Acta Med Scand [Suppl] 601: 9-52
3. Banting FG, Best CB, Collip JB, Cambell WR, Fletcher AA (1922) Pancreatic extract in the treatment of diabetes mellitus. Can Med Assoc J 2: 141-146
4. Gepts W (1965) Pathologic anatomy of the pancreas in juvenile diabetes mellitus. Diabetes 14: 619-633
5. Foulis AK, Stewart JA (1984) The pancreas in recent-onset Type 1 (insulin-dependent) diabetes mellitus: insulin content of islets, insulitis and associated changes in the exocrine acinar tissue. Diabetologia 26: 456-461
6. Bottazzo GF, Dean BM, McNally JM, McKay EH, Swift PGF, Gamble DR (1985) In situ characterization of autoimmune phenomena and expression of HLA molecules in the pancreas in diabetic insulitis. N Engl J Med 313: 353-360
7. Rahier J, Goebbels RM, Henquin JC (1983) Cellular composition of the human diabetic pancreas. Diabetologia 24: 366-371
8. Lacy PE, Wright PH, Silverman JL (1963) Eosinophilic infiltration in the pancreas of rats injected with anti-insulin serum. Fed Proc 22: 60
9. Renold AE, Soeldner JS, Steincke J (1964) Immunologic studies with homologous and heterologous pancreatic insulin in the cow. Ciba Foundations Colloquia 15: 122
10. Like AA, Rossini AA (1976) Streptozotocin-induced pancreatic insulitis: new model of diabetes mellitus. Science 193: 415-417
11. Craighead JE (1975) The role of viruses in the pathogenesis of pancreatic disease and diabetes mellitus. Prog Med Virol 19: 161-214
12. Notkins AL (1977) Virus-induced diabetes mellitus. Brief review. Arch Virol 54: 1-17
13. Nerup J, Andersen OO, Bendixen G, Egeberg J, Poulsen JE (1973) Antipancreatic, cellular hypersensitivity in diabetes mellitus. Antigenic activity of fetal calf pancreas and correlation with clinical type of diabetes. Acta Allergol 28: 223-230
14. Bottazzo GF, Florin-Christensen A, Doniach D (1974) Islet cell antibodies in diabetes mellitus with autoimmune polyendocrine deficiencies. Lancet II: 1279-1283
15. Lernmark Å, Freedman ZR, Hofmann C, Rubenstein AH, Steiner DF, Jackson RL, Winter RJ, Traisman HS (1978) Islet cell surface antibodies in juvenile diabetes mellitus. N Engl J Med 299: 375-380
16. Platz P, Jackson BK, Morling M, Ryder LP, Svejgaard A, Thomsen M, Christy M, Kromann H, Benn J, Nerup J, Green A, Hauge M (1981) HLA-D and DR-antigens in genetic analysis of insulin-dependent diabetes mellitus. Diabetologia 21: 100-115

17. Barbosa J, Chavers B, Dunsworth T, Michael A (1982) Islet cell antibodies and histocompatibility antigens (HLA) in insulin-dependent diabetes and their first degree relatives. Diabetes 31: 585-588
18. Owerbach D, Lernmark Å, Platz P, Ryder LP, Rask L, Peterson PA, Ludvigson J (1983) HLA-D region β-chain DNA endonuclease fragments differ between HLA-DR identical healthy and insulin-dependent diabetic individuals. Nature 303: 815-817
19. Gepts W (1964) The cytologic pathology of the islets of Langerhans in juvenile diabetes. In: Brolin SE, Helman B and Knutson H (eds) The structure and metabolism of the pancreatic islets. Pergamon, Oxford, pp 513-519
20. Mancini AM, Costanzi G, Zampa GA (1964) Human insulin antibodies detected by immunofluorescence techniques. Lancet I: 726
21. Lendrum R, Walker JG (1975) Serum antibodies in human pancreatic disease. Gut 16: 365-371
22. MacCuish AC, Jordan J, Campbell CJ, Duncan LJP, Irvine WJ (1974) Antibodies to islet-cell in insulin-dependent diabetics with coexistent auto-immune disease. Lancet II: 1529-1533
23. Lendrum R, Walker G, Gamble DR (1975) Islet-cell antibodies in juvenile diabetes mellitus of recent onset. Lancet I: 880-883
24. Lendrum R, Walker GJ, Cudworth AG, Theophanides C, Pyke DA, Bloom A, Gamble DR (1975) Islet-cell antibodies in diabetes mellitus. Lancet II: 1273-1276
25. MacLaren NK, Huang SW, Fogh J (1975) Antibody to cultured human insulinoma cells in insulin-dependent diabetes. Lancet I: 997-1000
26. MacLaren NK (1977) Etiology and pathogenesis of insulin-dependent diabetes. Report from National Institute of Arthritis. Metab Dig Dis: 1-48
27. Lernmark Å (1974) The preparation of, and studies on, free cell suspensions from mouse pancreatic islets. Diabetologia 10: 431-438
28. Dobersen MJ, Scharff JE, Ginsberg-Fellner F, Notkins AL (1980) Cytotoxic autoantibodies to β-cells in the serum of patients with insulin-dependent diabetes mellitus. N Engl J Med 303: 1493-1498
29. Van de Winkel M, Smets G, Gepts W, Pipeleers DG (1982) Islet cell surface antibodies from insulin-dependent diabetics bind specifically to pancreatic B-cells. J Clin Invest 70: 41-49
30. Lernmark Å, Bækkeskov S (1981) Islet cell antibodies - theoretical and practical implications. Diabetologia 21: 431-435
31. Bottazzo GF, Pujol-Borell R, Doniach D (1981) Humoral and cellular immunity in diabetes mellitus. Clin Immunol Allergy 1: 139-159
32. Bækkeskov S, Nielsen JH, Marner B, Bilde T, Ludvigsson J and Lernmark Å (1982) Autoantibodies in newly diagnosed diabetic children immunoprecipitate specific human pancreatic islet cell protein. Nature 298: 167-169
33. Palmer JP, Asplin CM, Clemons P, Lyen K, Tatpati O, Raghu PK, Paquette TL (1983) Insulin antibodies in insulin-dependent diabetics before insulin treatment. Science 222: 1337-1339
34. McConnell I, Munro A, Waldmann H (1981) Autoimmune disease in the immune system - a course on the molecular and cellular basis of immunity, 2nd edn. Blackwell, London, pp 273
35. Ayoub EM, Barret DJ, MacLaren NK, Krischer JP (1986) Association of class II human histocompatibility leukocyte antigens with rheumatic fever. J Clin Invest 77: 2019-2026
36. Weiss M, Ingbar SH, Winblad S, Kaspar DL (1983) Demonstration of a saturable binding site for thyrotropin in *Yersinia enterocolitica*. Science 219: 1331-1333
37. Waldmann TA, Broder S (1982) Polyclonal B-cell activators in the study of the regulation of immunoglobulin synthesis in the human system. Adv Immunol 48: 196-200
38. Walls KW, Smith JW (1979) Serology of parasite infections. Int J Parasitol 10: 329-340
39. Perrin LH, Mackey LJ, Lambert PH (1985) Immunology of malaria. In: Rosse WF (ed) Clinical immunology update. Elsevier, New York, pp 234-264
40. Forsgren A, Sjöquist J (1966) Protein A from *S. aureus*. Pseudo-immune reaction with human-globulin. J Immunol 97: 822-827
41. Björck L, Kronvall G (1984) Purification and some properties of streptococcal protein G, a novel IgG-binding reagent. J Immunol 133: 969-974
42. Vergani D (1986) Complement. Diabetic Med 3: 306-311
43. Todd I, Bottazzo GF (1985) Laboratory investigation of autoimmune endocrine diseases. Clin Immunol Allergy 5: 613-638

44. Bottazzo GF, Dean BM, Gorsuch AN, Cudworth AG, Doniach D (1980) Complement-fixing islet-cell antibodies in type-I diabetes: possible monitors of active beta-cell damage. Lancet I: 668-672
45. Srikanta S, Rabizadeh A, Omar MAK, Eisenbarth GS (1985) Assay for islet cell antibodies. Protein A-monoclonal antibody method. Diabetes 34: 300-305
46. Kobayashi T, Sugimoto T, Itoh T, Kosaka K, Tanaka T, Suwa S, Sato K, Tsuji K (1986) The prevalence of islet cell antibodies in Japanese insulin-dependent and non-insulin-dependent diabetic patients studied by indirect immunofluorescence and by a new method. Diabetes 35: 335-340
47. Brogren CH, Lernmark Å (1982) Islet cell antibodies in diabetes mellitus. J Clin Endocrinol Metab 11: 409-430
48. Eisenbarth GS (1986) Type I diabetes mellitus. A chronic autoimmune disease. N Engl J Med 314: 1360-1368
49. Lernmark Å (1985) Molecular biology of type 1 (insulin-dependent) diabetes mellitus. Diabetologia 28: 195-203
50. Bottazzo GF, Gleichmann H (1986) Immunology and diabetes workshops: report on the first international workshop on the standardisation of cytoplasmic islet cell antibodies. Diabetologia 29: 125-126
51. Madsen OD, Landin Olsson M, Bille G, Sundkvist G, Lernmark Å, Dahlqvist G, Ludvigsson J (1986) A two-colour immunofluorescence test with a monoclonal human proinsulin antibody improves the assay for islet cell antibodies. Diabetologia 29: 115-118
52. Eisenbarth GS, Morris MA, Scearce RM (1981) Cytotoxic antibodies to cloned rat islet cells in serum of patients with diabetes mellitus. J Clin Invest 67: 403-408
53. Yokono K, Shii K, Hari J, Yaso S, Imamura Y, Ejiri K, Ishihara K, Fujii S, Kazumi T, Taniguchi H, Baba S (1984) Production of monoclonal antibodies to islet cell surface antigens using hybridization of spleen lymphocytes from non-obese diabetic mice. Diabetologia 26: 379-385
54. Matsuba I, Marner B, Nerup J, Lernmark Å (1987) Detection of islet cell autoantibodies in newly diagnosed diabetic patients using insulin-producing Syrian hamster cells. Diabetes Res 4: 103-107
55. Grant Am, Harrison DE, Moysey L, Smith D, Ashcroft SJH (1985) Detection of islet cell surface antibodies using cloned beta cells and comparison of their incidence with that of islet cell cytoplasmic antibodies. Diabetes Res 2: 225-229
56. Pujol-Borrell R, Kouhry EL, Bottazzo GF (1982) Islet cell surface antibodies in Type 1 (insulin-dependent) diabetes mellitus: use of human fetal pancreas cultures as substrate. Diabetologia 22: 89-95
57. Contreas G, Madsen OD, Vissing H, Lernmark Å (1987) A simple assay for the detection of antibodies to endocrine islet cell surface antigens. J Immunol Methods 95: 135-139
58. Huen A, Haneda M, Freedman Z, Lernmark Å, Rubenstein AH (1983) Quantitative determinations of islet cell surface antibodies using ^{125}I-protein A. Diabetes 32: 460-465
59. Kanatsuna T, Bækkeskov S, Lernmark Å, Ludvigsson (1983) Immunoglobulin from insulin-dependent diabetic children inhibits glucose-induced insulin release. Diabetes 32: 520-524
60. Svenningsen A, Dyrberg T, Gerling I, Lernmark Å, Mackay P, Rabinovitch A (1983) Inhibition of insulin release after passive transfer of immunoglobulin from insulin-dependent diabetic children to mice. J Clin Endocrinol Metab 57: 1301-1304
61. Lernmark Å, Sehlin J, Täljedal I-B, Kromann H, Nerup J (1978) Possible toxic effects of normal and diabetic patients serum on pancreatic beta-cells. Diabetologia 14: 25-31
62. Idahl L-Å, Sehlin J, Täljedal I-B, Thornell L-E (1980) Cytotoxic activation of complement by mouse pancreatic islet cells. Diabetes 29: 636-642
63. Bendtzen K, Mandrup-Poulsen T, Nerup J, Nielsen JH, Dinarello CA, Svenson M (1986) Cytotoxicity of human pI 7 interleukin-1 for pancreatic islets of Langerhans. Science 232: 1545-1547
64. Rittenhouse HG, Oxender DL, Pek S, Ar D (1980) Complement-mediated cytotoxic effects on pancreatic islets with sera from diabetic patients. Diabetes 29: 317-322
65. Rabinovitch A, MacKay P, Ludvigsson J, Lernmark Å (1984) A prospective analysis of islet cell cytotoxic antibodies in insulin-dependent diabetic children: transient effects of plasmapheresis. Diabetes 33: 224-228

66. Toguchi Y, Ginsberg-Fellner F, Rubinstein P (1985) Cytotoxic islet cell surface antibodies (ICSA) in patients with type I diabetes and their first-degree relatives. Diabetes 34: 855-860
67. Marner B, Lernmark Å, Ludvigsson J, MacKay P, Matsuba I, Nerup J, Rabinovitch A (1985) Islet cell antibodies in insulin-dependent (Type I) diabetic children treated with plasmapheresis. Diabetes Res 2: 231-236
68. Smets G, Gepts W (1986) Selective complement fixation by pancreatic B-cells after binding to islet cell surface antibodies. J Endocrinol Invest 9: 43-49
69. Maruyama T, Takei I, Matsuba I, Tsuruoka A, Taniyama M, Ikeda Y, Kataoka K, Abe M, Matsuki S (1984) Cell-mediated cytotoxic islet cell surface antibodies to human pancreatic beta cells. Diabetologia 26: 30-33
70. Lernmark Å, Bækkeskov S, Dyrberg T, Gerling I, Marner B, Papadopoulos G, Svenningsen A, Binder C, Christy M, Nerup J, Mandrup-Poulsen T (1984) Pathogenesis of type I diabetes mellitus. In: Labrie F, Proulx L (eds) Endocrinology. Elsevier, Amsterdam, pp 92-96
71. Michaelis D, Rjasanowski I, Hehmke B, Kohnert K-D, Hildmann W, Keilacker H, Richter KV (1985) Lack of strong association between residual human C-peptide secretion and islet cell antibodies, complement-dependent antibody-mediated cytotoxicity, and HLA antigens in newly diagnosed type I diabetics. Biomed Biochim Acta 44: 99-106
72. Charles AM, Suzuki M, Waldeck N, Dodson LE, Slater L, Ong K, Kershnar A, Buckingham B, Golden M (1983) Immune islet killing mechanisms associated with insulin-dependent diabetes: in vitro expression of cellular and antibody-mediated islet cell cytotoxicity in humans. J Immunol 130: 1189-1194
73. Weringer EJ, Like AA (1985) Immune attack on pancreatic islet transplant in the spontaneously diabetic Biobreeding/Worcester (BB/W) rat is not MHC restricted. J Immunol 134: 2383-2386
74. Bækkeskov S, Dyrberg T, Lernmark Å (1984) Autoantibodies against a M_r 64000 islet cell protein precede the onset of spontaneous diabetes. Science 224: 1348-1350
75. Bækkeskov S, Bruining S, Srikanta T, Mandrup-Poulsen T, Beaufort C, Eisenbarth GS, Lernmark Å (1986) Antibodies to a M_r 64000 human islet cell protein in the prediabetic period od IDDM patients. Ann NY Acad Sci 475: 415-417
76. Kanatsuna T, Bækkeskov S, Lernmark Å, Ludvigsson J (1983) Immunoglobulin from insulin-dependent diabetic children inhibits glucose-induced insulin release. Diabetes 32: 520-524
77. Arslanian SA, Becker DJ, Rabin B, Atchinson R, Eberhardt M, Cavender D, Dorsman J, Drash AL (1985) Correlates of insulin autoantibodies in newly diagnosed diabetic children with insulin-dependent diabetes before insulin therapy. Diabetes 34: 926-930
78. Wilkin T, Armitage M, Casey C, Pyke DA, Hoskins PJ, Rodier M, Diaz JL, Leslie RDG (1985) Value of insulin autoantibodies as serum markers for insulin-dependent diabetes mellitus. Lancet I: 480-482
79. Atkinson MA, MacLaren NK, Riley WJ, Winter WE, Fisk DD, Spillar RP (1986) Are insulin autoantibodies markers for insulin-dependent diabetes mellitus? Diabetes 35: 894-898
80. Soeldner JS, Tuttleman M, Srikanta S, Ganda OP, Eisenbarth GS (1985) Insulin-dependent diabetes mellitus and autoimmunity: islet cell autoantibodies, insulin autoantibodies and beta-cell failure. N Engl J Med 313: 893-894
81. Kaplan DR, Colca JR, McDaniel ML (1983) Insulin as a surface marker on isolated cells from rat pancreatic islets. J Cell Biol 97: 433-437
82. Bækkeskov S, Kanatsuna T, Klareskog L, Nielsen DA, Peterson PA, Rubenstein AH, Steiner DF, Lernmark Å (1981) Expression of major histocompatibility antigens on pancreatic islet cells. Proc Natl Acad Sci USA 78: 6456-6460
83. Faustman D, Hauptfeld V, Davie JM, Lacy PE, Schreffler DC (1980) Murine pancreatic-cells express H-2K and H-2D but not Ia antigens. J Exp Med 151: 1563-1568
84. Dean BM, Walker R, Bone AJ, Baird JD, Cooke A (1985) Pre-diabetes in the spontaneously diabetic BB/E rat: Lymphocyte subpopulations in the pancreatic infiltrate and expression of MHC class II molecules in endocrine cells. Diabetologia 28: 464-466
85. Contreas G, Lernmark Å, Mathiasen ER, Deckert T (1985) Immune complexes in insulin-dependent diabetes. Biomed Acta 44: 129-132
86. Borsey DQ, Di Mario U, Irvine WJ, Gray SR, Guy K, Weston J, Pentherer J, Duncan LJP (1982) Humoral immunity in Type 1 diabetes mellitus: a prospective study. J Clin Lab Immunol 5: 9-15

87. Pipeleers DG, Pipeleers-Marichal MA (1981) A method for the purification of single A, B and D cells and for the isolation of coupled cells from isolated rat islets. Diabetologia 20: 654-663
88. Pipeleers DG, In't Veld PA, Van de Winkel M, Maes E, Schmit FC, Gepts W (1985) A new in vitro model for the study of pancreatic A and B cells. Endocrinology 117: 806-816
89. Pipeleers D, van de Winkel M (1986) Pancreatic B cells possess defense mechanisms against cell-specific toxicity. Proc Natl Acad Sci USA 83: 5267-5271

Immune Interactions with Islet Cells: Implications for the Pathogenesis of Insulin-Dependent Diabetes Mellitus

J. Nerup, T. Mandrup-Poulsen, J. Mølvig and G. Spinas

Introduction

Occasionally a single scientific paper may signal a new era in the study of a disease. The 1965 paper by WILLY GEPTS was such a signal [1]. The (re)discovery of insulitis provided the impetus for new thoughts about the pathogenesis of insulin-dependent diabetes mellitus (IDDM) and for the emergence of a new research field: immunology of IDDM.

In his remarkable paper GEPTS emphasized several points pertinent to current research into the pathogenesis of IDDM: (a) Insulitis is found in the majority of recent-onset IDDM patients and is not, as previously thought, a rare finding. (b) The pathology of the islets of Langerhans in IDDM is heterogeneous. Most islets are devoid of B-cells and display no mononuclear cell (MNC) infiltration (pseudoatrophic islets); some contain normal or hypertrophic B-cells, but no mononuclear cells; and others present with a variable number of B-cells together with an MNC infiltration dominated by small lymphocytes and a few macrophages, but no plasma cells. Furthermore, it was hypothesized that the insulitis was the morphological expression of an immune attack against the B-cells.

In the subsequent papers [reviews 2, 3] it was shown that MNC infiltration was present only in islets containing B-cells and the overall picture of islet pathology in IDDM was interpreted to be compatible with a slowly progressing process. The extent of insulitis varies considerably among IDDM patients. One study [4] showed 15–75% of the islets to be affected, most pronouncedly in patients with very young age at onset.

Since IDDM does not become clinically manifest until about 90% of the B-cell mass is destroyed, the islet morphology at the time of diagnosis of IDDM represents the late stages of IDDM pathogenesis. Monoclonal antibody studies of pancreatic sections from newly diagnosed or recent-onset IDDM patients have shown the MNC infiltrate of the islets to contain cytotoxic/suppressor and helper subsets of T-lymphocytes, natural killer (NK)-cells, (K)-cells, and B-lymphocytes, but *no* macrophages or monocytes [5]. HLA-DR alpha-chain expression on B-cells was demonstrable in about 27% of the B-cell-containing islets [6] in this *end-stage* type of lesion.

The early features of islet morphology in human IDDM are unknown. However, admitting that what is being described may represent a secondary immune response, the islet pathology seen in biopsies from segmental pancreatic grafts transplanted between identical twins discordant for IDDM, taken at the time of recurrence of IDDM in the recipients, may reflect at least somewhat *earlier steps* in the pathogenetic process underlying IDDM. The MNC infiltrate in such islets was dominated by activated T-lymphocytes, cytotoxic/suppressor T-lymphocytes, *and* macrophages and monocytes. HLA-DR expression, not observed on endocrine cells, was prominent on islet endothelial cells. Furthermore, no islet IgG deposits were found [7].

Thus, differences seem to exist between islet morphology in the end-stage lesion typically seen in autopsy specimens from recent-onset IDDM-patients and the earlier lesions presumably studied during disease recurrence in transplanted IDDM twins. However, the pathogenetically more relevant *very early* or *initial* morphological features of IDDM in man are still unknown.

If the islet pathology of IDDM in the BioBreeding (BB) rat is at all relevant to human IDDM, it is worth noting that before typical insulitis develops in this animal, islet infiltration, mainly by macrophages, and B-cell destruction is seen [8, 9] together with HLA-DR expression on the islet vascular endothelium [10]. This may speak for a central role of the macrophage in the *early (initial?) stages* of B-cell destruction and pathogenesis of IDDM in the BB rat. That similar events may be relevant to IDDM pathogenesis in man is highly compatible with the possible role of a major macrophage product, interleukin-1 (IL-1) in B-cell destruction as described below.

Autoimmune Phenomena in IDDM

Inspired by the 1965 paper by GEPTS, a search began for autoimmune phenomena in IDDM. It was, however, not until 1971 that the first experimental demonstration of antipancreatic cell-mediated autoimmunity as a feature of IDDM was published [11]. Islet cell antibodies (ICA) were first described in 1974 [12], antibodies reacting with dispersed rat islet cells (ICSA) in 1978 [13] and antibodies reacting with a 64-kD protein of normal human and rat islet tissue (64-kD antibodies) in 1982 [14]. Furthermore, autoantibodies reacting with thyroid, adrenal cortex, and gastric mucosal epithelium were demonstrated more often in IDDM patients than in nondiabetic controls [15], as were insulin receptor antibodies [16], DNA and RNA antibodies [17], and circulating immune complexes [18]. This multitude of autoantibodies in IDDM patients is compatible with the demonstration of polyclonal B-lymphocyte activation in recent-onset IDDM patients [19]. Autoimmunity in IDDM has been extensively reviewed in ref. 20 (see also chapter 4 in this volume).

Islet Cell Autoantibodies as Effector Molecules in B-Cell Destruction

ICA [21], ICSA [22], 64-kD antibodies [23], and also insulin autoantibodies (IAA) [24] have been shown to be present years before onset of IDDM and to be associated (ICA) with an accelerated loss of residual B-cell function in newly diagnosed IDDM patients [25]. On this basis it has been suggested that ICA may be markers of ongoing B-cell destruction and thus predict the development of IDDM [26, 27]. In other words, a pathogenetic role of ICA is implied. Supporting this hypothesis is the finding that ICA-containing sera (predominantly ICSA-positive sera) from recent-onset IDDM patients, through complement-dependent antibody-mediated cytotoxicity (CAMC), may lyse xenogenic islet cell targets [29-33] in vitro. Furthermore, insulin release is inhibited from human islets exposed to islet cell antibodies [31], and transfer of large quantities of ICA from IDDM patients to immunosuppressed mice inhibited glucose-stimulated insulin release, but did not cause B-cell destruction [34].

However, a series of observations speak against a pathogenetic role of ICA. The predictive power of such antibodies for IDDM in first-degree relatives of IDDM probands is rather poor, since only about one-third of ICA-positive family members develop IDDM [35] and IDDM may develop in ICA-negative individuals [36]. The in vivo relevance of CAMC is doubtful, since it occurs with high frequency in healthy individuals [30]. In addition, transplacental transfer of ICA does not seem to lead to IDDM [37].

More convincing evidence is perhaps that cyclosporin-induced clinical remission in IDDM patients is completely unrelated to the presence or absence of ICA [38, 39] and that recurrence of diabetes in the transplanted twins mentioned above was not associated with IgG deposits in the islets of the grafts [7]. Finally, a primary pathogenetic role of ICA is difficult to reconcile with the heterogeneous islet morphology characteristic of recent-onset IDDM (see above). Probably a more uniform pathological picture would be expected if islet damage was induced by a circulating B-cell-cytotoxic antibody.

Cell-Mediated Immune Reactions as Effector Mechanisms in B-Cell Destruction

If antibodies are not responsible for the target cell killing in IDDM, the other obvious possibility is that B-cell destruction is performed by the action of cytotoxic T-lymphocytes.

Peripheral blood MNC (PBMNC) from recent-onset IDDM patients have been shown to be cytotoxic to rat islet cells [40] and rat islets [41] and to inhibit insulin release from isolated mouse islets [42, 43]. This effect has been shown with T-lymphocyte-enriched cell populations on mouse islets [44], but rat islet cell cytotoxicity was found to be similar when PBMNC populations with T-lymphocyte contents ranging from 5% to 60% were tested [40, 45].

However, evidence for cytotoxic effects on human B-cells is lacking. The studies mentioned, showing the effects of human IDDM patients' PBMNC on xenogenic islet targets, clearly demonstrate that the B-cell destruction or the inhibition of B-cell function described are not MHC-restricted (MHC = major histocompatibility complex). In other words, the effector cell is unlikely to be the cytotoxic T-lymphocyte. Transplantation experiments performed in the BB rat [46, 47] and the

NOD mouse [48] provide further evidence that B-cell destruction is not an MHC-restricted phenomenon: by grafting MHC-incompatible, culture-conditioned islets (cultured under conditions making them nonrejectable in an allograft situation in nondiabetic recipients) it was clearly shown that B-cell destruction in the grafts took place at the same time as in the host islets when diabetes occurred. Thus, in these animal models of IDDM, cytotoxic T-lymphocytes cannot be responsible for the B-cell destruction. If this applies to man, and no published evidence contradicts this, there is a need to look for effector mechanisms other than those mediated by antibodies and cytotoxic T-lymphocytes in IDDM pathogenesis in man.

Recently a T-lymphocyte line expressing the T-lymphocyte receptor complex has been reported to lyse tumor cells in a non-MHC-restricted fashion [49]. These "non-MHC-restricted cytotoxic T-lymphocytes" preferentially lyse NK-cell targets and may be identical with a subpopulation of NK-cells expressing the B-chain of the T-cell receptor [50, 51].

That NK-cells may be of interest in relation to beta-cell destruction is supported by the finding that NK-cells are probably the most important cytotoxic cell-type in the lymphopenic diabetic BB rat [52]. Furthermore, it has been suggested that B-cell cytotoxicity in acutely diabetic and diabetes-prone BB rat spleen cell populations is conferred by NK-cells [53]. This is supported by the observation that antibodies against NK-cell phenotypic markers prevent diabetes development in BB rats [54].

Also macrophages have been shown to be cytotoxic to or to inhibit insulin release from rodent islets in vitro [55, 56], and blocking of macrophage function by silica [57] prevents diabetes-prone BB rats from developing diabetes and protects islet allografts from rejection in nondiabetic recipients [58].

Whether NK-cells and/or macrophages are the cells primarily responsible for B-cell destruction in the earlier stages of IDDM pathogenesis in man is - for good reasons - unknown so far. However, they are both interleukin-1 (IL-1)-producing cells (NK-cells [59]) and IL-1 has been shown to potently interfere with B-cell function and survival.

A Role for IL-1 in B-Cell Destruction

The precise role of the MHC class II gene products in the qualitative and quantitative regulation of immune responsiveness is not known.

The initial event in a primary immune response involves the uptake, processing, and presentation of soluble antigen by the antigen-presenting cell (APC; Fig. 1). The antigen is recognized by the helper T-lymphocyte with the specific receptor (clonotype) for the antigen in question, provided that the antigen is presented in the context of compatible class II molecules. Triggering of the helper T-lymphocyte, however, is dependent on a third activation signal in the form of the monokine IL-1, produced and secreted by the activated APC. Only when the helper T-cell is primed by antigen, class II molecules, and IL-1 can a primary immune response be elicited. This is effected via the secretion of many different lympho-

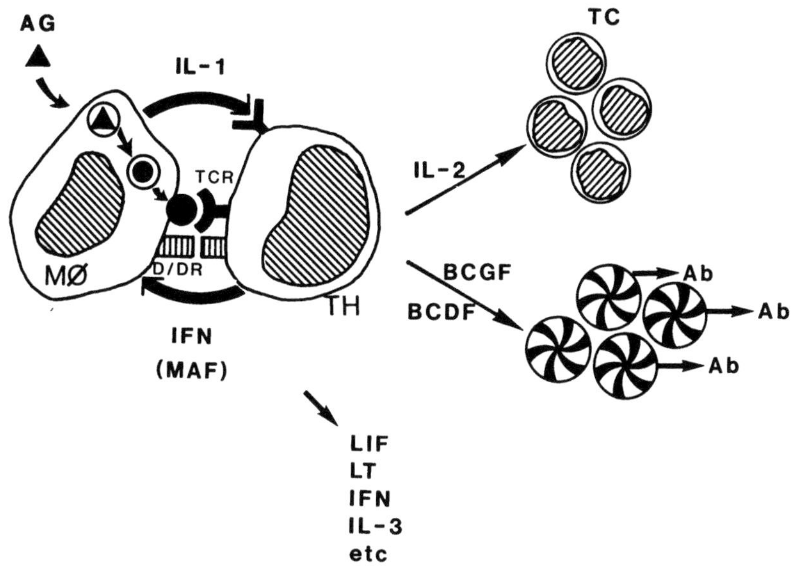

Fig. 1. Schematic representation of the activation of the immune response. For detailed explanation see text. *AG*, antigen; *MØ*, macrophage/antigen-presenting cell; *IL-1*, interleukin-1; *TCR*, T-lymphocyte receptor complex; *D/DR*, HLA-D/DR antigens; *IFN*, gamma-interferon; *MAF*, macrophage-activating factor; *TH*, helper T-lymphocyte; *IL-2*, interleukin-2; *TÇ*, cytotoxic T-lymphocyte; *BCGF*, B-cell growth factor; *BCDF*, B-cell differentiation factor; *Ab*, antibody; *LIF*, leukocyte migration inhibitory factor; *LT*, lymphotoxin; *IL-3*, interleukin-3

kines which are necessary for the clonal expansion of antigen-specific T- and B-lymphocytes and for the development of the inflammatory response in general (chemotaxis, vasodilatation, migration inhibition of recruited macrophages and neutrophils, etc.).

Together, monokines and lymphokines are termed cytokines. Cytokines are antigen-nonspecific, nonimmunoglobulin peptides synthesized and secreted by cells interacting in the immune response (i.e., T- and B-lymphocytes, monocytes, macrophages, dendritic cells etc.) [60]. These peptides are bioactive in picomolar concentrations, and exert their effects primarily over short distances between interacting cells, where high local concentrations can be achieved in the intercellular spaces, in analogy to neurotransmitters in neuromuscular junctions. This "paracrine" action of cytokines is contrasted by the "endocrine" hormone-like action on distant target organs of many cytokines, present in low concentrations in the circulation.

Theoretically, class II molecules could influence the immune response in a qualitative way by affecting antigen presentation or recognition, whereas an effect on monokine or lymphokine production would more likely lead to quantitative differences in host responsiveness to an antigen, since the amount of monokine/lymphokine produced could determine the magnitude of the immune response.

The concept of a possible immunoregulatory effect of HLA-D molecules mediated via cytokine production is particularly attractive in the context of IDDM pathogenesis, since cytokines have been suggested to act as immune effector molecules in this disease, as will be discussed in the following section.

As mentioned, the characteristic pathoanatomic finding associated with clinical onset of IDDM is MNC infiltration and B-cell destruction in the islets of LANGERHANS [1]. Interaction of infiltrating MNC may lead to secretion of cytokines up to high local concentrations in the endocrine pancreas.

Since islet cell antibodies and cytotoxic T-lymphocytes do not seem to be primarily responsible for B-cell destruction in IDDM, it was suggested that cytokines might adversely affect the function of the islet cells and that cytokines may participate in B-cell destruction in IDDM.

Since cytokines are produced by MNC in response to any antigen, and even in response to totally nonspecific stimuli, such as plant lectins, the effect of crude cell-free supernatants of peripheral blood MNC from healthy donors activated in vitro with lectin (PHA) or antigen (PPD) was tested on the function of isolated human and rat islets of LANGERHANS.

The glucose-induced insulin release, insulin content, and glucagon content of the islets were significantly reduced when human or rat islets were incubated with 50% conditioned media from activated MNC [61]. The inhibition of B-cell function was significant after 24 h incubation, and after 7 days incubation islets were disintegrated when examined in the light microscope. Further studies [62] revealed that the functional impairment of islet function was a dose-dependent effect of the cytokine preparation, and electron-microscopy of light-microscopically intact islets demonstrated a total dissolution of normal organelle and nuclear chromatin structure in all islet cells, but surprisingly nuclear and cytoplasmic membranes of these evidently dead cells were well preserved. By screening available purified cytokine preparations it was found that the tested lymphokines could not, but the monokine IL-1 could reproduce the effects of the crude MNC cytokine-rich supernatants [63]. Immunoadsorption with a monospecific polyclonal anti-IL-1 antibody removed the islet cytotoxic activity of the crude cytokine preparations, and human recombinant IL-1, but not human recombinant gamma-interferon or human recombinant tumor necrosis factor (TNF)-alpha mimicked the effects of crude and affinity-purified IL-1 [64]. Testing a chromatofocused native human IL-1 revealed that islet cytotoxicity was only found in the pI 7 fraction corresponding to the human IL-1 beta gene product [64], but not in the pI 5 IL-1 alpha fraction.

When the activity of native IL-1 or recombinant IL-1 beta was tested on rat islets and murine thymocytes in parallel, it was found that the dose responses were very similar [64], suggesting that in vitro IL-1 has adverse effects on islet cells in concentrations that activate immune cells. The sensitivity of rat B-cells to IL-1 effects is comparable to or higher than murine thymocytes and rat islets in organ culture provide an additional assay system for IL-1 [65].

The sensitivity of human islets to IL-1 effects showed great variation between individual pancreatic isolates [62], apparently unrelated to age, sex, or HLA type of the pancreatic donor.

A blind study of ultrastructural changes in rat and human islets exposed to IL-1 from 30 min to 24 h was undertaken [66]. Within 30 min ultrastructural changes were detectable in human and rat B-cells exposed to the lowest dose of IL-1 that would maximally inhibit insulin secretion (approximately 25 U/ml). Within 24 h of exposure to IL-1 electron-microscopic changes were seen only in islet B-cells. These findings demonstrate that the IL-1-mediated cytotoxic effect is very rapid and B-cell-selective.

What Is IL-1?

IL-1 is a 17.5-kD polypeptide produced primarily by phagocytic and connective tissue cells, e.g., blood monocytes, tissue macrophages, dendritic cells, cells of LANGERHANS, endothelial cells, mesangial cells, neutrophils, fibroblasts, epithelial cells, astrocytes, and microglial cells [67, 68]. This pleiotropic hormone has multiple biological effects both on immune cells and on distant nonimmune tissues [69]. Since IL-1 has both "paracrine" and "endocrine" effects, IL-1 might be involved in the destruction of islet B-cells in different ways.

How IL-1 affects glucose-induced insulin release and exerts its cytotoxic, B-cell-selective action is unknown. We hypothesized [66], that IL-1 induces free radical formation ($\acute{O}_2^-$ or hydroxyl groups) in the B-cells, as it is known to do in neutrophils [70], eosinophils (Dinarello personal communication), and endothelial cells [71]. It has been known for years that B-cells are exquisitely sensitive to free radicals [72]. In other words, IL-1 may destroy B-cells in a way similar to that of alloxan.

Requirements for Pathogenetic Models of IDDM in Man

As documented in this review, the process, i.e., the *initial pathogenetic effector mechanism,* that destroys B-cells in IDDM is *non-MHC-restricted.* However, IDDM - and hence most likely the B-cell destructive process - is certainly *MHC-linked* since about 95% of all IDDM-patients are HLA-DR3 and/or DR4-positive [73]. Furthermore, the effector mechanism is *B-cell-specific.*

In addition, any hypothetical model of IDDM pathogenesis must explain how the B-cell destruction is *initiated* and how the B-cell destructive process may be *self-perpetuating* and *self-limiting.* The *heterogeneous histopathology* of the islets of Langerhans in recent-onset IDDM patients, as well as the *"immunological diversification"* (i.e., polyclonal B-lymphocyte activation and antibody formation and T-lymphocyte activation) seen in such patients, should also be explainable by the model. The model must also account for the fact that B-cell destruction may be a *slowly progressing process,* taking perhaps years to produce IDDM. Finally, the frequent clinical association of IDDM with other "autoimmune endocrinopathies" [15, 74], e.g., GRAVES' disease, primary myxedema, idiopathic ADDISON's disease, hypergonadotropic hypogonadism, and pernicious anemia, ought to be reconcilable with the model too.

IL-1 as the Effector Molecule in IDDM

IL-1 is a strong candidate for the effector molecule in B-cell destruction in human IDDM, in the animal models of IDDM (BB rat and NOD mouse), and during diabetes recurrence after transplantation: IL-1 production and action is not MHC-restricted and its cytotoxic effect on islet cells seems to be B-cell-specific in low (picomolar) concentrations. IL-1 is produced in situ in the insulitis process very early on. To explain the HLA association of IDDM we have suggested [75] that monokine production from macrophages and monocytes is under quantitative control of HLA-D/DR genes or genes in linkage disequilibrium with HLA-D/DR genes. In this context it is worth noting that TNF alpha (another macrophage product) and beta genes have been mapped into the HLA region on chromosome 6 [76].

On this background we suggested the following hypothesis for the etiopathogenesis of IDDM [75]:

- Release of beta-cell antigen, processed and presented by macrophages to T-helper lymphocytes initiates
- A self-perpetuating and self-limiting circuit of cytokine production of which IL-1 is beta-cell cytotoxic.
- IL-1 production is controlled in a quantitative way by HLA-D genes

Pathogenetic Models of IDDM

Figure 2 shows a model of IDDM pathogenesis which fulfils all requirements described previously. *Initiation, perpetuation,* and *limitation* of the B-cell destruction will depend upon B-cell antigen release. Anything that can produce antigen liberation from B-cells (e.g., virus, chemicals, IL-1) can initiate the process, provided antigen is taken up, processed, and presented by macrophages to a specifically reactive helper T-lymphocyte. Thus, *specificity* of the B-cell destructive process is T-lymphocyte-dependent. *Magnitude,* i.e., the extent and the rapidity by which the cellular infiltrate in the islets is being built up will be determined by the intensity of cytokine production when antigen-presenting macrophages and specifically reactive helper T-lymphocytes interact. B-cell destruction will go on as long as antigen is being released and will stop when antigen release stops.

The helper T-lymphocyte activated by the antigen-presenting macrophage will secrete lymphokines. One of these, gamma-interferon, will further stimulate other macrophages, monocytes, dendritic cells, and NK-cells in the cellular infiltrate to produce and secrete IL-1, which in turn may then destroy more B-cells. This would be a "paracrine" effect of IL-1. The result will be an islet devoid of B-cells and expansion of the specifically reactive helper T-lymphocyte clone. Nothing will happen to B-cells in islets where no initial B-cell destruction is taking place, or in islets where no specifically reactive helper T-lymphocytes are present. The *heterogeneous islet pathology* in recent-onset IDDM patients may be explained in this way.

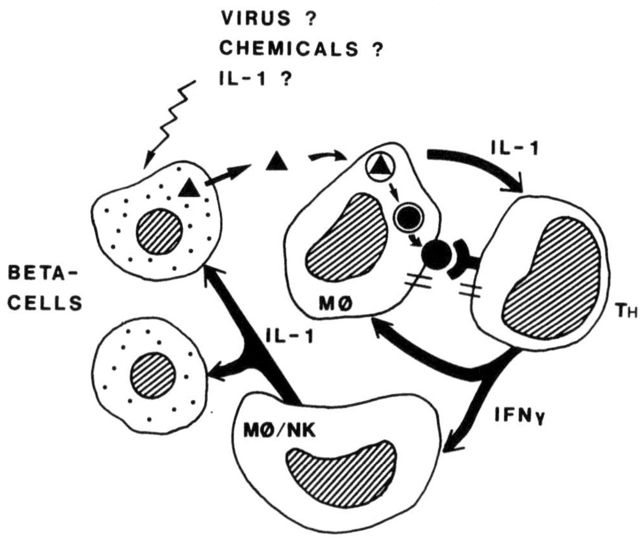

Fig. 2. Model of IL-1-mediated B-cell killing. For details see text. For explanation of abbreviations see legend to Fig. 1

This model implies that many B-cell-damaging mechanisms may initiate the process and that multiple hits may be necessary for the destruction of a sufficient number of islets to produce clinically manifest IDDM. That IDDM may result from a *slowly progressing* B-cell destruction, for a long time perhaps balanced by B-cell regeneration, may thus also be understandable. It follows that there is no need in this model to postulate the existence of specific environmental trigger(s) of IDDM.

According to this model, the magnitude of IL-1 production by the APC and other IL-1-producing cells (e.g., dendritic cells, NK-cells) will directly determine the extent of B-cell destruction. Thus, the B-cell killing by IL-1 is *MHC-nonrestricted* and *B-cell-specific.* The *HLA association,* i.e., the high frequency of HLA-DR3 and/or DR4 in IDDM, may then be explained by an HLA-D gene controlled quantitative effect on IL-1 production. The immunological diversification (see above) may be explained in this model simply by the release of several different antigenic components from the B-cells following the initial pathogenetic damage.

As seen in Fig. 2, the model suggests as a possibility that IL-1 may produce the initial B-cell damage and thus itself be a trigger of the perpetuating process. This implies that circulating levels of IL-1 - through what may be called an "endocrine" IL-1 effect - may be sufficient to exert the cytotoxic effects on the B-cells. Since any stressful event (infections, trauma, etc.) will lead to increased IL-1 production and increased systemic levels of IL-1, this possibility needs investigation.

Finally, a variant of this model may be considered. Figure 3 demonstrates how an "irrelevant" infection of the islet may supply a local IL-1 concentration high enough to bring about initial B-cell destruction and thereby provide the B-cell antigen release necessary for establishing the self-perpetuating destructive process.

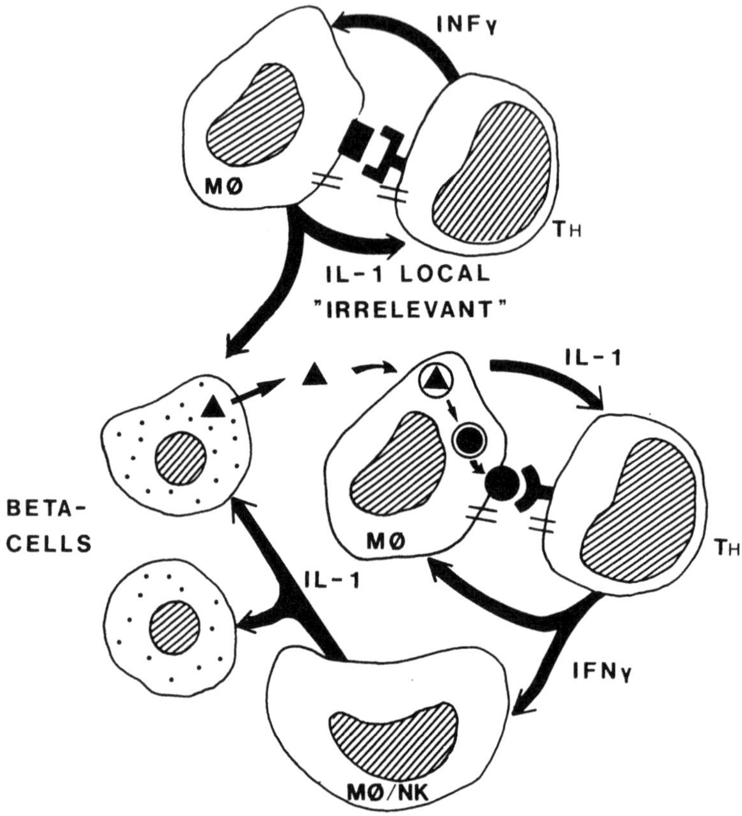

Fig. 3. Alternative model of IL-1-induced, IL-1-mediated B-cell killing. For details see text. For explanation of abbreviations see legend to Fig. 1

Conclusions

The mechanism(s) responsible for B-cell destruction in IDDM is clearly MHC-nonrestricted, but nonetheless MHC-associated and B-cell-specific. Recent observations attribute a central role in the initial destruction - i.e., in the pathogenetic mechanism in sensu strictu - to IL-1-producing cells. ICA and cytotoxic T-lymphocytes may well participate in the B-cell destruction, but are probably secondary in time and importance.

The pathogenetic model described (Fig. 2) is conceptually rather simple. It is, however, reconcilable with present experimental and clinical knowledge about IDDM. Importantly, it is directly accessible to experimental testing. Investigations to unravel the molecular mechanisms underlying IL-1's cytotoxic effects on B-cells (free radical induction?) are clearly needed and may lead to new approaches to the treatment of IDDM.

References

1. Gepts W (1965) Pathological anatomy of the pancreas in juvenile diabetes mellitus. Diabetes 14: 619-633
2. Gepts W (1983) Role of cellular immunity in the pathogenesis of type 1 diabetes. Curr Probl Clin Biochem 12: 86-99
3. Gepts W, LeCompte PM (1985). The pathology of type 1 (juvenile) diabetes. In: Volk BW, Arquilla ER (eds) The diabetic pancreas. Plenum, New York, pp 337-365
4. Junker K, Egeberg J, Kromann H, Nerup J (1977) An autopsy study of the islets of Langerhans in acute-onset juvenile diabetes mellitus. Acta Pathol Microbiol Scand (Sect A) 85: 699-706
5. Bottazzo GF, Dean BM, McNally JM, MacKay EH, Swift PGF, Gamble DR (1985) In situ characterization of autoimmune phenomena and expression of HLA molecules in the pancreas in diabetic insulitis. N Engl J Med 313: 353-360
6. Foulis AK, Farquharson MA (1982) Aberrant expression of HLA-DR antigens by insulin-containing β-cells in recent-onset Type I diabetes mellitus. Diabetes 35: 1215-1224
7. Sibley RK, Sutherland DER, Goetz F, Michael AF (1985) Recurrent diabetes mellitus in the pancreas iso- and allograft. A light and electron microscopic and immunohistochemical analysis of four cases. Lab Invest 53: 132-144
8. Kolb-Bachofen V, Kolb H (1983) New concept of insulitis and B-islet cell destruction. Diabetes 32 [suppl 1]: 22A
9. Kolb H, Kantwerk G, Treichel U, Kürner T, Kiesel U, Hoppe T, Kolb-Bachofen V (1986) Prospective analysis of islet lesions in BB rats. Diabetologia 29: 559A
10. Dean BM, Walker R, Bone AJ, Baird JD, Cooke A (1985) Pre-diabetes in the spontaneously diabetic BB/E rat: lymphocyte subpopulations in the pancreatic infiltrate and expression of rat MHC class II molecules in endocrine cells. Diabetologia 28: 464-466
11. Nerup J, Andersen OO, Bendixen G, Egeberg J, Poulsen JE (1971) Antipancreatic cellular hypersensitivity in diabetes mellitus. Diabetes 20: 424-427
12. Bottazzo GF, Florin-Christensen A, Doniach D (1974) Islet-cell antibodies in diabetes mellitus with autoimmune polyendocrine deficiences. Lancet II: 1279-1282
13. Lernmark Å, Freedman ZR, Hofman C, Rubinstein AH, Steiner DF, Jackson RL, Winter RJ, Traisman HS (1978) Islet-cell-surface antibodies in juvenile diabetes mellitus. N Engl J Med 299: 375-380
14. Bækkeskov S, Nielsen JH, Marner B, Bilde T, Ludvigsson J, Lernmark Å (1982) Autoantibodies in newly diagnosed diabetic children immunoprecipitate human pancreatic islet cell proteins. Nature 298: 167-169
15. MacCuish AC, Irvine WJ (1975) Autoimmunological aspects of diabetes mellitus. Clin Endocrinol Metab 4: 434-471
16. Maron R, Elias D, de Jongh BM, Bruining GJ, van Rood JJ, Shechter Y, Cohen IR (1983) Autoantibodies to the insulin receptor in juvenile onset insulin-dependent diabetes. Nature 303: 817-818
17. Huang S-W, Haedt LH, Rich S, Barbosa J (1981) Prevalence of antibodies to nucleic acids in insulin-dependent diabetics and their relatives. Diabetes 30: 873-874
18. Irvine WJ, Al-Khateeb SF, DiMario U, Feek CM, Gray RS, Edmond B, Duncan LJP (1977) Soluble immune complexes in the sera of newly diagnosed insulin-dependent diabetics and in treated diabetics. Clin Exp Immunol 30: 16-21
19. Papadopoulos G, Petersen J, Andersen V, Lernmark Å, Marner B, Nerup J, Binder J (1984) Spontaneous in vitro immunoglobulin secretion at the diagnosis of insulin-dependent diabetes. Acta Endocrinol 105: 521-527
20. Scott J, Nerup J, Lernmark Å (1985) Immunologic factors in diabetes mellitus. In: Rosse WF (ed) Clinical immunology. Update reviews for physicians. Elsevier, Amsterdam, 53-85
21. Gorsuch AN, Spencer KM, Lister J, McNally JM, Dean BM, Bottazzo GF, Cudworth AG (1981) Evidence for a long prediabetic period in type 1 (insulin-dependent) diabetes mellitus. Lancet II: 1363-1365
22. Pujoll-Borell R, Hanafusa T, Cudworth AG, Bottazzo GF (1982) Islet-cell surface antibodies and the natural history of Type 1 (insulin-dependent) diabetes. Diabetologia 23: 194A

23. Bækkeskov S, Bruining J, Srikanta S, Mandrup-Poulsen T, de Beaufort C, Eisenbarth G, Nerup J, Lernmark Å (1986) Antibodies to a M_r 64,000 human islet cell protein in the prediabetic period of IDDM patients. Ann NY Acad Sci 475: 415-417
24. Srikanta S, Ricker T, McCulloch DK, Soeldner JS, Eisenbarth GS, Palmer JP (1986) Autoimmunity to insulin, beta cell dysfunction, and development of insulin-dependent diabetes mellitus. Diabetes 35: 139-142
25. Marner B, Agner T, Binder C, Lernmark Å, Nerup J, Mandrup-Poulsen T, Waldorff S (1985) Increased reduction in fasting C-peptide is associated with islet cell antibodies in type 1 (insulin-dependent) diabetic patients. Diabetologia 28: 875-880
26. Bottazzo GF, Dean BM, Gorsuch AN, Cudworth AG, Doniach D (1980) Complement-fixing islet-cell antibodies in type-I diabetes: possible monitors of active beta-cell damage. Lancet I: 668-672
27. Srikanta S, Ganda OP, Eisenbarth GS, Soeldner JS (1983) Islet-cell antibodies and beta-cell function in monozygotic triplets and twins initially discordant for type 1 diabetes mellitus. N Engl J Med 308: 322-325
28. Srikanta S, Ganda OP, Rabizadeh A, Soeldner JS, Eisenbarth GS (1985) First-degree relatives of patients with type 1 diabetes mellitus. Islet cell antibodies and abnormal insulin secretion. N Engl J Med 313: 461-464
29. Rittenhouse HG, Oxender DL, Pek S, Ar D (1980) Complement-mediated cytotoxic effects on pancreatic islets with sera from diabetic patients. Diabetes 317-322
30. Dobersen MJ, Scharff JE, Ginsberg-Fellner F, Notkins AL (1980) Cytotoxic autoantibodies to beta cells in the serum of patients with insulin-dependent diabetes mellitus. N Engl J Med 303: 1493-1498
31. Sai P, Boitard C, Debray-Sachs M, Pouplard A, Assan R, Hamburger J (1981) Complement-fixing islet cell antibodies from some diabetic patients alter insulin release in vitro. Diabetes 30: 1051-1057
32. Kanatsuna T, Lernmark Å, Rubinstein AH, Steiner DF (1981) Block in insulin release from column-perifused pancreatic beta-cells induced by islet cell surface antibodies and complement. Diabetes 30: 231-234
33. Kanatsuna T, Bækkeskov S, Lernmark Å, Ludvigsson J (1983) Immunoglobulin from insulin-dependent diabetic children inhibits glucose-induced insulin release. Diabetes 32: 520-524
34. Svenningsen A, Dyrberg T, Gerlin I, Lernmark Å, MacKay P, Rabinovitch A (1983) Inhibition of insulin release after passive transfer of immunoglobulin from insulin-dependent diabetic children to mice. J Clin Endocrinol Metab 57: 1301-1304
35. Spencer KM, Tarn A, Dean BM, Lister J, Bottazzo GF (1984) Fluctuating islet-cell autoimmunity in unaffected relatives of patients with insulin-dependent diabetes. Lancet I: 764-766
36. Srikanta S, Ganda OP, Jackson RA, Brink SJ, Fleischnick E, Yunis E, Alper C, Soeldner JS, Eisenbarth GS (1984) Pre-type 1 (insulin-dependent) diabetes: common endocrinological course despite immunological and immunogenetic heterogeneity. Diabetologia 27: 146-148
37. Tingle AJ, Lim G, Wright VJ, Dimmick JF, Hunt JA (1979) Transplacental passage of islet cell antibodies in infants of diabetic mothers. Pediatr Res 13: 1323-1325
38. Mandrup-Poulsen T, Nerup J, Stiller CR, Marner B, Bille G, Heinrichs D, Martell R, Dupre J, Keown PA, Jenner MR, Rodger NW, Wolfe B, Graffenried BV, Binder C (1985) Disappearance and reappearance of islet cell cytoplasmic antibodies in cyclosporin-treated insulin-dependent diabetics. Lancet I: 599-602
39. Feutren G, Papoz L, Assan R, Vialettes B, Karsenty G, Vexiau P, Charbonnel B, Rodier M, Lallemand A, Bach J-F (1986) Cyclosporine A in recent onset type 1 (insulin-dependent) diabetic patients: preliminary analysis of the French randomized trial at 6-9 months. Diabetologia 29: 536A
40. Charles MA, Suzuki M, Waldeck N, Dodson LE, Slater L, Ong K, Kershnar A, Buckingham B, Golden M (1983) Immune islet killing mechanisms associated with insulin-dependent diabetes: in vitro expression of cellular and antibody-mediated islet cell cytotoxicity in humans. J Immunol 130: 1189-1195
41. Lohmann D, Krug J, Lampeter EF, Bierwolf B, Verlohren H-J (1986) Cell-mediated immune reactions against B cells and defect of suppressor cell activity in type 1 (insulin-dependent) diabetes mellitus. Diabetologia 29: 421-425

42. Boitard C, Debray-Sachs M, Pouplard A, Assan R, Hamburger J (1981) Lymphocytes from diabetics suppress insulin release in vitro. Diabetologia 21: 41-46
43. Quiniou-Debrie MC, Debray-Sachs M, Dardenne M, Czernichow P, Assan R, Bach JF (1985) Anti-islet cellular and humoral immunity, T-cell subsets, and thymic function in type 1 diabetes. Diabetes 34: 373-379
44. Boitard C, Chatenoud L-M, Debray-Sachs M (1982) In vitro inhibition of pancreatic B cell function by lymphocytes from diabetics with associated autoimmune diseases: a T cell phenomenon. J Immunol 129: 2529-2531
45. Negishi K, Waldeck N, Chandy G, Buckingham B, Kershnar A, Fisher L, Gupta S, Charles MA (1986) Natural killer cell and islet killer cell activities in type 1 (insulin-dependent) diabetes. Diabetologia 29: 352-357
46. Weringer EJ, Like AA (1985) Immune attack on pancreatic islet transplants in the spontaneously diabetic Biobreeding/Worcester (BB/W) rat is not MHC restricted. J Immunol 134: 2384-2386
47. Prowse SJ, Bellgrau D, Lafferty KJ (1986) Islet allografts are destroyed by disease occurrence in the spontaneously diabetic BB rat. Diabetes 35: 110-114
48. Nomikos IN, Prowse SJ, Carotenuto P, Lafferty KJ (1986) Combined treatment with nicotinamide and desferrioxamine prevents islet allograft destruction in NOD mice. Diabetes 35: 1302-1304
49. Lanier LL, Phillips JH (1986) Evidence for three types of human cytotoxic lymphocytes. Immunol Today 7: 132-134
50. Yanagi Y, Caccia N, Kronenberg M, Chin B, Roder J, Rohel D, Kiyohara, Lauzon R, Toyonaga B, Rosenthal K, Dennert G, Acha-Orbea H, Hengartner H, Hood L, Mak TW (1985) Gene rearrangement in cells with natural killer activity and expression of the beta-chain of the T-cell antigen receptor. Nature 314: 631-633
51. Moingeon P, Ythier A, Goubin G, Faure F, Nowill A, Delmon L, Rainaud M, Forestier F, Daffos F, Bohuon C, Hercend T (1986) A unique T-cell receptor complex expressed on human fetal lymphocytes displaying natural-killer-like activity. Nature 323: 638-640
52. Woda BA, Biron CA (1986) Natural killer cell number and function in the spontaneously diabetic BB/W rat. J Immunol 137: 1860-1866
53. MacKay P, Jacobson J, Rabinovitch A (1986) Spontaneous diabetes mellitus in the BioBreeding/Worcester rat. Evidence in vitro for natural killer cell lysis of islet cells. J Clin Invest 77: 916-924
54. Like AA, Biron CA, Weringer EJ, Byman K, Sroczynski E, Guberski DL (1986) Prevention of diabetes in Biobreeding/Worcester rats with monoclonal antibodies that recognize T lymphocytes or natural killer cells. J Exp Med 164: 1145-1159
55. Debray-Sachs M, Boitard C, Assan R, Hamburger J (1981) Are "activated" macrophages cytotoxic against normal cells? Transplant Proc 13: 1111-1113
56. Schwitzer RW, Leiter EH, Evans R (1984) Macrophage-mediated cytotoxicity against cultured pancreatic islet cells. Transplantation 37: 539-544
57. Oschilewski U, Kiesel U, Kolb H (1985) Administration of silica prevents diabetes in BB rats. Diabetes 34: 197-199
58. Nash JR, Everson NW, Wood RFM, Bell PRF (1980) Effect of silica and carrageenan on the survival of islet allografts. Transplantation 29: 206-208
59. Scala G, Allavena P, Djeu JY, Kasahara T, Ortaldo JR, Herberman RB, Oppenheim JJ (1984) Human large granular lymphocytes are potent producers of interleukin-1. Nature 309: 56-59
60. Bendtzen K (1985) Lymphokines in inflammation. In: Venge P, Lindbom A (eds) Inflammation - basic mechanisms, tissue injuring principles, and clinical models. Almqvist and Wiksell, Stockholm, pp 187-217
61. Mandrup-Poulsen T, Bendtzen K, Nielsen JH, Bendixen G, Nerup J (1985) Cytokines cause functional and structural damage to isolated islets of Langerhans. Allergy 40: 424-429
62. Mandrup-Poulsen T, Bendtzen K, Nerup J, Egeberg J, Nielsen JH (1986) Mechanisms of pancreatic islet cell destruction. Dose-dependent cytotoxic effect of soluble blood mononuclear cell mediators on isolated islets of Langerhans. Allergy 41: 250-259
63. Mandrup-Poulsen T, Bendtzen K, Nerup J, Dinarello CA, Svenson M, Nielsen JH (1986) Affinity-purified human interleukin 1 is cytotoxic to isolated islets of Langerhans. Diabetologia 29: 63-67

64. Bendtzen K, Mandrup-Poulsen T, Nerup J, Nielsen JH, Dinarello CA, Svenson M (1986) Cytotoxicity of human pI7 interleukin-1 for pancreatic islets of Langerhans. Science 232: 1545-1547
65. Bendtzen K, Barington T, Mandrup-Poulsen T, Pedersen JG, Svenson M (1986) Measurement of human IL-1 by LIF induction, pancreatic islet-cell cytotoxicity, and bone resorption. Lymphokine Res 5: S93-S98
66. Mandrup-Poulsen T, Egeberg J, Nerup J, Bendtzen K, Nielsen JH, Dinarello CA (1987) Ultrastructural study of time-course and cellular specificity of interleukin-1 mediated islet cytotoxicity. Acta Pathol Microbiol Immunol Scand (C) Acta path. microbiol. immunol. scand. Sect C, 95: 55-63
67. Dinarello CA (1984) Interleukin-1. Rev Infect Dis 6: 51-95
68. Dinarello CA (1984) Interleukin-1 and the acute-phase response. N Engl J Med 311: 1413-1418
69. Dinarello CA (1986) Interleukin-1: amino acid sequences, multiple biological activities and comparison with tumor necrosis factor (Cachectin). In: Cruse JM, Lewis RE, Jackson M (eds) The year in immunology, vol 2. Karger, Basel, pp 68-89
70. Klempner MS, Dinarello CA, Henderson WR, Gallin JI (1979) Stimulation of neutrophil oxygen-dependent metabolism by human leukocytic pyrogen. J Clin Invest 64: 996-1002
71. Matsubara T, Ziff M (1986) Increased superoxide anion release from human endothelial cells in response to cytokines. J Immunol 137: 3295-3298
72. Malaisse WJ (1982) Alloxan toxicity to the pancreatic B-cell. A new hypothesis. Biochem Pharmacol 31: 3527-3534
73. Svejgaard A, Jakobsen BK, Platz P, Ryder LP, Nerup J, Christy M, Borch-Johnsen K, Parving H-H, Deckert T, Mølsted-Pedersen L, Kühl C, Buschard K, Green A (1986) HLA associations in insulin-dependent diabetes: search for heterogeneity in different groups of patients from a homogeneous population. Tissue Antigens 28: 237-244
74. Nerup J (1974) The clinical and immunological association of diabetes mellitus and Addison's disease. In: Bastenie PA, Gepts W (eds) Immunity and autoimmunity in diabetes mellitus. Excerpta Medica, Amsterdam, pp 149-152
75. Nerup J, Mandrup-Poulsen T, Mølvig J (1987) Thc HLA-IDDM association: implications for etiology and pathogenesis of IDDM. In: De Fronzo RA, Skylev JS (eds) Diabetes/Metabolism Rev 3: 779-802
76. Spies T, Morton CC, Nedospasov SA, Fiers W, Pious D, Strominger JL (1986) Genes for the tumor necrosis factors α and β are linked to the human major histocompatibility complex. Proc Natl Acad Sci USA 83: 8699-8702

Viral Interactions with Pancreatic B-Cells*

E. H. Leiter and G. L. Wilson

Introduction

It has long been hypothesized that viruses play an important role in the etiology of some forms of insulin-dependent diabetes mellitus (IDDM). This hypothesis began to develop following the initial report of an association between community outbreaks of mumps and the occurrence of IDDM [38] and was supported by the discovery of a seasonal variation in the incidence of new cases of IDDM [27]. Subsequent studies have suggested correlations between rubella [21, 50, 73] cytomegalovirus [43], reovirus [109] and group B Coxsackie virus [28] infections and IDDM. Additionally, the description of B-cell death associated with insulitis, as eloquently described by Gepts [31] has been considered to be consistent with the pathogenesis of an ongoing viral infection.

Interactions Between B-Cells and Lytic Viruses

Coxsackie Virus Infections in Humans

Specific evidence that human viruses could cause diabetes was provided by Yoon and coworkers [107]. These investigators isolated a Coxsackie B4 virus from the pancreas of a young boy who died in acute diabetic ketoacidosis. This virus, when injected into mice, produced a diabetes-mellitus-like syndrome that was characterized by insulitis and B-cell necrosis. In another less well characterized report, Champsaur et al. [10] isolated a Coxsackie B5 virus from the feces of a child that developed IDDM a few days after a viral infection. This virus also produced abnormal glucose tolerance in infected mice. Finally, Ahmad and Abraham [1] isolated a Coxsackie B5 virus from the heart, lung, and feces of a 10-day-old infant who died of myocarditis. Histological evaluation of the pancreas from this child revealed inflammation and destruction of approximately 50% of the B-cells with complete sparing of the acinar cells.

---

* This work was supported by research grants AM 17631, AM 27722, and AM 36175 from the National Institute of Arthritis, Diabetes, Digestive, and Kidney Diseases to EHL and by research grants ES 03456 and a Research Career Development Award ES 00150 from the National Institute of Environmental Health Sciences to GLW.

Until recently, the abrupt onset of clinical symptoms of IDDM was considered to be evidence for a viral cause of this disease. However, the finding that at least some forms of IDDM have a slow progressive pathogenesis has lead to a change in the concept of how viruses may play a role in this disease [19]. Rather than precipitating IDDM by overt B-cell damage resulting from infection with lytic viruses, it has been proposed that viruses may trigger the development of autoimmune processes that lead ultimately to the clinical manifestations of IDDM. Alternatively, it is conceivable that B-cell tropic viruses can augment immunological processes and hasten the onset of clinical symptoms. Indirect evidence for this has been supplied by the observations of GEPTS [32] of pseudoatrophic islets, containing A-cells and D-cells but lacking B-cells, in cases of acute IDDM of apparent recent onset. If IDDM is a heterogeneous disease with more than one distinct etiologic pathway, as has been postulated by several investigators [44, 86], then any one of the three scenarios for a viral etiology could be applicable in individual cases. Direct evidence that IDDM is a heterogeneous condition has recently been provided by the Pittsburgh IDDM Study [18]. This investigation showed that there was considerable heterogeneity in the presenting characteristics of patients with IDDM that could be correlated with HLA-DR type. Individuals that were HLA-DR4 were found to have a more severe presentation of clinical symptoms and were more likely to have a recent history of viral infection.

Encephalomyocarditis-Virus-Induced Diabetes

To date, most of the insight into the pathogenesis of virus-induced diabetes has been provided by the study of encephalomyocarditis (EMC) virus. This virus is a cardiovirus belonging to the Picornaviridae, and is closely related to the Coxsackie group B viruses. A diabetogenic EMC virus was originally obtained from swine in Panama [66]. Two strains of the EMC virus were isolated. These strains were found to differ both in organ tropism and pathogenicity in adult mice. One strain, designated "E," is highly neurotropic and produces extensive acinar cell necrosis in the pancreas with little islet cell involvement. The other strain, designated "M," produces mild myocarditis but has little effect on the central nervous system [11]. This strain was capable of inducing a disease resembling IDDM in some inbred strains of mice [12, 13, 14]. Pathologic lesions in the pancreases of diabetes-susceptible mice included B-cell degranulation and contraction within the islets of LANGERHANS and coagulation necrosis [14, 45]. Neither other islet cells nor acinar cells appeared to be infected. A mononuclear cell invasion, or insulitis, surrounded most virus-infected islets [101, 102]. Viral antigens could be demonstrated by immunofluorescence in affected B-cells during the acute phase of infection. A direct correlation could be made between the amount of B-cell destruction resulting from the lytic properties of the virus and the overt manifestation of diabetes in infected mice [40].

Genetic Factors Affecting EMC Virus Infection

As work with EMC virus proceeded, it became apparent that other inbred strains were resistant to this diabetogenic effect even though the animals did sustain a viral infection [5, 6]. Therefore, it was concluded that genetic factors played an integral role in this virus-induced diabetes. Studies based on crosses between diabetes-prone and -resistant mice showed that susceptibility was controlled by one or more recessive genes [84, 106]. The exact gene product or products controlling the outcome of the infection have yet to be elucidated. It has been proposed that a genetically determined increase or decrease in the number of viral receptors might be the critical determinant for susceptibility to the diabetogenic properties of the virus [9, 106]. However, several studies do not support this hypothesis. Cultured B-cells from susceptible CD-1 mice and resistant C57BL/6J mice were equally susceptible to the lytic effects of the M strain of EMC virus [104] and produced relatively equal amounts of virus following infection [105]. Additionally, in vivo studies by DEFOE and colleagues [16] demonstrated that transplanted pancreases from diabetes-susceptible (DBA/2J) and -resistant (C57BL/6J) mice were equally susceptible to infection by the diabetogenic strain of EMC virus when grafted into F1 hybrids.

Another genetically-controlled factor which dramatically affects the outcome of infection is the gender of the animal. It was discovered that male mice were more susceptible to the diabetogenic effects of the virus than were females [22]. Castration rendered males more resistant [22, 34, 65]. Administration of testosterone to male castrates restored susceptibility to precastration levels. Testosterone treatment also increased the susceptibility in females of some strains of mice to EMC-virus-induced diabetes [22, 34]. The mechanism by which testosterone deprivation protects against the diabetogenic effects of EMC virus remains to be elucidated. However, alteration of the immune response to the virus is a strong possibility. Differences have been noted between the cellular and humoral immune responses of male and female mice of the same strain [71, 95, 97]. These differences were abolished by castration.

A final way that genetic factors can influence the outcome of infection with EMC viruses has been illustrated by studies of the obese gene *(ob/ob)* on the diabetes-resistant C57BL/6J background. In these experiments, mice homozygous *(ob/ob)* for the obesity gene were susceptible to the diabetogenic effects of the M strain of EMC virus [15]. Heterozygous littermates (*ob*/+) and normal controls (+/+) were resistant to the diabetogenic effects of this virus. Although the reason for the increased susceptiblity to virus-induced diabetes resulting from genetically induced obesity remains obscure, immune alteration is a viable possibility. In this regard, it is of interest to note that C57BL/6J *ob/ob* mice have been found to be deficient in natural killer cells [8].

Variants of the M Strain of EMC Virus

Studies of the composition of the M strain of EMC virus have found it to contain a mixture of variants which differ in their diabetogenic properties. Two of these variants (designated "D" and "B") have been separated by plaque isolation and extensively characterized [108]. Each variant possessed unique tissue tropisms with different sites of replication within the same inbred strain of mouse [35]. However, the two variants were serologically indistinguishable from one another. The D variant exhibited a high degree of B-cell tropism and was extremely diabetogenic in susceptible strains. Conversely, the B variant caused little, if any, B-cell damage and was not diabetogenic. Analysis of the genomes of the two variants, using hybridization and thermal elution techniques, showed that the RNAs were homologous. However, when T1 digests of the RNAs were fingerprinted, the B variant was found to be missing one oligonucleotide that was 20-25 nucleotides long [76]. No major differences were found in the structural proteins of the two viruses, making it unlikely that the two viruses differ at the level of receptor recognition.

Interferon in EMC Virus Infections

A likely hypothesis for the difference in action of the two variants is that the B variant provokes a more substantial host defense response which is capable of controlling the infection. This concept was supported by the finding that the B variant was capable of inducing a greater interferon response in diabetes-susceptible mice than did the D variant [108]. The onset of interferon production was quicker and of greater magnitude in response to the B variant. These investigations suggested that this difference in interferon kinetics was responsible for blocking the diabetogenic effects of the D variant when the B variant was coinfected or given prior to infection with the D variant. The interferon system was further implicated by studies which showed that mice treated with antibody to interferon after infection with the B variant developed mild diabetes. Collectively, these results suggest that when the interferon response was attenuated, the B variant was capable of critically infecting B-cells. An interesting extension of this work has recently been described by GAINES et al. [25]. Following infection with the D variant, diabetes-resistant C57BL/6J mice were found to generate a significant interferon response against the D variant, with peak levels ($>5\times10^4$ international units) found in the serum at 24 h following infection. Additional studies showed that when mice were treated with antibody to interferon at the time of infection and 3 days later, mild diabetes resulted. Histological examination of the islets from these mice revealed severe lesions confined to the B-cells which were correlated with a significant reduction in pancreatic insulin concentration. It has been noted previously that various inbred strains of mice differ in the quantity of interferon produced following infection with the same virus. Some strains have been designated as high producers and others as low producers [17]. C57BL/6J mice were found to be high producers of interferon in response to infection with a variety of other viruses. Therefore, although the B-cells of the C57BL/6J mice were susceptible to infection by the D variant, interferon production in these animals appeared to be sufficient to attenuate the infection. This finding supported earlier in vivo [16] and in vitro [104] studies suggesting that B-cells from C57BL/6J mice possessed sufficient numbers of receptors to allow critical infection. The finding that interferon was an important determinant controlling the outcome of the infection extended previous in vitro studies which showed that B-cells from C57BL/6J mice were more sensitive to the inhibitory effect of interferon on virus replication than were those from diabetes-prone CD-1 mice [105]. In regard to the protective effect of interferon, GOULD and coworkers [36] recently demonstrated that at 4 days post-infection with the D variant the addition of alpha-, beta- or gamma-interferon exacerbated the development of diabetes in C57BL/6J and ICR Swiss mice. Based on these findings, it can be concluded that although a substantial interferon response early in the infection can attenuate the infection of B-cells, an interferon response at a later stage may modulate vital secondary immune functions such as macrophage activation and cell-mediated and humoral immunity, necessary for the long-term control of the infection. It has been well established that interferons can influence the state of the immune system [94]. Similar results have been obtained from infections with other picornaviruses. Studies of Coxsackie-B3-induced myocarditis have shown that the administration of interferon or poly I:C, an inducer of interferon, could protect against these virus-induced lesions only if they were given within 24 h of the virus infection. Conversely, if interferon was administered 72 h after infection, the development of myocardial lesions was accelerated [61].

Pathogenesis of EMC Virus Infection

Work with other inbred strains of mice that are resistant to the diabetogenic effects of the D variant have shown that the mechanisms of resistance may be diverse [26]. In contrast to the findings with C57BL/6J mice, the D variant had a completely different pathogenesis in diabetes-resistant C3H/HeJ and C3HeB/FeJ mice. Infection of these mice with the D variant produced massive acute pancreatitis with little islet cell involvement. This exocrine tropism was a gender-specific phenomenon, females being more resistant to the exocrine destruction. Castration of male C3H/HeJ mice, using a protocol that had been reported to block the diabetogenic effects of this virus in susceptible animals, did not prevent the development of this acinar lesion. The B variant of EMC virus did not induce acinar cell destruction in the C3H/HeJ mouse, nor was it diabetogenic. However, preinfection with the B variant 3 days prior to infection with the D variant did protect against the development of the exocrine lesion. Coinfection with equal doses of the two variants also protected against this lesion, as did coinfection with a lower dose of B variant. Therefore, the host response that was generated against the B variant appeared to be responsible for the protection from the D variant exocrine destruction. Due to the short time-frame, it was unlikely that this protection was the result of an antibody response. Rather, these data were more consistent with an interferon response generated against the B variant that would inhibit replication of the D variant. These studies demonstrated that a plaque-isolated virus that was very diabetogenic in some inbred strains of mice produced a completely different pancreatic pathology in other inbred strains. In contrast to the findings with diabetes-resistant C57BL/6J mice, C3H/HeJ and C3HeB/FeJ mice did not appear to possess receptors on their B-cells. However, sufficient receptors were present on the acinar cells to allow for their critical infection. Based on this exocrine tropism it would seem more appropriate to refer to the D variant as virulent rather than diabetogenic, and the B variant as avirulent.

Immunological Responses to EMC Virus Infection

As a result of the growing body of evidence implicating immunopathologic mechanisms in the etiology of human IDDM, the role of immune mechanisms in EMC-virus-induced diabetes has been the subject of intense interest. Initial studies by JANSEN et al. [47] using the M strain of EMC virus suggested that there was an immunological contribution to the target cell destruction. These investigators reported that X-irradiation of DBA/2J mice protected them from EMC-virus-induced diabetes. However, these animals could not be studied for longer than 6 days due to very high mortality. Other studies have suggested a role for T-lymphocytes in the pathogenesis of EMC-virus-induced diabetes. BUSCHARD et al. [7] and JANSEN et al. [48] using different strains of athymic nude mice *(nu/nu)*, reported that these animals were resistant to the diabetogenic effects of EMC virus, whereas their immunocompetent littermates (*nu*/+) became diabetic. More recently, DEFOE et al. [16] have reported that antilymphocyte globulin protected EMC-virus-infected mice from diabetes. All these studies indicated a major role for T-lymphocytes as part of the immune process that is operative in EMC-virus-induced diabetes. However, work by other investigators is in conflict with the autoimmune hypothesis. Studies with the immunosuppressive chemicals cyclophosphamide [16], ASTA 5122 [48], and cyclosporin A [37, 99] were unable to demonstrate the inhibition of EMC-virus-elicited diabetes. Indeed, work with cyclosporin A showed that this compound increased the diabetogenic effects of EMC virus both at early and late intervals after infection. In an effort to resolve these conflicting observations, YOON et al. [111] recently reinvestigated the role of immune functions in the pathogenesis of EMC-virus-induced diabetes. Specifically, the susceptibility of athymic nude mice, thymectomized mice, immunosuppressed mice, and the segregation of H-2 haplotypes in crosses of resistant and susceptible mice were assessed following infection with the D variant. The studies on the F1 and backcross progeny of susceptible and resistant strains of mice failed to reveal an association between susceptibility and the major histocompatibility locus. Immunosuppression by antilymphocyte serum did not prevent the induction of a D-variant-induced diabetes. Athymic nude mice infected with the D variant showed a diabetogenic response nearly identical to that of heterozygous littermates. Passive transfer of lymphocytes from mice made diabetic with the D variant into normal mice failed to produce diabetes. Based on these findings, it was concluded by YOON and colleagues that the development of EMC-virus-induced diabetes is due to the direct destruction of B-cells by the virus, and that the contribution of the immune system in this disease is minimal. However, a subsequent report by HUBER et al. [42] demonstrated that the pathogenesis of EMC-virus-induced diabetes differed among inbred strains of mice, and that on the proper genetic background autoimmune mechanisms may be operative. These investigators studied the pathogenesis of EMC-virus-induced diabetes in DBA/2J and BALB/cByJ mice following infection with a variant of the M strain which had been purified using a critical dilution technique. Interestingly, in this study a correlation could be made between increased virus concentrations in the pancreas and increased hyperglycemia in DBA/2J mice but not in BALB/cByJ. In agreement with previous studies, T-lymphocyte depletion of DBA/2J mice, in this case by thymectomy and bone marrow reconstitution, failed to alter the incidence or severity of hyperglycemia in comparison to intact animals. However, when BALB/cByJ mice were made T-lymphocyte-deficient, hyperglycemia was reduced substantially. Therefore, it was apparent that at least two genetically influenced pathogenic mechanisms existed that lead to the development of diabetes in susceptible mice. In some strains of mice, hyperglycemia resulted exclusively from a viral infection that led to the direct lysis of B-cells. This mechanism was apparently operative in the SJL/J mice studied by YOON et al. [111], and the DBA/2J mice studied by HUBER et al. [42]. Alternatively, viral damage could be compounded by immunological events, as appeared to be the case with BALB/cByJ mice. These findings supported the concept that there is considerable variation in the response of diabetes-susceptible and -resistant mice to infection with EMC virus.

EMC Virus Infection in Combination with Other Diabetogenic Agents

A final way that EMC viruses can influence the development of diabetes in mice is by augmenting the diabetogenic effects of other agents. TONIOLO et al. [98] were able to produce diabetes in strains of mice resistant to the diabetogenic effects of the D variant by injecting the mice with a subdiabetogenic dose (1 mg/mouse) of the B-cell toxin streptozotocin, followed 12 days later by infection with the D variant. This treatment was particularly effective in AKR/J mice, with 100% of treated animals becoming diabetic. Other studies by BLAY et al. [4] have demonstrated that infection with the nondiabetogenic B variant of EMC virus in combination with treatment with a subdiabetogenic dose of streptozotocin can cause diabetes in ICR Swiss or CD-1 mice. Induction of diabetes was dependent upon the interval between the two insults. Streptozotocin treatment followed by infection with the B variant 4 days later induced diabetes in the mice. When mice were infected with the B variant before treatment with streptozotocin, diabetes did not occur. Based on these findings, it appears reasonable to speculate that viruses could augment immunological processes directed against beta cells in a similar manner as B-cell cytotoxic agents.

Persistent Vs Latent Viral Infections

Viral infection of B-cells does not necessarily trigger an immediate cell lysis. A persistent or a latent infection can result if lytic viruses infect semipermissive or nonpermissive target cells, or if nonlytic viruses infect permissive cells. The differences between persistent and latent viral infections have recently been reviewed by SOUTHERN and OLDSTONE [91]. Both types of infection are characterized by a marked reduction of viral release over time, the major distinction being that some release of infectious virus (or expression of viral antigen on the cell surface) continues in a persistent, but not in a latent infection. The reduced level of viral gene expression (permissive infection) or silenced expression (latent infection) is a mechanism whereby the virus avoids clearance by the host's immune system. In either situation, a long-term association between virus and host cell implies that the viral nucleic acid becomes stabilely incorporated into the host cell. Even though the host cell does not show cytopathic change, levels of differentiated function (e.g., insulin biosynthesis and secretion in the case of the B-cell) may be reduced. Examples of persistent or latent viral infections that may interact with autoimmune or environmental factors to compromise B-cell function are discussed below.

Diabetic Consequences of Subclinical Virus Infections

Congenital Rubella Syndrome in Man

The congenital rubella syndrome (CRS) in humans seems to be an example of how a persistent virus infection, initiated in the fetus, could culminate in diabetes in later life (for review [78]). Fetuses of women contracting German measles (the infectious agent is rubella, an RNA-containing member of the Togaviridae) during the first trimester of pregnancy are at high risk of congenital malformations, including the triad of deafness, cataracts, and heart disease. An unusually high percentage of CRS patients develop glucose intolerance or overt diabetes (the majority developing IDDM) in later life. The diabetes generally requires 5-20 years to develop in individuals who have also inherited the necessary diabetes susceptibility genes linked to HLA-DR loci [87]. A persistent expression of the virus has been reported in pancreases of some CRS children [64]. However, rubella is not a particularly lytic virus. Since CRS patients often exhibit polyendocrine disorders, including thyroiditis, and autoantibodies against both islet cell surface and thyroid microsomal antigens have been reported [34], the persistent virus expression by endocrine cells may be the environmental agent required to trigger tissue destruction by autoimmune mechanisms in individuals with the requisite autoimmune predisposing HLA-DR genes [87]. The possibility that such an autoimmune attack could result from a molecular mimicry between viral antigens and structures on endocrine cells will be discussed later. T-lymphocytes are believed by many to be the mediators of B-cell destruction in IDDM. What events could induce T-lymphocytes to lyse specifically B-cells that herefore had been recognized as "self" by the patient's immune system? Persistent abnormalities of T-lymphocyte subsets in young adults with a history of congenital rubella infection suggest that the dysfunction of the immune system permitting the autoimmune reactivity in that syndrome could itself stem from virus infection [75].

Rubella Virus: An Autoimmune Trigger of Diabetes?

A very promising animal model has recently been developed by Rayfield and Yoon [82] in which neonatal golden Syrian hamsters were infected with a diabetogenic rubella strain selected by repeated passage in neonatal hamster islet cell cultures. Within 7-10 days, the infected animals developed hyperglycemia and hypoinsulinemia, indicative of direct viral lysis of B-cells. Nevertheless, insulin continued to be secreted over a 15-week period, albeit at a reduced level, indicating residual B-cell function. Rubella antigens were found in the B-cells, and rubella virus could be isolated 7 days postinfection. Islet cell cytoplasmic antibodies were detected in almost half of the infected group within a month following infection, and leukocytic infiltrates in islets became increasingly common with time. These authors also reported that infection of hamster fetuses in utero produced congenital anomalies similar to CRS in humans. Rubella infection of rat insulinoma (RIN m5F) cells in culture did not lead to lysis, only to a decrease in insulin secretion and cAMP content [80]. Since rubella infection in vivo led to a progressive loss of B-cells accompanied by induction of anti-islet antibodies and insulitis, rubella may indeed act as an environmental trigger of autoimmunity following establishment of a persistent infection. It should be considered that in the hamster model described above, the relatively short period required for pathogenesis probably reflected the fact that the virus was preselected for growth in B-cells.

RNA viruses (EMC, Mengo, and Coxsackie) adapted for growth in cultured B-cells replicate rapidly in pancreatic B-cells of susceptible strains of mice, and generally elicit diabetes by direct lysis of B-cells rather than by establishment of a persistent infection capable of triggering an autoimmune response. However, mice infected with reovirus, another RNA virus (Reoviridae) widely disseminated in the human population, may provide a more representative model of how a viral infection serves as only one of a number of mediators of subclinical diabetogenic stress. Infection of suckling SJL/J mice with reovirus type 3 adapted for growth in B-cells did not produce sufficient B-cell destruction to produce overt hyperglycemia, but glucose tolerance was impaired in many of the mice 3 weeks postinfection [69]. When suckling SJL/J mice were inoculated with the Lang strain of reovirus type 1, impaired glucose tolerance was accompanied by induction of autoantibodies against cytoplasmic antigens in islet cells, pituitary somatotropes, and gastric mucosal cells [69, 70]. Treatment of infected mice with antilymphocyte serum reversed the endocrinopathies [70]. Similarly, as discussed previously, diabetogenesis induced by the M strain of EMC virus in BALB/cByJ inbred mice entailed an interaction between virus-infected cells and the host's immune system [42]. Thus, there is little reason to doubt that persistent infections in certain virus-host combinations, or alternatively, acute infections producing a subclinical level of B-cell destruction, can stimulate an autoimmune response against B-cells as well as against other types of endocrine cells (e.g., somatotropes in the pituitary).

Diabetogenic Effects of Persistent Virus Infection: Other Examples

Although the hamster model of rubella-induced diabetes described above appears to reflect a situation in which the virus triggers organ-specific autoimmunity, there are other examples of persistent virus infection in which glucose intolerance is engendered by alteration of the B-cell's metabolism as assessed by its ability to synthesize and/or release insulin. The most notable examples are provided by diabetogenic variants of two RNA viruses, lymphocytic choriomeningitis virus (LCM virus, Arenaviridae), and Venezuelan encephalitis virus (VE virus, Togaviridae, arbovirus group).

Inoculation of newborn BALB/WEHI mice with LCM virus (strain WE and Armstrong strain 1371) produced a persistent infection of pancreatic B-cells without causing their injury or destruction; nevertheless, glucose intolerance could be demonstrated at 90 days of age [68]. Morphologic examination showed that the B-cells continued to express LCM virus at their surfaces, and that the islets had undergone hypertrophy [83].

Similar impairment of B-cell function in the absence of extensive cell lysis may be elicited by VE virus. Golden Syrian hamsters infected with the TC-83 variant of VE virus did not show long-term morphologic alterations in the pancreatic islets, yet exhibited a sustained impairment in glucose tolerance [77]. Isolated pancreatic islets from such hamsters exhibited a diminution in glucose-stimulated insulin release that was correctable by cAMP or by phosphodiesterase inhibitors [81]. Stimulation of insulin gene transcription by glucose, as well as inhibition of insulin mRNA degradation, may entail the generation of cAMP [67, 103]. Whether the defect in B-cell cAMP generation reflected an effect of viral protein(s) on host cell adenyl cyclase is unknown. The virus-induced defect in insulin release was not the result of a nonspecific membrane change inasmuch as insulin secretory responses to alpha-ketoisocaproic acid were normal. Interestingly, the secretory defect was correctable by tolbutamide, a compound frequently used to stimulate insulin secretion from islets of non-insulin-dependent diabetes mellitus (NIDDM) patients [79]. Viruses are usually discussed in the context of the etiopathogenesis of IDDM, but are seldom discussed in the context of NIDDM, in which obesity rather than autoimmunity is a prevalent associated factor. Nevertheless, the studies with LCM virus and VE virus outlined above suggest that certain persistent virus infections could play a role in both types of diabetes. If virus proteins shared antigenic sequences with either insulin or its receptor, anti-idiotypic antibodies directed against the antiviral antibodies might cross-react with either the "mirrored" sequence on the insulin or the insulin receptor molecule. Either situation could lead to insulin resistance; evidence that such molecular mimicry can exist between viruses, insulin, or insulin receptors will be discussed later.

Indirect Mechanisms of Diabetes Induction by Virus

The classic "slow virus" diseases such as kuru and Jakob-Creutzfeldt syndrome affect the central nervous system. Although the studies reviewed above have been conducted with viruses selected for pancreatic tropism by growth in cultured B-cells, many of these viruses still retain tropisms for other tissues as well, especially those of the central nervous system. Thus, some of the anomalies in B-cell function following infection could have a neurochemical basis. Viral lesions in certain hypothalamic regions can produce severe perturbations of B-cell function; an excellent example was provided by intracranial inoculation of canine distemper virus (Paramyxoviridae family, a morbillivirus antigenically related to measles virus) into young adult Swiss albino mice (NCS/R). Approximately 26% of the mice that did not die of acute encephalitis developed severe obesity accompanied by marked hyperplasia of the islet cell mass within 6-20 weeks postinfection, and catecholamine biosynthesis in the brain was altered [62]. Of interest in this regard was a recent report that intracerebral infection of 6-week-old Syrian golden hamsters with scrapie agent produced abnormal glucose tolerance without any obvious changes in pancreatic islet hormone content [93]. The above examples illustrate that persistent or latent infection by a neurotropic virus may produce a deterioration in glucose homeostasis without apparent direct damage to the pancreatic B-cells.

Diabetogenic Consequences of Latent Viral Infections

Activation of Endogenous Virus Genomes: Murine Retroviruses (Retroviridae)

The majority of the animal models for study of virus-host interactions in diabetogenesis have utilized mice or hamsters infected with exogenous virus. However, the genomes of many mammalian species also contain endogenous viral or virus-like genes transmitted through the germ line. These genes may be expressed in early development and silenced during the course of differentiation, but reactivated following infection by an exogenous virus. These endogenous viruses are oncoviruses (so named because of their demonstrated roles in tumorigenesis). The virion genome is RNA, but the proviral gene integrated into the host genome is a DNA transcript produced by the RNA-dependent DNA polymerase ("reverse transcriptase"). Because the replication cycle of these viruses entails a reverse transcription of RNA to DNA, they are commonly referred to as retroviruses. The molecular biology of the Retroviridae is extensively reviewed in the two volumes edited by Weiss et al. [100]. The genome of replication competent retroviruses consists of a *gag* gene coding for the virus core protein (group-specific antigens), a *pol* gene coding for the polymerase, and an *env* gene coding for the envelope glycoprotein required for viral budding from the cell surface. The 5′ and 3′ ends of retroviral genomes are delimited by characteristic long terminal repeat regions. Strains of inbred mice carry variable numbers of copies per haploid genome of three types of retroviruses: type C [approximately 0-10 copies of ecotropic virus (grow only in mouse cells) and 30-50 copies of xenotropic virus (grow only in cells of heterologous species)], type B (0-10 copies), and intracisternal type A particles (over 1000 copies). Oncogenic type C viruses are usually recombinants between eco- and xenotropic (dualotropic) viruses [20].

Cytopathic Retroviruses

Research on the cellular effects of mouse retroviruses has mainly concentrated on the generation of malignant or transformed cellular growth either by murine type C leukemia and sarcoma viruses, or the type B mouse mammary tumor viruses. Until the recent discovery that HTLV-III, a type C human T-lymphotropic virus, triggered the acquired immunodeficiency syndrome (AIDS) by destroying helper T-lymphocytes, most researchers had concentrated on the oncogenic properties of the retroviruses rather than their potential to produce cytopathic effects in differentiated cells. Predating the isolation of HTLV-III was the isolation of a neurotropic type C virus from wild mice causing lower limb paralysis [29]; destruction of central nervous system neurons was associated with extensive replication of type C retrovirus within the rough endoplasmic reticulum, a completely aberrant site for type C virus, which normally self-assembled at its budding site at the plasma membrane.

Mouse pancreas appeared to be a very conducive site for expression of endogenous retroviral genes, and this expression was enhanced in pancreatic disease states, including duct cell adenocarcinoma [52] B-cell adenoma [88], hereditary diabetes [55], and spontaneous necrosis of exocrine pancreatic cells [51]. Activation of type C virus was observed in the exocrine pancreas of moribund (encephalitic) ICR mice infected with VE virus [39]. Following multidose streptozotocin treatment of male CD-1 mice, LIKE and ROSSINI [60] reported an induction of an aberrant type C virus budding into the rough endoplasmic reticulum of B-cells 2-3 days prior to development of insulitis. Of a panel of inbred strains compared to outbred CD-1 males for sensitivity to induction of hyperglycemia and insulitis by multidose streptozotocin, only the C57BL/KsJ strain was comparably sensitive [86]. In this latter strain, IAP but not type C viruses were induced in the B-cells [2]. However, no direct evidence links heightened sensitivity of these two strains specifically to heightened levels of retroviral expression in B-cells [2].

Retroviral Gene Expression Without Virus Formation

Retroviral genes can be expressed even in the absence of formation of a complete virion; for example, the major envelope glycoprotein of type C virus, gp70, can be expressed on lymphoid and epithelial cell surfaces of mouse strains which do not

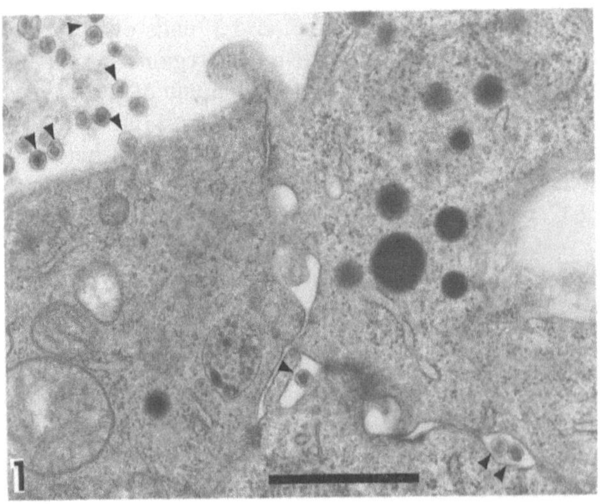

Fig. 1. Expression of a latent type C retroviral genome in an established rat epithelial cell line (RC4B/C) established from an anterior pituitary adenoma. Retroviral particles *(arrowheads)* are budding into the interstitial spaces between the cells growing in aggregate culture. The *horizontal bar* represents 1 μm

produce retrovirus such as 129/J [49]. In lupus-prone strains of mice, gp70 from a xenotropic retroviral genome is shed into the serum at high concentrations and is strongly immunogenic [46].

Unlike the mouse type C retroviruses, the endogenous rat type C virus is not commonly observed from tissues of normal or tumor-bearing rats, but is frequently present after prolonged culture of both normal and neoplastic rat cell lines [96]. Figure 1 shows shedding of an endogenous rat type C virus from a cell line derived from rat pituitary adenoma (RC4B/C). No particles were seen in the parent tumor or in this ultrastructurally well-differentiated cell line prior to the 5th year in vitro. The appearance of cell-surface-budding type C particles between the 5th and 6th year in culture correlated with the acquisition of ability of the cells to survive frozen storage and a decreased cell cycle time. No evidence of a contaminating mouse eco- or xenotropic C type virus was found.

Intracisternal Type A Particles

Intracisternal type A particles (IAPs) represent the most enigmatic retrovirus associated with murine diabetes. IAPs are normally expressed in oogenesis and in early embryogenesis The 73 000-dalton core protein (p73) may be a differentiation antigen, because when IAPs show a stage-specific appearance in 2- to 8-cell stage preimplantation embryos, p73 is expressed at the cell surface [41]. IAPs are not infectious, since they lack an *env* gene product and therefore cannot bud extracellularly but only intracisternally into the rough endoplasmic reticulum. If p73, indeed, is a differentiation antigen normally expressed prior to the constitution of an immune surveillance system, then its expression by B-cells in adult hyperglycemic mice might lead to its perception as a neoantigen. This, in turn, could lead to an autoimmune reaction against B-cells.

Like and Chick [59] first observed these particles in electron micrographs of prenecrotic and necrotic B-cells of the genetically C57BL/KsJ-*db/db* mouse. Subsequent biochemical and immunocytochemical studies established that these particles were IAPs [53, 54]. In a study analyzing the response of different inbred strains of mice to the *db* mutation, only those strains constitutively expressing B-cell IAPs developed severe diabetes [54]. Both the transcription and translation of the IAP genome in B-cells of diabetes-susceptible, but not diabetes-resistant strains, were inducible by elevated glucose concentration [57]. Abrogation of female resistance to the diabetogenic action of the *db* mutation in C3HeB/FeJ mice following outcross to the C3H. SW/SnJ strain was associated with coinduction of an aberrant (intracisternal budding) type C virus and IAPs [55]. This link between induction of novel retrovirus and B-cell destruction, as well as the presence of the virus in prenecrotic C-cells, suggested that retroviruses played an active role in pathogenesis and were not simply reflections of necrosis. Structurally aberrant and internally budding type C particles were also observed in prenecrotic cells of the nonobese diabetic (NOD) mouse, a model of autoimmune IDDM; and a viral role in induction of B-cell autoimmunity was suggested [24]. In addition to the type C virus, IAPs were also expressed in the prenecrotic NOD B-cells (Fig. 2). Indeed, autoantibodies against p73 have been found in serum of normal and geneti-

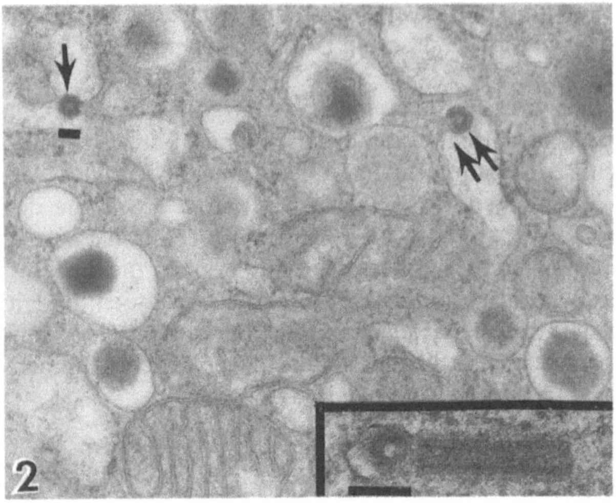

Fig. 2. Expression of both intracisternal type A *(single arrow)* and intracisternally budding type C *(double arrow)* particles in a B-cell of a 14-week-old NOD strain male. The type C particle is distinguished from the type A particle by the presence of an additional unit membrane structure. The inset shows an aberrant cylindrical form of an intracisternal type C particle seen in both cross- and sagittal sections. The *horizontal bars* represent 0.1 μm

cally diabetic mice and in serum of NOD mice shortly before the onset of hyperglycemia [90]. Insulin autoantibodies have also been detected by ELISA assay in the sera of both NOD and *db/db* mice.

Reactivity Between Autoantibodies and Retroviral Antigens

The most compelling evidence to date that endogenous retroviral antigens may play a role in glucose intolerance syndromes has been the surprising finding that a common epitope on insulin and p73 can be recognized by the autoantibodies found in diabetic mice (Table 1). Indeed, a monoclonal anti-insulin antibody derived from an autoimmune NOD mouse (kindly supplied by Dr. C. Boitard, Paris, France) was also found to bind to p73 in ELISA (D. V. Serreze and E. H. Leiter, unpublished observation). While the homology between insulin and the much larger p73 molecule is presumably small, there may be considerably more homology between p73 and the product of a different cellular gene coding for IgE-binding protein. T-lymphocyte genes coding for soluble factors binding the Fc portions of IgE are apparently fusion products of portions of the IAP *gag* and *pol* genes [63]. Thus, more extensive protein sequence homology could exist between IAP proteins and IgE-binding proteins of both mice and rats. Accordingly, it is not surprising that serum from NOD or *db/db* mice containing autoantibodies against insulin and p73 also bound IgE-binding protein [90]. The pathogenic significance of these autoantibodies remains unclear. Combining the *db* and a severe combined immunodeficiency mutation allowed us to examine genetically diabetic mice with no functional T- and B-lymphocytes and thus no autoantibodies. Such mice,

Table 1. Cross-reactivity of autoantibodies against insulin and p73 as measured by ELISA

Serum donor[a]	Serum dilution	Ligand on ELISA plate					
		Insulin Absorbed with			p73 Absorbed with		
		None	Insulin	p73	None	Insulin	p73
NOD	1/800	0.702	0.240 (66%)	0.319 (55%)	0.814	0.498 (39%)	0.540 (34%)
C57BL/KsJ-*db/db*	1/400	0.345	0.089 (74%)	0.095 (73%)	0.660	0.402 (39%)	0.495 (25%)

Data represent mean optical densities at 405 nm of replicate samples in an alkaline-phosphatase-based ELISA system, using a ligand of either porcine insulin (500 ng/well) or purified IAP core protein (p73, 10 ng/well). Absorptions were performed overnight in ice using either porcine insulin at 2 μg/ml or p73 at 1 μg/ml. Numbers in parentheses show percent absorption
[a] The NOD donor was an aglycosuric 42-week-old female, the genetically diabetic (C57BL/KsJ-*db/db*) donor a 28-week-old female

nevertheless, exhibited B-cell necrosis and developed diabetes, albeit at a slower rate [58]. Consequently, it appears likely that autoantibodies against retroviruses are not prerequisites for B-cell destruction in this model. Whether retroviral mRNAs compete with B-cell housekeeping or luxury (e.g., insulin) mRNAs, leading to functional degeneration, remains to be elucidated. C57BL/KsJ(BKs), but not C57BL/6J (B6), B-cells in culture responded to high glucose by induction of IAP gene transcription and p73 synthesis [57]. This stimulation by glucose of both insulin and p73 mRNA transcription in cultured BKs islets had no obvious deleterious effects on insulin biosynthesis in comparison to B6 [57]. On the other hand, this differential response to glucose may be of significance in vivo when islets are subjected to hyperglycemic stress. Fifty BKs islets graftes intrasplenically into BKs recipients previously made hyperglycemic by streptozotocin were eliminated within 11 days, whereas 50 B6 islets grafted into hyperglycemic B6 hosts were not eliminated [57].

Molecular Mimicry Between Virus and Host Proteins

The preceding example of autoantibodies from diabetic mice recognizing a common epitope on insulin and p73 has amply illustrated that products of viral genes may share antigenic sites with products of normal cellular genes, a phenomenon referred to as molecular mimicry. This phenomenon would explain the finding that a monoclonal (auto)antibody from lymphocytes transformed by Epstein-Barr virus could cross-react with antigens in a wide variety of tissues [30]. When 600 monoclonal antiviral antibodies made against 11 different viruses were screened against 14 different organs from normal uninfected mice, 3.5% were reactive, some in multiple organs including pancreatic islets [89]. The most striking example of molecular mimicry by an infective virus triggering organ-specific autoimmunity was recorded by FUJINAMI and OLDSTONE [23], who observed a sequence homology between eight amino acids in the hepatitis B virus polymerase (HBVP) and the encephalitogenic site of myelin basic protein. Injection of the HBVP sequence into rabbits induced production of antimyelin antibodies and generated an inflammatory response in the central nervous system. The important implications of this study were that induction of cross-reactivity would not necessarily require an infectious agent to replicate, only to immunize. Once the autoimmune phenomenon had been initiated, clearance of the infectious agent would be of little consequence to the final outcome, i.e., overt disease. Given that only 20 amino acids are employed to produce the tens of thousands of proteins in an organism, the probability of two similar sequences capable of serving as antigenic determinants appearing by chance in two unrelated molecules is not insignificant [92]. Fujinami and Oldstone [23] speculate that autoimmunity occurs when viral determinants are sufficiently similar to host configurations capable of inducing autoimmune disease, but remain sufficiently different to break the organism's tolerance to self-antigen. Just as molecular mimicry exists between p73 and insulin, there also appears to be a shared epitope between the insulin receptor and $pp60^{SRC}$, the protein kinase encoded by the *src* (onco) gene of an avian retrovirus [72]. Anti-idiotypic antibodies have been mentioned previously. It has been suggested by Plotz [74] that autoantibodies are primarily anti-idiotypes formed by the host against part of an antiviral antibody which in turn is cross-reactive with a structure of the host. Accordingly, an anti-idiotype against an anti-insulin could cross-react with the insulin receptor [89], and anti-idiotype against an antibody to insulin receptor might react with the insulin-producing B-cell. The former could lead to impaired glucose tolerance, and the latter possibly could lead to antibody-dependent cell-mediated cytotoxicity against B-cells.

Conclusions

Although viral infections occasionally appear to be the causative agent in IDDM, such clear-cut cases are relatively rare. Analysis of the temporal relation between the appearance of high titers of neutralizing antiviral antibodies, the appearance of anti-islet cell autoantibodies, and onset of diabetes have given conflicting results (for the controversies regarding Coxsackie virus, see ref. no. 3). Given our increasing understanding of the complexities of host-virus interactions and the complexities of the pathogenesis of IDDM, determination of the order of appearance of anti-islet and antiviral antibodies in the serum of a prediabetic patient may not be the critical means of establishing whether a given virus was or was not a mediator of diabetogenic stress. As more structural homologies between products of viral and cellular genes are identified with the aid of computers searching sequence data banks, we may understand by how many different mechanisms a transient exposure to virus might induce functional alteration or destruction of the B-cells. Childhood exposure to potentially diabetogenic viruses ubiquitous in the environment is a fact of life. These viruses probably represent only one source of a number of "provocations" that stress the B-cells either directly or through the nervous system or, alternatively, alter the function of regulatory and/or effector cells of the immune surveillance system. In most cases, viral provocation alone is probably not sufficient for IDDM induction. As suggested by certain of the mouse models of virus-induced diabetes, disease induction in humans probably requires that the host be of a diabetes-susceptible genetic constitution such that autoimmune reactivity against B-cells could develop. Whether viruses trigger these autoimmune processes, merely augment a preexisting condition, or both remains to be determined.

Acknowledgements. The authors would like to thank JAN WILSON and REXANN WARREN for their help in preparing this manuscript.

References

1. Ahmad N, Abraham AA (1982) Pancreatic isleitis with Coxsackie virus B5 infection. Human Pathol 13: 661-662
2. Appel MC, Rossini AA, Williams RM, Like AA (1978) Viral studies in streptozotocin-induced pancreatic insulitis. Diabetologia 15: 327-336
3. Barrett-Conner E (1985) Is insulin-dependent diabetes mellitus caused by Coxsackie B infection? A review of the epidemiologic evidence. Rev Infect Dis 7: 207-215
4. Blay RA, Bigley NJ, Giron DJ (1985) A murine model of insulin-dependent diabetes mellitus resulting from the cumulative effects of the nondiabetogenic strain of encephalomyocarditis virus and a single low dose of streptozotocin. Diabetes 31: 288-1292
5. Boucher DL, Notkins AL (1973) Virus-induced diabetes mellitus. I. Hyperglycemia and hypoinsulinemia in mice infected with encephalomyocarditis virus. J Exp Med 137: 1226-1239
6. Boucher DL, Hayashi Y, Rosenthal J, Notkins AL (1975) Virus induced diabetes. I. Influence of sex and strain of the host. J Infect Dis 131: 462-466
7. Buschard K, Rygaard J, Lund E (1976) The inability of a diabetogenic virus to induce diabetes in athymic nude mice. Acta Pathol Microbiol Scand 84: 299-303
8. Clark EA, Windsor NT, Struge J, Stanton TH (1980) Mutations that influence natural killer cell-mediated cytotoxicity in rodents. In: Huberman RB (ed) Natural cell-mediated immunity against tumors. Academic, New York, pp 417-429
9. Chairez R, Yoon JW, Notkins AL (1978) Virus-induced diabetes mellitus. X. Attachment of encephalomyocarditis virus and permissiveness of cultured pancreatic beta cells to infection. Virol 85: 606-611
10. Champsaur H, Dussaix E, Samolyk D, Fabre M, Bach C, Assan R (1980) Diabetes and coxsackie B5 infection. Lancet 1: 251 (letter)
11. Craighead JE (1966) Pathogenicity of the M and E variants of the encephalomyocarditis (EMC) virus. I. Myocardiotropic and neurotropic properties. Am J Pathol 48: 333-345
12. Craighead JE, McLane MF (1968) Diabetes mellitus: induction in mice by encephalomyocarditis virus. Science 162: 913-914
13. Craighead JE, Steinke J (1971) Diabetes mellitus-like syndrome in mice infected with encephalomyocarditis virus. Am J Pathol 63: 119-134
14. Craighead JE, Kanich RE, Kessler JB (1974) Lesions of the islets of Langerhans in encephalomyocarditis virus-infected mice with a diabetes mellitus-like disease. Am J Pathol 74: 287-294
15. D'Andrea BJ, Wilson GL, Craighead JE (1981) Effect of genetic obesity in mice on the induction of diabetes by encephalomyocarditis virus. Diabetes 30: 451-454
16. Defoe DC, Naji A, Plotkin SA, Barker CF (1980) Susceptibility to diabetogenic virus: host versus pancreatic factors. J Surg Res 28: 338-347
17. De Maeyer-Guignard JE, Dandoy F, Bailey DW, De Maeyer E (1986) Interferon structural genes do not participate in quantitative regulation of interferon production by If loci as shown in C57BL/6 mice that are congenic with BALB/c mice at the alpha interferon gene cluster. J Virol 58: 743-747

18. Eberhardt MS, Wagener DK, Orchard TJ, LaPorte RE, Cavender DE, Rabin BS, Atchison RW, Kuller LH, Drash AL, Becker DJ (1985) HLA heterogeneity of insulin-dependent diabetes mellitus at diagnosis. Diabetes 34: 1247-1252
19. Eisenbarth GS (1986) Type I diabetes mellitus: a chronic autoimmune disease. N Engl J Med 314: 1360-1368
20. Elder JH (1984) On the role of recombinant retroviruses in murine leukemia. In: Notkins AL, Oldstone MBA (eds) Concepts in viral pathogenesis. Springer, Berlin Heidelberg New York, pp 86-93
21. Forrest JM, Menses MA, Burgess JA (1971) High frequency of diabetes mellitus in young adults with congenital rubella. Lancet 2: 332-334
22. Friedman SB, Grota LJ, Glasgow LA (1972) Differential susceptibility of male and female mice to encephalomyocarditis virus. Effects of castration, adrenalectomy, and administration of sex hormones. Infect Immun 5: 637-644
23. Fujinami RS, Oldstone MBA (1985) Amino acid homology between the encephalitogenic site of myelin basic protein and virus: mechanism for autoimmunity. Science 230: 1043-1045
24. Fujino-Kurihara H, Fujita H, Hakura A, Nonaka K, Tarui S (1985) Morphological aspects on pancreatic islets of non-obese diabetic (NOD) mice. Virchows Arch 49: 107-120
25. Gaines KL, Kayes SG, Wilson GL (1987) Factors affecting the infection of the D variant of encephalomyocarditis virus in the B cells of C57BL/6J mice. Diabetologia 30: 419-425
26. Gaines KL, Kayes SG, Wilson GL (1986) Altered pathogenesis in encephalomyocarditis virus (D variant)-infected diabetes-susceptible and -resistant strains of mice. Diabetologia 29: 313-320
27. Gamble DR, Taylor KW (1969) Seasonal incidence of diabetes mellitus. Br Med J 3: 627-630
28. Gamble DR, Kinsley ML, Fitzgerald MG, Bolton R, Taylor KW (1969) Viral antibodies in diabetes mellitus. Br Med J 3: 627-630
29. Gardner MB, Henderson BE, Officer JE, Rongey RW, Parker JC, Oliver C, Estes JD, Huebner RJ (1973) A spontaneous lower motor neuron disease apparently caused by indigenous type-C RNA virus in wild mice. JNCI 51: 1243-1254
30. Garzelli C, Taub FE, Scharff JE, Prabhakar BS, Ginsberg-Fellner F, Notkins AL (1984) Epstein-Barr virus-transformed lymphocytes produce monoclonal antibodies that react with antigens in multiple organs. J Virol 52: 722-725
31. Gepts W (1965) Pathologic anatomy of the pancreas in juvenile diabetes mellitus. Diabetes 14: 619-633
32. Gepts W (1984) The pathology of the pancreas in human diabetes. In: Andreani D, DiMario U, Federlin KF, Heding LG (eds) Immunology in diabetes. Kimpton, London, pp 21-34
33. Ginsberg-Fellner F, Witt ME, Yagihashi S, Dobersen MJ, Taub F, Fedun B, McEvoy RC, Roman SH, Davies TF, Cooper LZ, Rubinstein P, Notkins AL (1984) Congenital rubella as a model for type 1 (insulin dependent) diabetes mellitus: increased prevalence of islet cell surface antibodies. Diabetologia [Suppl] 27: 87-89
34. Giron DJ, Patterson RR (1982) Effect of steroid hormones on virus-induced diabetes mellitus. Infect Immun 37: 820-822
35. Gould CL, Trombley ML, Bigley NJ, McMannama KG, Giron DJ (1984) Replication of diabetogenic and nondiabetogenic variants of encephalomyocarditis (EMC) virus in ICR Swiss mice. Proc Soc Exp Biol Med 175: 449-453
36. Gould CL, McMannama KC, Bigley NJ, Giron DJ (1985a) Exacerbation of the pathogenesis of the diabetogenic variant of encephalomyocarditis virus in mice by interferon. J Interferon Res 5: 33-37
37. Gould CL, McMannama KG, Bigley NJ, Giron DJ (1985b) Virus-induced murine diabetes: enhancement by immunosuppression. Diabetes 34: 1217-1221
38. Gunderson E (1927) Is diabetes of infectious origin? J Infect Dis 41: 197-202
39. Harrison AK, Murphy FA (1975) Murine oncornavirus activation in the pancreas during infection with Venezuelan equine encephalitis virus. JNKI 55: 917-923
40. Hayashi K, Boucher DW, Notkins AL (1974) Virus-induced diabetes mellitus. II. Relationship between beta cell damage and hyperglycemia in mice infected with the encephalomyocarditis virus. Am J Pathol 75: 91-102
41. Huang TTF, Calarco AG (1981) Evidence for the cell surface expression of intracisternal A particle associated antigens during early mouse development. Dev Biol 82: 338-392

42. Huber SA, Babu PG, Craighead JE (1985) Genetic influences on the immunologic pathogenesis of encephalomyocarditis (EMC) virus-induced diabetes mellitus. Diabetes 34: 1186-90
43. Hultquist G, Nosvall S, Sundstrom C (1973) Insulitis in cytomegalovirus infection in a newborn infant. Upsala J Med Sci 78: 139-144
44. Irvine WJ, McCallum CJ, Gray RS, Campbell CJ, Duncan LJP, Farquhar JW, Vaughan H, Morris PJ (1977) Pancreatic islet-cell antibodies in diabetes mellitus correlated with the duration and type of diabetes, coexistent autoimmune disease and HLA type. Diabetes 26: 138-147
45. Iwo K, Bellomo SC, Mukai N, Craighead JE (1983) Encephalomyocarditis virus-induced diabetes in mice: long-term changes in the structure and function of the islets of Langerhans. Diabetologia 25: 35-44
46. Izui S, Elder JH, McConahey PJ, Dixon FJ (1981) Identification of retroviral gp70 antibodies involved in circulating immune complexes in NZB × NZW mice. J Exp Med 153: 1151-1160
47. Jansen FK, Muntefering H, Schmidt WAK (1977) Virus-induced diabetes and the immune system. I. Suggestion that appearance of diabetes depends on immune reactions. Diabetologia 13: 545-549
48. Jansen FK, Thurneyssen O, Munterfering H (1979) Virus-induced diabetes and the immune system. II. Evidence for an immune pathogenesis of the acute phase of diabetes. Biomedicine 31: 1-2
49. Johnson DA, Elder JH (1983) Antibody directed to determinants of a Moloney virus derived MCF gp70 recognizes a thymic differentiation antigen. J Exp Med 159: 1751-1756
50. Johnson GM, Tudor RB (1970) Diabetes mellitus and congenital rubella infection. Am J Dis Child 120: 453-455
51. Leiter EH, Cunliffe-Beamer T (1977) Exocrine pancreatic insufficiency syndrome in CBA/J mice III. Pathological and genetic analysis. Gastroenterol 73: 260-266
52. Leiter EH, Malinoski F, Eppig JJ (1978) An epithelial cell line with chronic polyoma infection established from a spontaneous mouse pancreatic adenocarcinoma. Cancer Res 38: 969-977
53. Leiter EH, Bedigian HG (1979) Intracisternal type A particles in genetically diabetic mice: identification in pancreas and induction in cultured B-cells. Diabetologia 17: 175-185
54. Leiter EH, Kuff EL (1984) Intracisternal type A particles in murine pancreatic B cells: immunocytochemical demonstration of increased antigen (p73) in genetically diabetic mice. Am J Pathol 114: 46-55
55. Leiter EH (1985) Type C retrovirus production by pancreatic B-cells: association with accelerated pathogenesis in C3H-*db/db* ("diabetes") mice. Am J Pathol 119: 22-32
56. Leiter EH, Yoon J-W, Kuff EL (1985) Spontaneous autoantibody production against insulin and retrovirus distinguishes C57BL/KsJ from C57BL/6J mice. Diabetes 34 [Suppl 1]: 80A
57. Leiter EH, Fewell JW, Kuff EL (1986) Glucose induces intracisternal type A retroviral gene transcription and translation in pancreatic B-cells. J Exp Med 163: 87-100
58. Leiter EH, Prochazka M (1987) Effect of immunodeficiency on diabetogenesis in genetically diabetic *(db/db)* mice. J Immunol 138: 3224-3229
59. Like AA, Chick WL (1970) Studies in the diabetic mutant mouse. II. Electron microscopy of pancreatic islets. Diabetologia 6: 216-242
60. Like AA, Rossini AA (1976) Streptozotocin-induced pancreatic insulitis: new model of diabetes mellitus. Science 193: 415-417
61. Lutton CW, Gauntt CJ (1985) Ameliorating effect of IFN-B and anti-IFN-B on Coxsackie virus B3-induced myocarditis in mice. J Interferon Res 5: 137-146
62. Lyons MJ, Faust IM, Hemmes RB, Buskirk DR, Hirsch J, Zabriskie JB (1982) A virally induced obesity syndrome in mice. Science 216: 82-85
63. Moore KW, Jardieu P, Mietz JA, Trounstine ML, Kuff EL, Ishizaka K, Martens CL (1986) Rodent IgE-binding factor genes are members of an endogenous retrovirus-like gene family. J Immunol 136: 4283-4290
64. Monif GRG, Avery GB, Korones SB, Sever JL (1965) Post-mortem isolation of rubella virus from three children with rubella-syndrome defects. Lancet I: 723-725
65. Morrow PL, Freedman A, Craighead JE (1980) Testosterone effect on experimental diabetes mellitus in encephalomyocarditis (EMC) virus-infected mice. Diabetologia 18: 247-249
66. Murnane TG, Craighead JE, Mondragon H, Shelokov A (1960) Fatal disease of swine due to encephalomyocarditis virus. Science 131: 498-499

67. Nielsen DA, Welsh M, Casadaban MJ, Steiner DF (1985) Control of insulin gene expression in pancreatic B-cells and in an insulin-producing cell line, RIN-5F cells. I. Effects of glucose and cyclic AMP on the transcription of insulin mRNA. J Biol Chem 260: 13585-13589
68. Oldstone MBA, Southern P, Rodriquez M, Lampert P (1984) Virus persists in B-cells of islets of Langerhans and is associated with chemical manifestations of diabetes. Science 224: 1440-1443
69. Onodera T, Toniolo A, Ray UR, Jenson AB, Knazek RA, Notkins AL (1981) Virus induced diabetes mellitus. XX. Polyendocrinopathy and autoimmunity. J Exp Med 153: 1457-1473
70. Onodera T, Ray UR, Melez KA, Suzuki H, Toniolo A, Notkins AL (1982) Virus induced diabetes mellitus: autoimmunity and polyendocrine disease prevented by immunosuppression. Nature 27: 66-68
71. Paavonen T, Anderson LC, Aldercreutz H (1981) Sex hormone regulation of in vitro immune response. J Exp Med 154: 1935-1945
72. Perrotti N, Grunberger G, Richert ND, Taylor SI (1986) Immunological similarity between the insulin receptor and the protein encoded by the *src* oncogene. Endocrinology 118: 2349-2354
73. Plotkin SA, Kaye R (1970) Diabetes and congenital rubella. Pediatrics 46: 650-651
74. Plotz PH (1983) Autoantibodies are anti-idiotype antibodies to antiviral antibodies. Lancet II: 824-826
75. Rabinowe SL, George KL, Laughlin R, Soeldner JS, Eisenbarth GS (1986) Congenital rubella: monoclonal antibody defined T cell abnormalities in young adults. Am J Med 81: 779-782
76. Ray U, Aulakh G, McClintock PR, Yoon JW, Notkins JW (1983) Virus-induced diabetes: difference in the RNA finger prints of diabetogenic and nondiabetogenic variants of encephalomyocarditis virus. J Gen Virol 64: 947-950
77. Rayfield EJ, Gorelkin L, Curnow RT, Jahrling PB (1976) Virus-induced pancreatic disease by Venezuelan encephalitis virus. Alterations in glucose tolerance and insulin resistance. Diabetes 25: 623-631
78. Rayfield EJ, Yoon J-W (1981) Role of viruses in diabetes. In: Cooperstein SJ, Watkins D (eds) The islets of Langerhans: biochemistry, physiology, and pathology. Academic, New York, pp 428-451
79. Rayfield EJ, Seto Y, Walsh S, McEvoy RC (1981) Virus-induced alterations in insulin release in hamster islets of Langerhans. J Clin Invest 68: 1172-1181
80. Rayfield EJ, Kelly KJ (1985) A direct mechanism by which rubella virus impairs insulin secretion. Diabetes 34 [Suppl 1]: 271A
81. Rayfield EJ, Kelly KJ (1986) Virus-induced alterations in cyclic adenosine monophosphate generation in hamster islets of Langerhans. J Clin Invest 77: 958963
82. Rayfield EJ, Kelly KJ, Yoon J-W (1986) Rubella virus-induced diabetes in the hamster. Diabetes 35: 1278-1281
83. Rodriguez M, Garrett RS, Raitt M, Lampert PW, Oldstone MBA (1985) Virus persists in B cells of islets of Langerhans and infection is associated with chemical manifestations of diabetes. Am J Pathol 121: 497-504
84. Ross ME, Onodera T, Brown KS, Notkins AL (1976) Virus-induced diabetes mellitus. IV. Genetic and environmental factors influencing the development of diabetes after infection with the M variant of encephalomyocarditis virus. Diabetes 25: 190-197
85. Rossini AA, Appel MA, Williams RM, Like AA (1977) Genetic influence of the streptozotocin-induced insulitis and hyperglycemia. Diabetes 26: 916-920
86. Rotter JI, Rimoin DL (1978) Heterogeneity in diabetes mellitus. Diabetes 27: 599608
87. Rubinstein P, Walker ME, Fedun B, Witt ME, Cooper LZ, Ginsberg-Fellner F (1982) The HLA system in congenital rubella patients with and without diabetes. Diabetes 31: 1088-1091
88. Sass B, Vernon ML, Peters RL, Kelloff GJ (1978) Mammary tumors, hepatocellular carcinomas, and pancreatic islet changes in C3H-A^{vy}mice. JNCI 60: 611-621
89. Sege K, Peterson PA (1980) Anti-idiotypic antibodies raised against anti-insulin antibodies cross-react with the insulin receptor. In: Irvine WJ (ed) Immunology of diabetes. Teviot, Edinburgh, pp 195-204
90. Serreze DV, Leiter EH, Kuff EL, Jardieu P, Ishizaka K (1988) Molecular mimicry between

insulin and retroviral antigen p73: development of cross reactive autoantibodies in sera of NOD and C57BL/KsJ-*db/db* mice. Diabetes, in press
91. Southern P, Oldstone MBA (1986) Medical consequences of persistent viral infection. N Engl J Med 314: 359-367
92. Srinivasappa J, Saegusa J, Prabhakar BS, Gentry MK, Buchmeier MJ, Wiktor TJ, Koprowski H, Oldstone MBA, Notkins AL (1986a) Molecular mimicry: frequency of reactivity of monoclonal antiviral antibodies with normal tissues. J Virol 57: 397-401
93. Srinivasappa J, Asher DM, Pomeroy KY, Yoon J-W, Gajdusek DC, Notkins AL (1986b) Virus-induced diabetes mellitus: slow viruses. Symposium program. In: Jaworski MA, Mollnar GD, Rajotte RV, Singh B (eds) Elsevier Science, Amsterdam The Immunology of diabetes mellitus meeting. Edmonton, pp 33
94. Stewart WE (1979) The interferon system. Springer, Berlin Heidelberg New York, pp 199-200
95. Talal N (1976) Disordered immunologic regulation and autoimmunity. Transplant Rev 31: 240-263
96. Teich N (1984) Taxonomy of retroviruses. In: Weiss R, Teich N, Varmus H, Coffin J (eds) RNA tumor viruses, vol 1, 2nd edn. Cold Spring Harbor Publications, Cold Spring Harbor, pp 25-207
97. Terres G, Morrison SL, Habicht GS (1968) A quantitative difference in the immune response between male and female mice. Proc Soc Exp Biol Med 127: 664-668
98. Toniolo A, Onodera T, Yoon JW, Notkins JW (1980) Induction of diabetes by cumulative environmental insults from viruses and chemicals. Nature 288: 383-385
99. Vialettes B, Baume D, Charpin C, De Maeyer-Guignard J, Vague P (1983) Assessment of viral and immune factors in EMC virus-induced diabetes. Effects of cyclosporin A and interferon. J Clin Lab Immunol 10: 35-40
100. Weiss R, Teich N, Varmus H, Coffin J (eds) (1984) RNA tumor viruses. Molecular biology of tumor viruses, 2 vols, 2nd edn. Cold Spring Harbor Publications, Cold Spring Harbor, pp 1-1233
101. Wellmann KF, Amsterdam D, Brooks JE, Volk BW (1972) Fine structure of pancreatic islets of mice infected with the M variant of the encephalomyocarditis virus. Diabetologia 8: 349-357
102. Wellmann KF, Amsterdam D, Brooks JE, Volk BW (1975) Glucose tolerance and pancreatic ultrastructure in mice with long-term diabetes induced by EMC virus (M variant). Proc Soc Exp Biol Med 148: 261-262
103. Welsh M, Nielsen DA, Mackrell AJ, Steiner DF (1985) Control of insulin gene expression in pancreatic B cells and in an insulin-producing cell line, RIN5F cells II. Regulation of insulin mRNA stability. J Biol Chem 260: 13590-13594
104. Wilson GL, D'Andrea BJ, Bellomo SC, Craighead JE (1980) Encephalomyocarditis virus infection of cultured murine pancreatic B cells. Nature 285: 112-113
105. Wilson GL, Bellomo SC, Craighead JE (1983) Effect of interferon on encephalomyocarditis virus infection of cultured mouse pancreatic B cells. Diabetologia 24: 38-41
106. Yoon J-W, Notkins AL (1976) Virus-induced diabetes mellitus. VI. Genetically determined host differences in the replication of encephalomyocarditis virus in pancreatic B cells. J Exp Med 143: 1170-1185
107. Yoon J-W, Austin M, Onodera T, Notkins AL (1979) Virus-induced diabetes mellitus: isolation of a virus from the pancreas of a child with diabetic ketoacidosis. N Engl J Med 300: 1173-1179
108. Yoon J-W, McClintock PR, Onodera T, Notkins AL (1980) Virus-induced diabetes mellitus. XVIII. Inhibition by a non-diabetogenic variant of encephalomyocarditis virus. J Exp Med 152: 878-891
109. Yoon J-W, Selvaggio S, Onodera T, Wheeler J, Jenson AB (1981) Infection of cultured human pancreatic B cells with reovirus type 3. Diabetologia 20: 462-467
110. Yoon J-W, London WT, Curfman BL, Brown RL, Notkins AL (1985) Coxsackie B4 produces transient diabetes in nonhuman primates. Diabetes 35: 712-716
111. Yoon J-W, McClintock PR, Bachurski CJ, Longstreth JD, Notkins AL (1985) Virus-induced diabetes mellitus: no evidence for immune mechanisms in the destruction of beta cells by the D-variant of encephalomyocarditis virus. Diabetes 34: 922-925
112. Yoon J-W, Ray UR (1986) Perspectives on the role of viruses in insulin-dependent diabetes. Diabetes Care 8: 39-44

Death of the Pancreatic B-Cell*

D. G. Pipeleers, P. A. In't Veld and M. Van De Winkel

Introduction

Insulin-dependent diabetes is the clinical definition for a condition of absolute insulin deficiency which leads to ketosis when no exogenous insulin is administered (LEFÈBVRE, this volume). The syndrome was attributed to an insufficient number of pancreatic B-cells after it became clear that newly diagnosed cases contained at least a five-fold smaller B-cell mass than normal controls [1-5]. Little is known about the events which lead to such quantitative deficit. Clarification of the underlying mechanisms has been hindered by two major obstacles. The first is the inability to measure the pancreatic B-cell mass in vivo, which prevents the detection of the disease at an earlier stage and hence its follow-up in the light of extrapancreatic events. Secondly, it has been impossible so far to screen for agents which impair the growth or survival of the pancreatic B-cells or their precursor cells. During recent years, both issues have been investigated in man and in rodents with a genetic predisposition for insulin-dependent diabetes. It was shown that abnormal glucose tolerance curves can precede the onset of clinical diabetes and may thus serve as a more sensitive parameter for a reduced B-cell mass [6-8]. It remains nevertheless questionable whether this functional test can be employed as a reliable index for the actual number of pancreatic B-cells. Observations in recent-onset diabetic patients also suggested a heterogeneous origin of the disease, but succeeded only in exceptional cases in identifying an agent which was primarily responsible for the killing of B-cells [9-11]. Common in many patients were the signs of immune reactions against the islet cells [1, 12-16], which nourished the view that autoimmune mechanisms are actively implicated in the destruction of islet B-cells (FOULIS and BOTTAZZO, LERNMARK et al., both this volume). The concept that diabetes may have an autoimmune origin has been further supported by studies in rodents with spontaneous diabetes (LIKE, this volume). One should nevertheless keep in mind that it is still uncertain whether the immune phenomena observed in man correspond to primary or secondary, to early or late events in the development of the disease. Neither is it known whether the reduced number of B-cells at clinical onset is entirely the result of destructive processes in the pancreatic islet, or whether it represents also the consequence of a disturbed growth in the endocrine cell population. In another chapter in this book, SWENNE and HEL-

* The authors' experimental work has been supported by grants from the Belgian Fonds Geneeskunding Wetenschappelijk Onderzoek (3.0066.84 and 3.0059.86) and the Belgian Ministerie voor Wetenschapsbeleid (gekonc. aktie 86/91-102).

LERSTRÖM discuss the possible involvement of islet cell growth in the pathogenesis of diabetes. Their work clearly demonstrates how in vitro studies contribute to our knowledge concerning this determinant of the total B cell mass. The present chapter will illustrate how in vitro experiments on islet cells can broaden the insights into the mechanisms leading to the death of pancreatic B cells.

The Process of Cytotoxicity

Cell death can result from exposure to cytotoxic agents of endogenous or exogenous origin. The process leading to the destruction of cells can be sequenced in three phases of variable length, intensity, and impact on the final damage (Table 1). In the first phase, the cells interact with the aggressor depending on the dose and the persistence of the agent as well as on its recognition by the target cells. The second phase starts with the appearance of (a) factor(s) which can initiate damage to the cellular constituents. The target cells may be able to influence the rate of production, inactivation, or clearance of those factors, and can thus be expected to participate in this episode of the cytotoxic process. In the third phase, the initiating compounds induce molecular alterations in cellular constituents which can result in structural changes and cell death. At this stage, the target cell may exhibit the capability to counteract the injuring process by correcting or repairing the initial insult. The episode over which defense reactions are effective is called the reversible phase of cell injury [17].

At the present time, we are able to recognize only the end-point of damaging processes to islet B-cells in man. It is therefore not surprising that virtually no information exists on the nature of the preceding events, and that no experimental evidence is available to extrapolate the described general model of cytotoxicity to the pathogenesis of diabetes. There are on the other hand no indications to discard, a priori, a model which has been valid in many other cytotoxic interactions [17, 18]. That the destruction process in human diabetes can be extended over months or years [19] may certainly create the conditions wherein the pancreatic B-cells can counteract the cytotoxic events. The mere fact that not all islets are affected at the same time or to the same extent [20] can be an illustration of this phenomenon. Differences in environmental conditions may well modulate the sensitivity and/or the defense of the islet B-cells to cytotoxic agents.

Table 1. The process of cytotoxicity

Phase	Aggressor	Participation by pancreatic B-cells
1	Interaction	Recognition
2	Generation of initiating factors	Regulation of production, inactivation, clearance
3	Damage to cellular constituents	Repair and defense reactions

In Vitro Model of Islet B-Cell Toxicity

The sequence of events observed in other cell systems raises the question of whether pancreatic B-cells also exhibit the ability to actively participate in or counteract the events leading to their own destruction. An affirmative answer may indicate new approaches to the prevention of the disease. The issue can be examined in experimental models of B-cell toxicity. Over the past decades, numerous in vivo and in vitro studies have focused on the diabetogenic action of alloxan and streptozotocin [21]. This work clearly demonstrated the B-cell toxic effect of both drugs and suggested mechanisms through which they may exert their destructive action [22-27]. It was also shown that the cytotoxicity of the two substances could vary with the prevailing glucose or nicotinamide levels [21, 28-31]. However, the experimental design did usually not permit a distinction of different phases in the process of B-cell death. Moreover, the toxicity to B-cells was often evaluated through indirect or insensitive parameters, such as a decrease in insulin secretory activity or a rise in plasma glucose levels. The cellular heterogeneity of the in vitro preparations made it also difficult to investigate whether and to which extent pancreatic B-cells or their environment participated in the sequence of events. The development of techniques for the purification of single pancreatic B-cells and for their maintenance in vitro [32-35] has created the opportunity to investigate the process of B-cell death in more detail.

Autofluorescence-activated sorting of islet cells prepares single, pure, and living B-cell suspensions from the adult rat pancreas [34, 35]. The isolated cells are attached to the poly-L-lysine coated bottom of polystyrene microtiter cups and cultured for several days or weeks. During culture, the cells remain single so that their survival can be easily quantified by vital staining techniques. Neutral red is a low-molecular-weight dye which is actively taken up by living cells where it accumulates in intracellular organelles. Freshly purified B-cells stain deeply red within minutes following administration of neutral red, both at room temperature and at 37 °C. After a 24-h culture period in RPMI-1640, more than 90% of the poly-L-lysine attached B-cells retained their ability to stain positively with the dye. Besides illustrating the viability of the purified B-cell preparation, this figure indicates that an in vitro model can be used to directly assess and quantify the survival or death of pancreatic B-cells. The simultaneous availability of pure islet non-B-cells offers an opportunity to examine the B-cell specificity of the observed toxic effects [32].

The experimental procedure can be adjusted so that various sequences in the process of B-cell toxicity can be distinguished (Fig. 1). Preincubation of the cells in media of different composition will indicate whether the sensitivity of the target cells to a particular cytotoxic agent can be altered. The interaction of the compound can be examined for varying dosages, exposure times, and temperatures, and can be compared for cells in varying states of functional activity. When, after removing the cytotoxic compound, the cells are cultured in media of different composition, it will become evident whether environmental conditions influence the degree and the rapidity of cell death. It is indeed well known that cell death not always follows cell damage, and that, if it does, it often occurs several hours or days after the initial attack [17, 18]. The in vitro model thus permits to investigate whether cell damage can be accelerated or counteracted by the target cell.

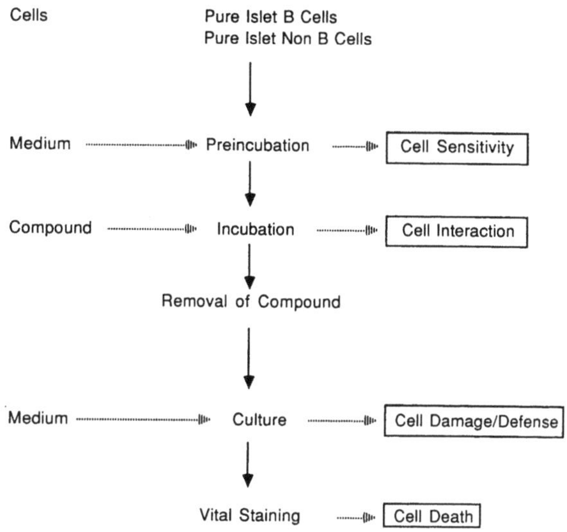

Fig. 1. In vitro model for the study of events involved in the death of pancreatic B-cells

The present chapter will focus on the possible participation of the pancreatic B-cell in the process which leads to its own destruction. Conform to the discussed model of cytotoxicity, we will successively review the evidence favoring such participation at the time of recognition of toxic agents, of generation of initiating factors, and of repair or defense reactions.

Selective Recognition of Toxic Agents

In insulin-dependent diabetes, the markedly low number of pancreatic B-cells is usually not accompanied by a reduced number of other islet cell types. This classical histologic finding is thought to result from a B-cell selective destruction by viral, immune, or chemical agents. Our in vitro model can be employed to screen for toxic agents which interact directly and selectively with B-cells. This property is illustrated by experiments using chemical agents which are known for their diabetogenic action in man and in laboratory animals [36-38].

When purified B-cells are exposed for 3 min to alloxan or to streptozotocin, they undergo a dose-dependent death within 24 h (Fig. 2). When islet non-B-cells are submitted to identical conditions, no cellular destruction is noted (Fig. 2). That glucagon- and somatostatin-containing islet cells survive in alloxan- and in streptozotocin-diabetic rodents has been known for many years; the present results demonstrate that this survival is not a feature of a particular subpopulation of these cell types, but rather a general characteristic of the entire A- and D-cell population, at least at the drug concentrations tested.

Several mechanisms have been proposed to explain the B-cell selectivity of alloxan and streptozotocin [21, 22-27, 39]. It has been suggested that the cell speci-

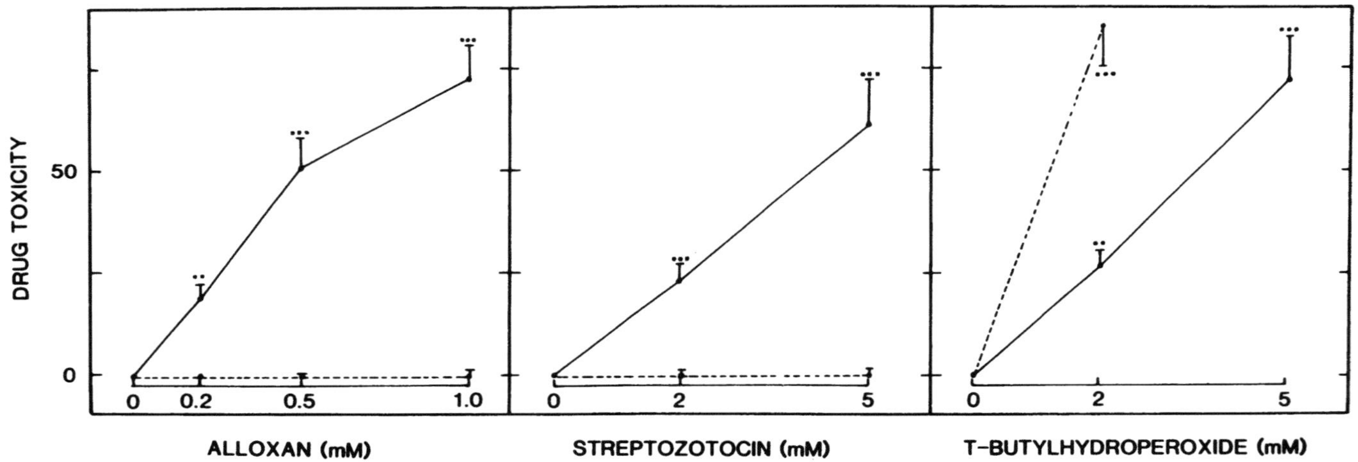

Fig. 2. Toxicity of alloxan, streptozotocin and *t*-butylhydroperoxide in islet B-cells (——) and islet non-B-cells (- - -). The cells were preincubated for 15 min without glucose before being exposed to the drugs for 3 min (alloxan, streptozotocin) or 5 min (*t*-butylhydroperoxide). After washing, the cells were cultured for 20 h at 5.6 m*M* glucose and the percent neutral red negative cells counted. Net toxicity was calculated by comparison with the control condition which underwent a similar procedure without exposure to a drug [see ref. 32]. The data express mean net toxicity ± SEM calculated from three to nine separate experiments. The statistical significance of differences with the control condition was determined by unpaired Student's t testing. $^{**}p < 0.01$; $^{***}p < 0.001$

ficity of the drug action results from its rapid accumulation in pancreatic B-cells [40, 41]. Once present in the cells, the two poisons probably induce cytotoxic events in a manner which is not specific for the cell type. Thus, alloxan - which is rapidly incorporated by islet B-cells but not by the other islet cells [41] - damages only the insulin-containing B-cells in an islet preparation [37]. On the other hand, *t*-butylhydroperoxide, another producer of highly toxic hydroxyl radicals, penetrates various cell types without any tissue specificity. It is therefore not surprising that this compound killed islet B cells as well as islet non-B-cells (Fig. 2). Since the various islet cell types appear equally sensitive to peroxides, it seems likely that the B-cell selectivity of certain peroxide generating agents results from either a cell selective recognition and uptake of these compounds or from an intracellular milieu which favors the build-up of toxic oxygen radicals during cellular handling of the drugs. This second mechanism will be further discussed in the following sections.

The antiprotozoal drug pentamidine has been found to affect the function of the insulin-containing B-cells in patients treated for *Pneumocystis carinii* pneumonitis [38]. When the compound was administered to isolated islet preparations, it suppressed the secretory capability of B-cells but not of A- and D-cells [42, 43]. Chromium release and trypan blue exclusion tests indicated the existence of islet cell necrosis [42], which, according to electron microscopy, appeared more prominent for the islet B-cells than for the other cell types [43]. To assess whether pentamidine exerts a direct and cell-specific toxicity upon islet B-cells, the survival of purified islet B and non B-cell preparations was measured after exposure to the pharmacologic compound. For concentrations up to 10^{-3}M and incubation times up to 15 min, the drug did not impair the survival of islet cells during a subsequent culture of 20 h (Fig. 3). Longer exposure periods resulted in damage of the B-cells, suggesting that the state of insulin deficiency which develops in patients treated with this compound, is caused by a cytotoxic action of the drug at the level of the pancreatic B-cells. When the in vitro exposure to pentamidine was restricted to 90 min, cell death was observed only in B-cells and not in other islet cell types (Fig. 3). Chemotherapy in patients is, however, expected to lead to longer interaction periods, which could mean that the in vivo cytotoxicity will not be restricted to the insulin-containing B-cells. A 20-h incubation with pentamidine is indeed sufficient to cause damage to both islet B-cells and non-B-cells (Fig. 3). There exists so far no sufficient evidence to consider the agent as a new diabetogenic drug which can be used to produce laboratory models of insulin-dependent diabetes. According to the in vitro experiments, a single administration of the compound may achieve a diabetogenic action if sufficiently high levels are reached and maintained for 90 min. However, as long as it remains uncertain whether these conditions will keep the other cell types and tissues intact, the drug cannot be considered as a tool for developing new in vivo models of diabetes.

The purified islet cell preparations also permitted the detection of immune components which are recognized by insulin-containing B-cells and not by other islet cell types. After Lernmark et al. described the occurrence of islet cell surface antibodies in recently diagnosed insulin-dependent diabetes [15], we demonstrated that most patients younger than 30 years exhibited antibodies which bound to islet B-cells but not to the other islet cell types [44]. This selective recognition resulted

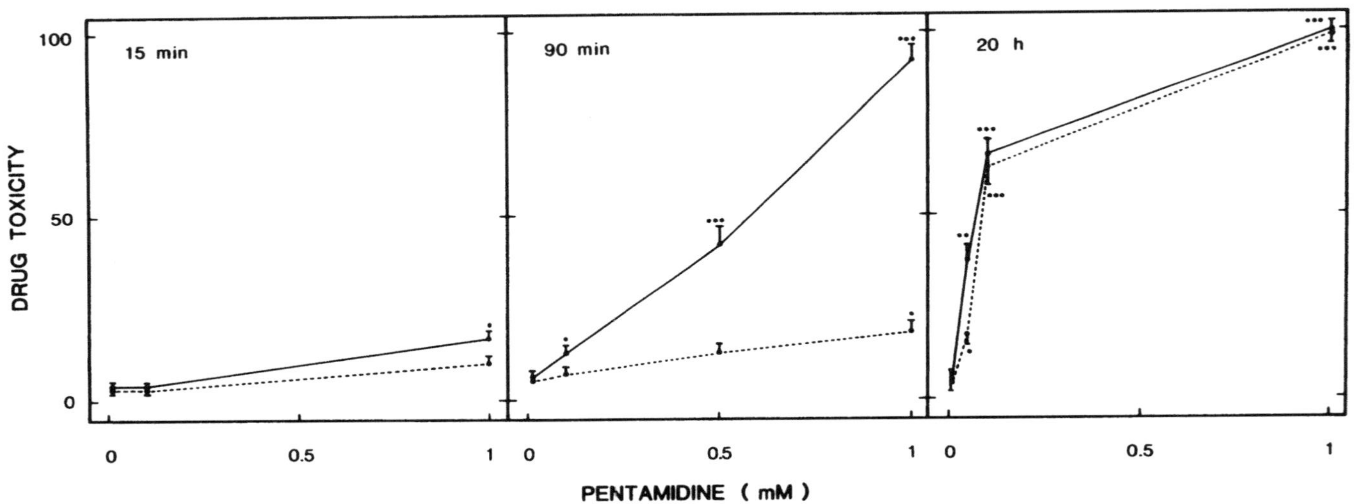

Fig. 3. Toxicity of pentamidine in islet B-cells (——) and islet non-B-cells (- - -). The experimental design was identical to that described in Fig. 1. The period of drug exposure was 15 min (left), 90 min (middle), or 20 h (right). Data were calculated and expressed as outlined in Fig. 1 ($n = 4$). $^{*}p < 0.05$; $^{**}p < 0.01$; $^{***}p < 0.001$

in selective death of B-cells when complement was added to the immunoglobulin-treated islet cells [32, 45]. The presence of such antibodies can, so far, be considered only as a sign of an autoimmune reaction against the islet B-cells, and not as the in vivo vector for the immune destruction of the cells. The infiltration of mononuclear cells in the pancreatic islets at the time of, or prior to the disappearance of B-cells [1, 20, 46] may indicate that cell-mediated immune mechanisms induce the destruction process. Compatible with this possibility is the fact that peripheral lymphocytes from insulin-dependent diabetic patients are cytotoxic for islet cells [47] or inhibit their function [48]. NERUP and MANDRUP-POULSEN have provided evidence for the concept that cytokines released from infiltrating leukocytes can cause the death of pancreatic B-cells [49-54]. They first demonstrated that cytokine-rich supernatants from blood mononuclear cells suppressed insulin release from cultured rat islets dose-dependently [49, 50], and provoked, after 6 days, a disintegration of the islet tissue, with severe damage being noted in both A- and B-cells [50]. The effects were attributed to interleukin-1 [51, 52] as this compound reproduced the observed phenomena; this cytokine was furthermore shown to specifically affect the pancreatic B-cells when the exposure was limited to 5 min [53]. On the basis of these findings, NERUP and MANDRUP-POULSEN postulate that interleukin-1 is responsible for a selective destruction of islet B-cells in human diabetes [54]. They suggest that the polypeptide generates free oxygen radicals to which the pancreatic B cells would then be particularly sensitive [54]. In our model of pure islet cells, we have not yet been able to demonstrate rapid cytotoxic effects of interleukin-1 upon the pancreatic B-cells. Under the circumstances wherein alloxan - a well-known generator of superoxide and hydroxyl radicals - destroys the islet B-cells, interleukin-1 did not impair the survival of the cells for exposure times up to 90 min. Further work on purified B-cells is thus clearly needed before this cytokine can be considered as a direct and B-cell-selective toxic agent which kills the cells via the generation of oxygen radicals.

The Generation of Initiating Factors

In human diabetes, the factors which initiate damage to the pancreatic B-cells are usually unknown. As the purpose of this section is to examine whether the target B-cells can influence the generation of initiating factors, it is not crucial to investigate the human situation for this particular issue. Instead, experimental models can be selected where more information exists on the mechanisms leading to the death of pancreatic B-cells. The alloxan-induced toxicity has been best analyzed in terms of the intracellular events which culminate in B-cell destruction, and therefore appears appropriate for the present discussion.

Alloxan is cytotoxic as a result of its oxidative action upon cellular constituents [22, 55, 56]. The oxidative damage is caused by a depletion in reduced cofactors and by the generation of highly reactive oxygen radicals (Fig. 4). The compound induces these damaging conditions when its rapid reduction to dialuric acid is followed by an immediate reoxidation and a new redox cycle. The pancreatic B-cell can participate actively in this part of the cytotoxic process. The cell may in the

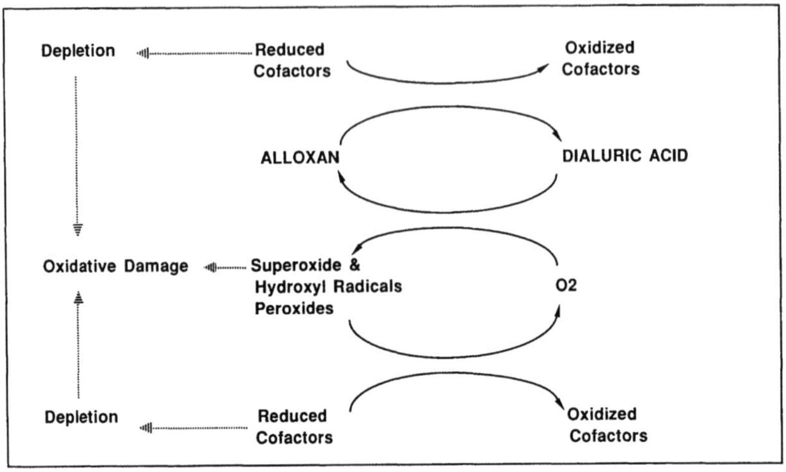

Fig. 4. The generation of factors initiating damage after exposure to alloxan

first place create favorable intracellular conditions for rapid redox transitions between alloxan and dialuric acid, thus amplifying the generation of initiating factors. A property like this may contribute to the cell-selective expression of the alloxan toxicity. A second mode of participation may come from the cellular handling of the initiating factors, namely the depletion in reduced cofactors and the generation of oxygen radicals (Fig. 4). According to MALAISSE et al., the enzymatic scavenging of peroxides is lower in islet tissue than in liver, exocrine pancreas, and kidney [57]. Thus, pancreatic B-cells may, more than other cell types, permit an accumulation of highly reactive oxidants [55, 57]. It is also conceivable that the cells can adopt functional states in which reduced factors are more rapidly depleted than in other cells. At low extracellular glucose concentrations, for example, the cells contain two- to threefold less NAD(P)H than at high sugar levels (Table 2). Under this condition, an oxidative agent such as alloxan further decreases the cellular NAD(P)H content, probably to levels which become incompatible with cell survival (Table 2). In contrast, virtually no decline in NAD(P)H content was noted in B-cells which had been exposed to alloxan in a high-glucose medium, and these cells were also markedly less sensitive to the drug's toxic action (Table 2). The fact that the cellular NAD(P)H levels parallel the cells' sensitivity to alloxan was further illustrated by comparing alloxan-induced toxicity in B-cells which were selected on the basis of their NAD(P)H content. In this experiment, B-cells were incubated for 15 min at 10 m*M* glucose and then analyzed for their NAD(P)H-related fluorescence intensity. Between 55% and 70% of the B-cells increased their NAD(P)H content two- to fourfold under this condition (Fig. 5). Addition of 0.2 m*M* alloxan to these glucose-responsive cells did not provoke cell death over the following 7-day culture period. The 30%–40% B-cells which were collected at the basal NAD(P)H levels were markedly more sensitive to the destructive effects of the drug (60%–80% dead cells) at the end of the 7 days' culture.

The study of the effects of alloxan on pure B-cells has demonstrated that the target B-cell can actively participate in the generation of factors which initiate cell

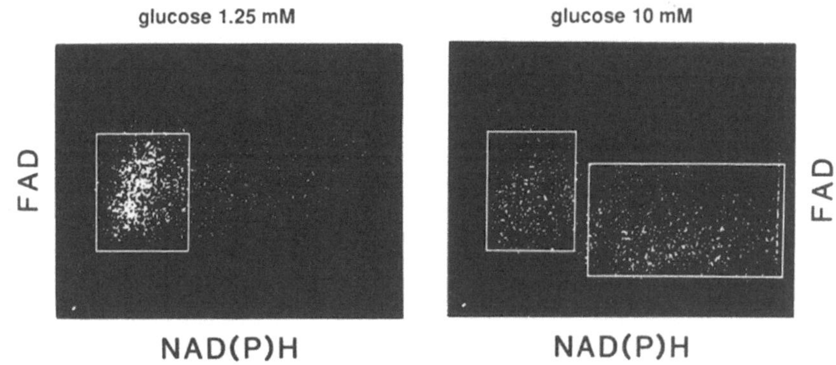

Fig. 5. FACS analysis of single purified B-cells incubated at 1.25 m*M* or 10 m*M* glucose. The cells were examined for their FAD and NAD(P)H fluorescence intensities. At 1.25 m*M* glucose, 90% of the cells were clustered within the values set by the rectangle. Raising the glucose concentration to 10 m*M* decreased FAD and increased NAD(P)H content in 55%-70% of the B-cells, while the remaining cells displayed the same values as measured at the low glucose level. The B-cell subpopulations with altered and with unchanged redox states were isolated by cell sorting, the separation windows set as indicated by the *rectangles*. The isolated subpopulations were then compared for their respective sensitivity to oxidative damage

Table 2. Effects of alloxan upon pancreatic B-cells

Test condition	Cellular NAD(P)H, % control fluorescence intensity (VC)	Toxicity, % dead cells (no. of experiments)	*p*
No glucose			
Control	100 (29)	0	
Alloxan 0.5 m*M*	64 (34)	51.0 ± 6.1 (9)	
20 m*M* glucose			
Control	251 (39)	0	
Alloxan 0.5 m*M*	238 (31)	9.0 ± 3.2 (4)	< 0.001

Isolated B-cells were preincubated for 15 min with or without 20 m*M* glucose and then exposed for 3 min to alloxan before their NAD(P)H fluorescence intensity was measured in the cell sorter. Results are expressed in arbitrary units; the variation coefficient (VC) is calculated as a percentage. Cells were also cultured at 5.6 m*M* glucose to determine drug toxicity. Toxicity is expressed as mean ± SEM. Statistical significance of differences with the corresponding condition preincubated without glucose is calculated by unpaired Student's t testing

[With permission from 32].

damage. The capability of the cells to rapidly reduce foreign molecules may facilitate the development of damaging conditions, in particular since [1] the B-cells appear less well equipped than other cell types to enzymatically scavenge oxygen radicals and [2] the cells can exhibit functional states wherein they are more rapidly depleted in reduced cofactors and therefore less apt to counteract oxidizing conditions. Other cell types are less avid to incorporate and reduce foreign substances, possess more potent enzymatic scavenging activities, or are less dependent on the nutrient status in terms of their reduced cofactor content. Hepatocytes con-

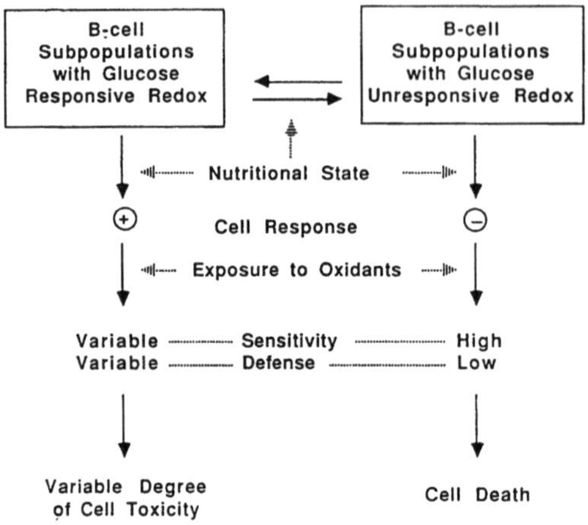

Fig. 6. Participation of target B-cells in the cytotoxic process induced by oxidants. Role of the functional heterogeneity in the B-cell population. The nutritional state will influence the redox state in glucose-responsive subpopulations, and hence determine their sensitivity to oxidative agents and subsequent defense reactions. The glucose-unresponsive subpopulations will be highly sensitive to oxidative interactions and develop minimal defense reactions

tain, for example, high glutathione levels which can protect cellular SH groups against oxidation and detoxify generated peroxides and reactive oxygen. The functional characteristics of the B-cells can thus favor the generation of initiating factors by oxidative agents. Alterations in functional activity can therefore be expected to modulate their participation in this part of the cytotoxic process. Glucose-stimulated cells interfere with the alloxan-induced oxidation, probably via the production of reducing equivalents. The nutritional status may thus determine to what extent an oxidative toxic agent generates factors that initiate cellular damage (Fig. 6). It should be noted that the pancreatic B-cell population is functionally heterogeneous, also with respect to its metabolic responsiveness to glucose [58]. Its metabolic state will thus depend not only on extracellular conditions such as the nutritional status, but also on the relative proportion of glucose-responsive cells and on their degree of glucose responsiveness (Fig. 6). The diabetogenicity of a B-cell poison such as alloxan is thus not merely a matter of drug concentration at the level of the target cell, but also of the genetic and environmental conditioning of the entire pancreatic B-cell population. Illustrations of this concept can be found in several reports on alloxan toxicity in vivo and in vitro [31, 59, 60]. Although not tested, it is likely that the target B-cells participate via similar mechanisms in cytotoxic processes induced by other chemical agents or by immune components, several of which are known to damage cells through the production of oxygen radicals [61, 62, 63].

Damage to Cellular Constituents

As soon as initiating factors are generated in the target cells, they may gain access to cellular constituents and alter their structure or configuration. In most cytotoxic conditions - be it hypoxia, complement activation, virally-induced lysis, or chemical poisoning - the initial injury can be corrected or repaired [17, 18]. The period over which cellular damage is reversible varies considerably with the nature and severity of the initiating factors as well as with the type of target cell. Once the damaged cells have entered the irreversible phase, several hours can pass before they reach the final stage of cell death as judged by morphologic criteria.

In analogy to other cell types, pancreatic B-cells can also proceed through a phase with reversible injuries after a viral, immune, or chemical attack. Their functional status may then determine the length of this episode and its final outcome, while environmental conditions can be expected to influence the cellular reactivity to the initial injury.

Using our in vitro model of islet cell toxicity, we were able to recognize such a reversible phase for each of the tested cytotoxic conditions. Two different methods can be employed for this purpose. The first one consists of an ultrastructural analysis of the aggressed cells whereby the classical features of a reversible or irreversible damage are sought (Table 3, Fig. 7). When B-cells are exposed to alloxan and then cultured for 20 h at 5.6 m*M* glucose, several cells present signs of a reversible injury while others are irreversibly damaged or dead; a third subpopulation is indistinguishable from normal control cells (Fig. 7). This morphologic observation supports the view that B-cell damage - even when of acute nature - can proceed through a reversible phase. Electron-microscopic techniques are, however, not suited to make any quantitative assessment of the damage inflicted on a total cell population and are therefore not the method of choice to assess precisely whether environmental conditions can regulate the reversibility of the cell lesions. A second, more appropriate method is based on measuring the ability of the plasma membranes to separate the extracellular from the intracellular milieu. Outward leakage of intracellular ions [64] or inward diffusion of high-molecular-weight dyes [65] has often been employed to quantify the percentage of cells with irreversible injuries. Another useful index for the degree of irreversible cell damage is pro-

Table 3. Ultrastructural signs of cell damage

Reversible phase	Irreversible phase
Alteration in cell shape with disappearing microvilli and developing cytoplasmic extensions (blebs)	Ruptured plasma membrane
Cell swelling with cytoplasmic edema and dilated endoplasmic reticulum	Gross swelling of cells with dissolution of organelles
Denser mitochondria	Gross swelling of mitochondria with vacuolization, lipid-rich aggregates, and disrupted cristae
Small aggregates of chromatin	Nuclear dissolution

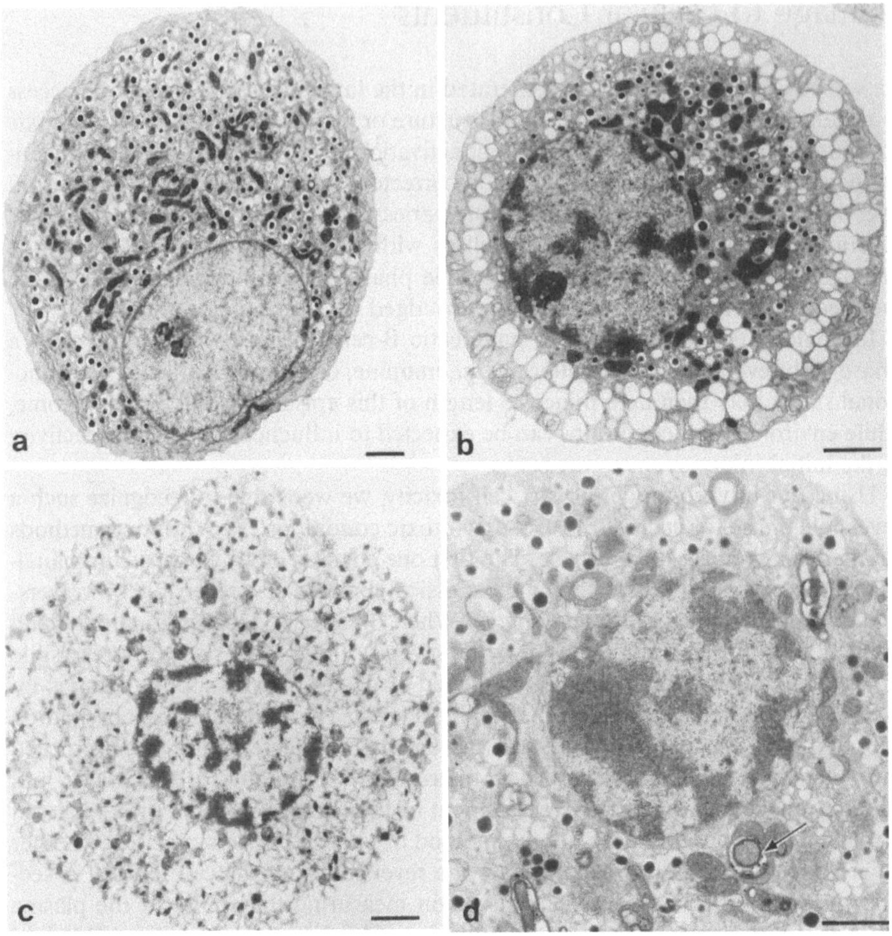

Fig. 7 a–d. Electron micrographs of isolated B-cells from control (**a**) and cytotoxic (**b–d**) conditions. The cells were cultured for 20 h following their exposure to 0.5 m*M* alloxan (**b, c**) or 0.5 m*M* pentamidine (**d**). Drug-treated cells exhibited either a normal ultrastructure (comparable to **a**), or an abnormal morphology with signs of reversible (**b**) or irreversible (**c, d**) cell damage. Characteristic reversible signs are the dilated endoplasmic reticulum, the denser mitochondria, and the chromatin aggregates (**b**). Classical irreversible signs include rupture of plasma membranes and dissolution of organelles and nuclear material (**c**). Irreversibility can also be predicted from the presence of vacuoles and disrupted cristae in swollen mitochondria (**d**) (bar 1 μm)

vided by tests which measure the ability of cells to accumulate low-molecular-weight dyes. The neutral red uptake test offers the advantage of a rapid and simple procedure whereby the irreversibly injured cells are readily detectable as unstained units. Cells which incorporate the dye are vital at the time of testing, but are not necessarily devoid of reversible signs of damage. The neutral red test thus provides an adequate method to examine whether environmental conditions can force aggressed pancreatic B-cells to counteract the transition to irreversible damage and hence to prevent destruction of the cells.

In our in vitro model, the cells were first exposed to cytotoxic agents for 3-10 min and finally cultured overnight in media of varying composition. Counting of the neutral red positive cells at the end of culture indicated to what extent the environment of aggressed B-cells could prevent the transition from reversible to irreversible injury. It was thus shown that media containing nicotinamide or increased glucose levels induced defensive reactions in aggressed B-cells [32]. The protective actions could be induced after the B-cells had undergone a cell-selective aggression, such as caused by alloxan, streptozotocin, or pentamidine, as well as after a non-selective interaction, such as *t*-butylhydroperoxide (Fig. 8) [32]. Depending on the cytotoxic condition, the vitamin or the sugar reduced the percentage of irreversibly damaged B-cells by 30%-70% when administered separately, and by even higher percentages when the two agents were combined. A high-glucose culture medium supplemented with nicotinamide also counteracted the destructive process in cells treated with surface antibodies plus complement, but its effect (22% less dead cells) was less pronounced than in chemically aggressed cells [32].

These observations clearly demonstrate that the destructive actions of B-cell toxic agents can vary with the functional state of the aggressed cells. Between the moment of cellular attack and that of irreversible damage, B-cells can actively influence the intracellular events which lead to their own destruction, with environmental conditions determining both nature and extent of the cellular reactivity. The notion that target cells can gear defense reactions against a cytotoxic process has already been documented in other cell systems [17, 18, 62, 65-68]. The fact that it also occurs in pancreatic B-cells further supports the concept that the functional status of this cell type should also be considered as an active component in the pathogenesis of insulin-dependent diabetes. It is not yet clear how glucose and nicotinamide stimulate the B-cells in their defensive reactivity against destructive events. The glucose-induced protection appeared cell-specific, as it could not be elicited in aggressed islet non-B-cells and as it could not be reproduced with nonmetabolized sugars such as galactose or fructose [32]. The effect of the sugar may consist in a repair of oxidative damage via reducing equivalents which are rapidly formed during glucose metabolism in pancreatic B-cells [69, 70]. It is also conceivable that glucose-stimulated B-cells survive aggression better as a result of an activated protein synthesis, as appears the case in neuronal survival [71]. Rapid glucose-induced alterations in calcium handling can also account for an increased resistance to damage, in analogy to the situation in isolated hepatocytes [72, 73]. Nicotinamide stimulated defense reactions in islet B-cells as well as in islet non-B-cells [32]. The vitamin was also found to induce repair in non-islet cells [74-76]. Its protective action seems to result from a restoration of NAD stores which are depleted after DNA injuries [26, 77]. In addition, the compound is also an effective scavenger of hydroxyl radicals [25]. Both glucose and nicotinamide have been previously shown to exert protective effects in vivo, the sugar against alloxan-induced diabetes [30, 31], the vitamin against the streptozotocin-induced form [28, 29] as well as against the immune-related disease [78]. In the latter in vivo studies, the protective substances were always administered prior to the cytotoxic agents, leaving unanswered the question of whether interventions at the level of the target B-cells can gear defensive reactivities in vivo so that a previous attack of chemical,

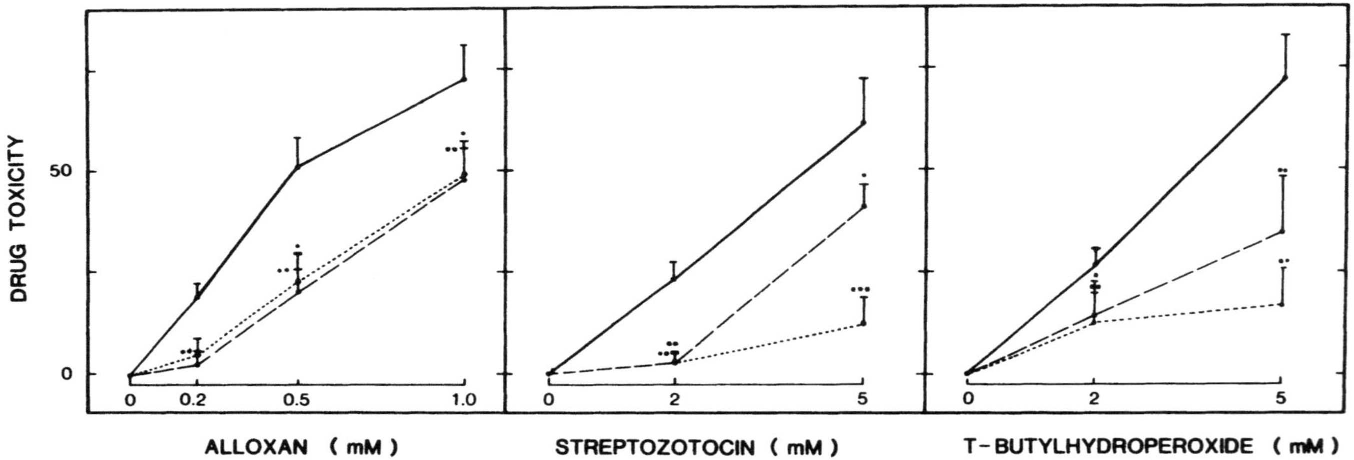

Fig. 8. Effect of culture conditions on the survival of islet B-cells which had been previously exposed to alloxan, streptozotocin, or *t*-butylhydroperoxide. After washing the control or drug-treated cells, they were cultured for 20 h at 5.6 m*M* glucose (——), 20 m*M* glucose (- - -), or 5.6 m*M* glucose plus 0.2 m*M* nicotinamide (· · · · ·). Data were calculated and expressed as outlined in Fig. 1 ($n = 3$-9). The statistical significance of differences with the corresponding condition cultured at 5.6 m*M* glucose was determined by unpaired t testing. *$p < 0.05$; **$p < 0.01$; ***$p < 0.001$ [32]

viral, or immune origin is completely counteracted and diabetes prevented. Such potential seems particularly important in cases where the destructive processes in the endocrine pancreas extend over prolonged periods [19].

Conclusion

In vitro studies on purified islet cells have discerned three phases in the cytotoxic process leading to the death of pancreatic B-cells. After cell-selective or -nonselective recognition of chemical or immune agents, the B-cells generate initiating factors which can induce damage to cellular constituents. During each phase, the target B-cells can participate actively in the course of cytotoxic events, accelerating or counteracting the development of reversible or irreversible injuries. It is concluded that the functional state of the pancreatic B-cells should be considered as a possible pathogenetic component in insulin-dependent diabetes.

Acknowledgement. The authors thank Nadine van Slycke for her excellent secretarial assistance.

References

1. Gepts W (1965) Pathologic anatomy of the pancreas in juvenile diabetes mellitus. Diabetes 14: 619-633
2. Maclean N, Ogilvie RF (1959) Observations on the pancreatic islet tissue of young diabetic subjects. Diabetes 8: 83-91
3. Stefan Y, Orci L, Malaisse-Lagae F, Perrelet A, Patel Y, Unger R (1982) Quantitation of endocrine cell content in the pancreas of nondiabetic humans. Diabetes 31: 694-700
4. Rahier J, Goebbels R, Henquin S (1983) Cellular composition of the human diabetic pancreas. Diabetologia 24: 366-371
5. Klöppel G, Drenck CR, Oberholzer M, Heitz PU (1984) Morphometric evidence for a striking B-cell reduction at the clinical onset of type 1 diabetes. Virchows Arch [A] 403: 441-452
6. Srikanta S, Ganda O, Glaeson R, Jackson R, Soeldner J, Eisenbarth G (1984) Pre-type I diabetes: linear loss of B-cell response to intravenous glucose. Diabetes 33: 717-720
7. Srikanta S, Ganda OP, Eisenbarth GS, Soeldner JS (1983) Islet cell antibodies and B-cell function in monozygotic triplets and twins initially discordant for type I diabetes mellitus. N Engl J Med 308: 322-325
8. Nakhooda A, Like A, Chappel C, Wei C, Marliss E (1978) The spontaneously diabetic Wistar rat (the 'BB' rat). Studies prior to and during development of the overt syndrome. Diabetologia 14: 199-207
9. Yoon J, Austin M, Onodera T, Notkins A (1979) Virus-induced diabetes mellitus: isolation of a virus from a child with diabetic ketoacidosis. N Engl J Med 300: 1173-1179
10. Helgason T, Jonasson MR (1981) Evidence for a food additive as a cause of ketosis-prone diabetes. Lancet II: 716-720
11. Karam J, Lewitt P, Young C, Nowlain R, Frankel B, Fujiya H, Freedman Z, Grdosky G (1980) Insulinopenic diabetes after rodenticide (Vacor) ingestion: a unique model of acquired diabetes in man. Diabetes 29: 971-978
12. Maclaren N, Huang S, Fogh J (1975) Antibody to cultured human insulinoma cells in insulin dependent diabetes. Lancet I: 997-999
13. Bottazzo G, Doniach D (1976) Pancreatic autoimmunity and HLA antigens. Lancet II: 800

14. Lernmark A, Freedman ZR, Hofmann C et al. (1978) Islet cell surface antibodies in juvenile diabetes mellitus. N Engl J Med 299: 375-380
15. Nerup J, Andersen OO, Bendixen G, Egeberg J, Poulsen J (1971) Antipancreatic cellular hypersensitivity in diabetes mellitus. Diabetes 20: 424-427
16. McCuish A, Jordan J, Campbell C, Duncan L, Irvine W (1974) Cell-mediated immunity to human pancreas in diabetes mellitus. Diabetes 23: 693-697
17. Bridges JW, Benford DJ, Hubbard SA (1983) Mechanisms of toxic injury. Ann NY Acad Sci 407: 42-63
18. Trump BF, Berezesky IK, Osorino-Vargas AR (1981) Cell death and the disease process. The role of calcium. In: Bowen ID and Lockskin RA (eds) Cell death in biology and pathology. Chapman and Hall, London, pp 209-242
19. Gorsuch AN, Spencer KM, Lister J, McNally JM, Dean EM, Botazzo GF, Lunworth AG (1981) Evidence for a long prediabetic period in type I (insulin-dependent) diabetes mellitus. Lancet II: 1363-1365
20. Foulis A, Stewart J (1984) The pancreas in recent-onset type I (insulin-dependent) diabetes mellitus: insulin content of islets, insulitis, and associated changes in the exocrine acinar tissue. Diabetologia 26: 456-461
21. Cooperstein SJ, Watkins D (1981) Action of toxic drugs on islet cells. In: Cooperstein SS, Watkins D (eds) The islets of Langerhans. Biochemistry, physiology and pathology. Academic, New York, pp 387-425
22. Heikkila RE, Winston B, Cohen E, Barden H (1976) Alloxan-induced diabetes. Evidence for hydroxyl radical as a cytotoxic intermediate. Biochem Pharmacol 25: 1085-1092
23. Grankvist K, Marklund S, Sehlin J, Täljedal IB (1979) Superoxide dismutase, catalase and scavengers of hydroxyl radical protect against the toxic action of alloxan on pancreatic islet cells in vitro. Biochem J 182: 17-25
24. Sandler S, Andersson A (1982) The partial protective effect of the hydroxyl radical scavenger dimethyl urea on streptozotocin induced diabetes in the mouse in vivo and in vitro. Diabetologia 23: 374-378
25. Wilson GL, Patton NJ, Mclord JM, Mullins DW, Mossman BT (1984) Mechanisms of streptozotocin- and alloxan-induced damage in rat B-cells. Diabetologia 27: 587-591
26. Uchigata Y, Yamamoto H, Kawamura A, Okamoto H (1982) Protection by superoxide dismutase, catalase, and poly (ADP-ribose) synthetase inhibitors against alloxan- and streptozotocin-induced islet DNA-strand breaks and against the inhibition of proinsulin biosynthesis. J Biol Chem 257: 6084-6088
27. Asayama K, English D, Slonim AE, Burr IM (1984) Chemiluminescence as an index of drug-induced free radical production in pancreatic islets. Diabetes 33: 160-163
28. Dulin W, Wyse B (1969) Reversal of streptozotocin diabetes with nicotinamide. Proc Soc Exp Biol Med 130: 992-994
29. Gunnarson R, Berne C, Hellerström C (1974) Cytotoxic effects of streptozotocin and N-nitroso methylurea on the pancreatic B-cells with special regard to the role of nicotinamide-adenine dinucleotide. Biochem J 140: 487-494
30. Bhattacharyya G (1953) Protection against alloxan diabetes by mannose and fructose. Science 117: 230-231
31. Scheynius A, Täljedal IB (1971) On the mechanism of glucose protection against alloxan toxicity. Diabetologia 7: 252-255
32. Pipeleers D, Van De Winkel M (1985) Pancreatic B-cells possess defense mechanisms against cell-specific toxicity. Proc Natl Acad Sci USA 83: 5267-5271
33. Pipeleers D, Pipeleers-Marichal M (1981) A method for the purification of single A, B and D cells and for the isolation of coupled cells form isolated islets. Diabetologia 20: 654-663
34. Van De Winkel M, Maes E, Pipeleers D (1982) Islet cell analysis and purification by light scatter and autofluorescence. Biochem Biophys Res Commun 107: 525-532
35. Pipeleers D, Schuit F, in't Veld P, Maes E, Hooghe-Peters E, Van De Winkel M, Gepts W (1985) Interplay of nutrients and hormones in the regulation of insulin release. Endocrinology 117: 824-833
36. Dunn JS, Sheehan HL, McLetchie NGB (1943) Necrosis of islets of Langerhans produced experimentally. Lancet I: 484-487
37. Rakieten N, Rakieten ML, Nadkarni MV (1963) Studies on the diabetogenic actions of streptozotocin. Cancer Chemother Rep 29: 91-98

38. Belehu A, Naap B (1982) Diabetes mellitus associated with pentamidine mesylate. Lancet I: 1463-1464
39. Colca JR, Kotagal N, Brooks CL, Lacy PE, Landt M, McDaniel ML (1983) Alloxan inhibition of a Ca^{2+}- and calmodulin-dependent protein kinase activity in pancreatic islets. J Biol Chem 258: 7260-7263
40. Tjäle H, Wilander E, Johansson E (1976) Distribution of labelled streptozotocin in mice: uptake and retention in pancreatic islets. J Endocrinol 69: 455-456
41. Gorus F, Malaisse W, Pipeleers D (1982) Selective uptake of alloxan by pancreatic B-cells. Biochem J 208: 513-515
42. Sai P, Boillot D, Boitard C, Debray-Sachs M, Reach G, Assan R (1983) Pentamidine, a new diabetogenic drug in laboratory rodents. Diabetologia 25: 418-423
43. Boillot D, In't Veld P, Sai P, Feutren G, Gepts W, Assan R (1985) Functional and morphological modifications induced in rat islets by pentamidine and other diamidines in vitro. Diabetologia 28: 359-364
44. Van De Winkel M, Smets G, Gepts W, Pipeleers D (1982) Islet cell surface antibodies from insulin-dependent diabetics bind specifically to pancreatic B cells. J Clin Invest 70: 41-49
45. Dobersen MJ, Scharff JE, Ginsberg-Fellner F, Notkins AL (1980) Cytotoxic autoantibodies to B-cells in the serum of patients with insulin-dependent diabetes mellitus. N Engl J Med 303: 1493-1498
46. Bottazzo GF (1984) B-cell damage in diabetic insulitis: are we approaching a solution? Diabetologia 26: 241-249
47. Charles MA, Suzuki M, Waldeck N et al. (1983) Immune islet killing mechanisms associated with insulin-dependent diabetes: In vitro expression of cellular and antibody mediated islet cell cytotoxicity in humans. J Immunol 130: 1189-1194
48. Boitard C, Chatenoud L, Debray-Sachs M (1982) In vitro inhibition of pancreatic B-cell function by lymphocytes from diabetics with associated autoimmune disease: a T cell. J Immunol 129: 2529-2539
49. Mandrup-Poulsen T, Bendtzen K, Nielsen J, Bendixen G, Nerup J (1985) Cytokines cause functional and structural damage to isolated islets of Langerhans. Allergy 40: 424-429
50. Mandrup-Poulsen T, Bendtzen K, Nerup I, Egeberg J, Nielsen J (1985) Mechanisms of pancreatic islet cell destruction: dose dependent cytotoxic effect of soluble blood mononuclear cell mediators on isolated islets of Langerhans. Allergy 41: 250-259
51. Mandrup-Poulsen T, Bendtzen K, Nerup J, Dinarello C, Svenson M, Nielsen J (1986) Affinity-purified human interleukin I is cytotoxic to isolated islets of Langerhans. Diabetologia 29: 63-67
52. Bendtzen K, Mandrup-Poulsen T, Nerup J, Nielsen J, Dinarello C, Svenson M (1986) Cytotoxicity of human pI interleukin-1 for pancreatic islets of Langerhans. Science 232: 1545-1547
53. Mandrup-Poulsen T, Spinas G, Prowse S, Hansen B, Jorgensen D, Nielsens J, Nerup J (1986) Interleukin 1 toxicity to islets in vitro: modulatory effects of islet donor characteristics and culture conditions. Diabetologia 29: 568 A
54. Nerup J, Mandrup-Poulsen T (1986) On the pathogenesis of insulin-dependent diabetes mellitus (IDDM). Transplant Proc XVIII: 1507-1508
55. Malaisse W (1982) Alloxan toxicity to the pancreatic B-cell. A new hypothesis. Biochem Pharmacol 31: 5527-5534
56. Grankvist K, Rooth P (1985) Alloxan does not increase mouse islets capillary permeability as judged by fluorescence microscopy in vivo. Acta Endocrinol [Suppl 273] 110: 33
57. Malaisse WJ, Malaisse-Lagae F, Sener A, Pipeleers DG (1982) Determinants of the selective toxicity of alloxan to the pancreatic B-cell. Proc Natl Acad Sci USA 79: 927-930
58. Pipeleers D (1987) Biosociology of the pancreatic B-cells. Diabetologia 30: 277-291
59. Maske H, Weinges K (1957) Untersuchungen über das Verhalten der Meerschweinchen gegenüber verschiedenen diabetogenen Noxen, Alloxan und Dithizon. Arch Exp Path Pharmakol 230: 406-411
60. Rossini A, Like A, Dulin W, Cahill G Jr (1977) Pancreatic B-cell toxicity by streptozotocin anomers. Diabetes 25: 1120-1124
61. Freeman BA, Crapo JD (1982) Biology of disease. Free radicals and tissue injury. Laboratory Invest 47: 412-426

62. Campbell AK, Morgan BP (1985) Monoclonal antibodies demonstrate protection of polymorphonuclear leucocytes against complement attack. Nature 317: 164-166
63. Oyanagui Y (1982) Macrophage-generated superoxide radicals: inflammation and tumor cell growth. In: Autor AP (ed) Pathology of oxygen. Academic, New York, pp 99-114
64. Idahl LA, Lernmark A, Sehlin J, Täljedal IB (1977) Alloxan cytotoxicity in vitro. Biochem J 162: 9-18
65. Grankvist K, Lernmark A, Täljedal IB (1979) Trypan blue as a marker of plasma membrane permeability in alloxan-treated mouse islet cells. J Endocrinol Invest 2: 139-145
66. Fariss MW, Pascoe GA, Reed DJ (1985) Vitamin E reversal of the effect of extracellular calcium on chemically induced toxicity in hepatocytes. Science 227: 751-753
67. Schlager S, Ohanian S, Borsos T (1978) Correlation between the ability of tumor cells to resist humoral immune attack and their ability to synthesize lipid. J Immunol 120: 463-471
68. Demple B, Halbrook J (1983) Inducible repair of oxidative DNA damage in *Escherichia coli*. Nature 304: 466-468
69. Malaisse WJ, Hutton JC, Kawazu S, Herchuelz A, Valverde I, Sener A (1979) The stimulus-secretion coupling of glucose-induced insulin release. Diabetologia 16: 331-341
70. Panten U, Christians I, von Kriegstein E, Poser W, Hasselblatt A (1973) Effects of carbohydrates upon fluorescence of reduced pyridine nucleotides from perifused isolated pancreatic islets. Diabetologia 9: 477-482
71. Weill CL, Greene DP (1984) Prevention of natural motorneurone cell death by dibutyryl cyclic GMP. Nature 308: 452-454
72. Acosta A, Sorensen EMB (1983) Role of calcium in cytotoxic injury of cultured hepatocytes. Ann NY Acad Sci 407: 78-92
73. Nicotera P, Hartzell P, Baldi C, Svensson S, Bellomo G, Orrenius S (1986) Cystamine induces toxicity in hepatocytes through the elevation of cytosolic Ca^{2+} and the stimulation of a nonlysosomal proteolytic system. J Biol Chem 261: 14628-14638
74. Berger NA, Sikorski GW (1980) Nicotinamide stimulates repair of DNA damage in human lymphocytes. Biochem Biophys Res Commun 95: 67-72
75. Warnick CT, Lazarus HM (1983) Protection from DNA damage during an ischemic cell injury. Biochem Biophys Res Commun 113: 996-1003
76. Schraufstatter I, Hyslop P, Hinshaw D, Spragg R, Sklar L, Cochrane C (1986) Hydrogen peroxide-induced injury of cells and its prevention by inhibitors of poly (APD-ribose) polymerase. Proc Natl Acad Sci USA 83: 4908-4912
77. Yamamoto H, Uchigata Y, Okamoto H (1981) Streptozotocin and alloxan induce DNA strand breaks and poly (ADP-ribose) synthetase in pancreatic islets. Nature 294: 284-286
78. Yamada K, Nonaka K, Hanafusa T, Miyozaki A, Toyoshima M, Tarni S (1982) Preventive and therapeutic effects of large-dose nicotinamide injections on diabetes associated with insulitis. An observation in nonobese diabetic (NOD) mice. Diabetes 31: 749-753

Disturbed Growth of the Endocrine Pancreas*

S. Falkmer and U. Askensten

Introduction

In the large neuroendocrine system, the islets of LANGERHANS belong to the third component [18], namely the classical endocrine glands of the human body. This endocrine parenchyma, like that of other neuroendocrine glands in the vertebrates, can be the subject of growth disturbances [25; 28]. Although a genuine aplasia of the islets of LANGERHANS has only exceptionally been reported in man [28], both hypoplastic/hyperplastic and genuinely neoplastic islet lesions do occur and form the underlying causes of several well-known clinical syndromes. The best examples of such diseases are (a) the hypoplastic condition diabetes mellitus; (b) the hyperplastic lesions in persistent neonatal hypoglycemia with hyperinsulinism and nesidioblastosis (PNHHN), and (c) the benign and malignant islet-cell neoplasms, where the hormone overproduction gives rise to a multitude of clinical syndromes [27]. Our review will focus on the hyperplastic disturbances of growth in endocrine pancreas, notably the pathogenesis and structural lesions in PNHHN. Here, we can offer some new observations on the ploidy of the hyperplastic insulin cells, as well as an account of some recent findings on the normal pre- and postnatal differentiation and maturation of the mammalian islet parenchyma.

Development of the Normal Endocrine Pancreas

Phylogenetic Background

As there are several recent rather comprehensive reviews on the evolution of the islets of LANGERHANS in the animal kingdom [15; 18; 51], the account of the phylogenetic background of the growth disturbances in the endocrine pancreas will be briefly summarized. If fairly strict criteria for the presence of any of the four main types of islet parenchymal cells - insulin, somatostatin, glucagon, and PP (the pancreatic polypeptide) - are used [15; 18], the following statements can be made (Fig. 1).

---

* This work was supported by grants from the Swedish Medical Research Council (Project No. 12x-718), the Swedish Diabetes Association, the Cancer Society of Stockholm, the King Gustaf V Jubilee Fund, and the Faculty of Medicine at the Karolinska Institute.

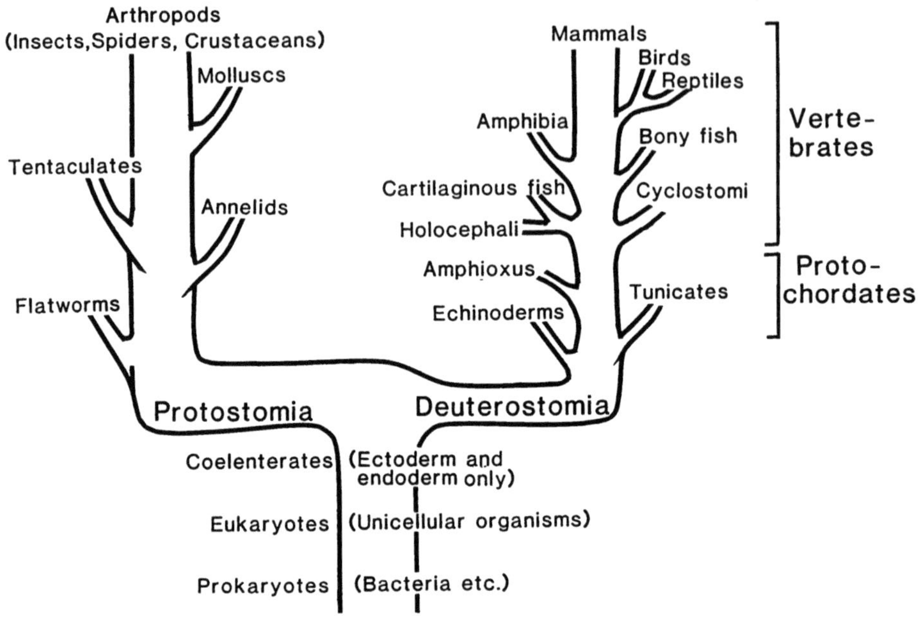

Fig. 1. Simplified survey of the evolution of the animal kingdom, where the animals above the coelenterates have been classified in two evolutionary lines, the protostomian and the deuterostomian, distinguished by means of their embryological features. More than 90% of the multicellular organisms belong to the protostomian line; only some of its major superclasses have been indicated here (15; 19)

Protozoa, Coelenterates, Protostomian and Deuterostomian Invertebrates

In prokaryote and eukaryote unicellular organisms, as well as in coelenterates, no islet-hormone-producing cells have been found so far [56]. However, even in rather "primitive" protostomian invertebrates, such as flatworms and annelids (Fig. 1), both somatostatin- and PP-immunoreactive nerve cells and fibers have been observed [19]. In the most highly developed species of this evolutionary line, namely the arthropods and molluscs (Fig. 1), all four islet hormones seem to be produced by neurons in the central nervous system [10], although there are some observations which indicate that an extraneuronal production of islet hormones may occur as well [56; 51]. It should be emphasized, however, that most of the evidence given above is based on results obtained from immunohistochemical investigations only and that no islet hormone from any protostomian invertebrate has been isolated, so far, so that its amino acid sequence has not yet been determined. The latter statement also holds true for the islet hormones of the deuterostomian invertebrates. Although there is good immunohistochemical evidence that the brain-gut axis distribution of the four islet hormones exists in the tunicates [51; 37], it has not been possible to isolate and identify any of them biochemically. Notwithstanding, all four islet-hormone-immunoreactive cells are here clearly not only of

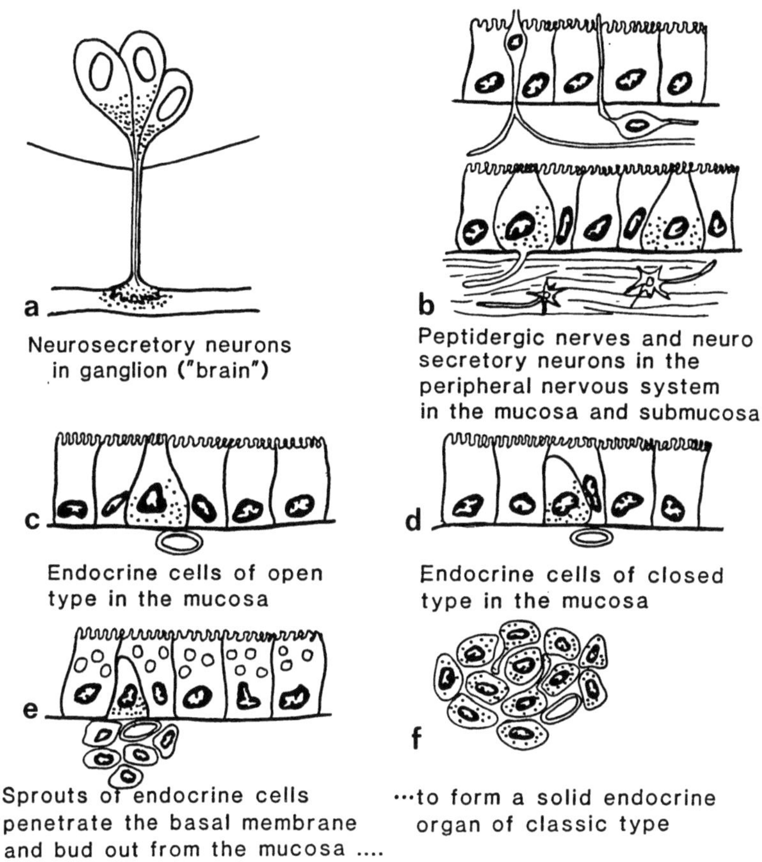

Fig. 2 a–f. Schematic outline of the phylogenetical development and a hypothetical mutual interrelationship between the three major parts of the whole neuroendocrine system: (**a, b**) the neurosecretory neuronal cells of the central and peripheral nervous system and their nerve fibers ("the peptidergic nervous system"), (**c, d, e**) the epithelial endocrine and paracrine cells of open or closed type in the mucosa of most hollow organs, in particular that of the alimentary tract, (**f**) the solid endocrine glands of classical type (e.g., the islets of Langerhans and the pituitary gland) (18)

neuronal nature but also of epithelial type, forming part of the disseminated neuroendocrine cell system in the mucosa of the alimentary tract [56; 51] (Fig. 2).

Vertebrates

It is not, however, until the developmental stage of the vertebrates that an islet organ appears for the first time in evolution [11]. Here a step-wise evolution can be discerned [15; 18]. The earliest islet parenchyma, i.e., that present in the Agnatha (cyclostomes, jawless fish; hagfishes, lampreys) is a grossly visible two-hormone organ, devoid of exocrine acinar pancreatic parenchyma, containing only insulin and somatostatin cells [11]. Here, the amino acid sequences of the two hormones (and other data as well) are established [6, 14, 20] and the structure of the two types of islet cells have been characterized rather comprehensively [51]. The insulin cells have left the gut mucosa but the other three islet hormone cells can still be found there. In the brain, no insulin or glucagon cells have been found; thus, a brain-gut axis only exists for the somatostatin and PP cells [12].

The next step in evolution is seen already in the most original Holocephalan cartilaginous fish. Here the first pancreatic gland with islets of Langerhans is found; now a three-hormone islet parenchyma exists, containing glucagon/glicentin cells in addition to insulin and somatostatin cells [11; 18; 48]. The PP cells remain as cells of open type in the gut mucosa or in the epithelium of the pancreatic ducts, at least in some Holocephalan species [18].

The well-known four-hormone islet parenchyma seen in mammals, is already present in the present-day cartilaginous fish and remains so throughout the vertebrates. In bony fish, amphibia, reptiles, birds, and mammals the general pattern is the same, although admittedly great variations exist. A typical example is the occurrence of grossly visible anatomical accumulations of islet parenchyma in certain animal groups, such as the Brockmann bodies ("the principal islets") in some bony fish [11; 47]. In particular, it is important to realize that a lobe rich in PP cells is present in the dorsal part of the head of the human pancreas [38]. This anatomical feature has a phylogenetic background; in the marine teleost (bony) fish, *Cottus scorpius* (the daddy sculpin), where there are two Brockmann bodies, one close to the spleen, the other just outside the pylorus and duodenum, the PP cells are concentrated in the pyloric/duodenal principal islet and are lacking in the splenic Brockmann body [47].

Summarizing Remarks

The main traits in the phylogenetic evolution of the islet parenchyma are summarized in Table 1 and Fig. 2. In conclusion, it can be stated that the islet parenchyma originally has a clear-cut neuronal origin, followed by a brain-gut axis stage with, inter alia, endocrine cells of open type in the gut mucosa, and ultimately - in the vertebrates - by a concentration of the islet hormone production in a particular endocrine gland, the islet of Langerhans (the "endocrine pancreas" of the mam-

Table 1. Summarizing survey of the occurrence of insulin cells in the three parts of the neuroendocrine system in multicellular animals

Animal group	Nervous system	Alimentary tract mucosa	Islet organ without pancreas	Pancreas with islets of Langerhans
Coelenterates	0	0	–	–
Protostomian invertebrates	+	?	–	–
Deuterostomian invertebrates	0	+	–	–
Agnathan vertebrates	0	0	+ +	–
Gnathostomian vertebrates	?	?	–	+ +

0, no immunohistochemical or biochemical evidence of any occurrence of insulin cells; ?, only limited evidence for the presence of insulin cells; +, good agreement between several immunohistochemical observations indicating the presence of insulin cells; + +, insulin isolated from endocrine B-cells and its molecular structure clarified; –, no such anatomical structure exists

mals). The insulin cells are the first to be concentrated in this special islet organ, followed by the somatostatin cells and the glucagon cells, whereas the PP cells are obviously the phylogenetically most recent type of the four islet parenchymal cells.

Ontogenetic Background

The embryological development of the islet parenchyma in man and in most other eutherian mammals does not closely follow the so-called HAECKEL's law or biogenetical rule ("ontogeny recapitulates phylogeny"); as a matter of fact, it is not the insulin and somatostatin cells that first appear in the earliest anlage of the endocrine pancreas, but the glucagon cells [52]. The PP cells are, however, also ontogenetically the "youngest" cell type in the fetal islets of Langerhans [1]. Thus, the ontogenetical order of appearance in mammals is (1) glucagon, (2) insulin, (3) somatostatin, (4) PP islet cells [15]. A comprehensive account of the differentiation and proliferation of islet cells during intrauterine life in mammals is given by HELLERSTRÖM et al. in the following chapter.

Argyrophil Insulin Cells

A particularly interesting feature of the embryonal endocrine mammalian pancreas is the appearance - already in the early developmental stages - of insulin-immunoreactive islet parenchymal cells that are argyrophil [52]. Normally, the insulin cells are nonargyrophil; so far, only islet cell neoplasms and actively regenerating islet parenchyma have been shown to contain argyrophil (Grimelius' silver nitrate procedure) cells [9; 13]. Recently, however, this cell type has also been found in postnatally immature islets of LANGERHANS (see below) and in the hyperplastic endocrine pancreas in patients suffering from PNHHN (see below). The fact that they appear already during the normal embryological development of the islet parenchyma in rabbits [52] supports the working hypothesis that argyrophil insulin cells are immature.

Neuroendocrine Features of Islet Parenchymal Cells

No clear-cut neuronal origin of the islet parenchymal cells, such as that observed in the phylogenetic evolution pattern of the endocrine pancreas (see above) has been ascertained; instead, the earliest islet progenitor cells appear to arise from the dorsal pancreatic bud of the gut groove [1]. However, there is some immunohistochemical evidence for a relationship between the islet parenchymal cells and neurons in the central nervous system. Thus, all four types of mammalian islet cells contain the enzyme neuron-specific enolase (NSE) and also the newly discovered neuronal peptide synaptophysin; this statement also applies to neoplastically transformed islet parenchymal cells [7; 54].

Neonatal Maturation and Reorganization of the Endocrine Pancreas

As stated in the following chapter, it has become increasingly evident during recent years that the endocrine pancreas undergoes a maturation process, not only before but also after birth [49]. This fact holds in particular for man [49] and for some ruminants [18; 53]. A detailed account of the course of islet cell maturation in the rat pancreas is given in the next chapter. As a supplement, some new aspects will be summarized on the transient appearance of the large hemorrhagic islets *(Blutinseln)* of lambs and calves, described as early as 1896 by LAGUESSE.

The Blutinseln of Newborn Ruminants

During the first week after birth the endocrine pancreas of lambs and calves undergoes a rather dramatic reorganization [5; 18]. At birth, large (0.2-2 mm in diameter) islet bodies, situated in the interstitial soft tissue, predominate the endocrine parenchyma. Already in the first few days of postnatal life, these islet bodies start to undergo regressive changes, characterized in particular by large hemorrhagic foci that during the following days become progressively larger, so that they can be seen by the naked eye (the ***Blutinseln***). These islet bodies consist of more than 90% argyrophil insulin cells (see above), ultrastructurally found to be equipped with spherical secretion granules and sometimes also with cilia and microvilli [53]. As the regressive lesions progress during the following week, this type of islet parenchyma soon disappears; at about 2 months of age there are virtually no remnants left. Instead, small islets of LANGERHANS of conventional mammalian type, located within the lobules of the acinar exocrine pancreas and present already at birth, constitute the endocrine pancreas of these young ruminants. Here, the insulin cells are all nonargyrophil [53].

Age Variations in the Cellular Composition of the Islets of Langerhans in Man

That a kind of postnatal maturation of the endocrine pancreas occurs also in man [49] - though admittedly not so dramatic as that in newborn ruminants - has become evident since the advent of modern morphometric techniques [58], combined with immunohistochemical procedures [40]. It is now known that in the neonatal period, and during several successive months of infancy, there is a markedly higher relative occurrence of somatostatin cells - about 30% - than in the islets of Langerhans of adults - about 5% - [39; 41]. It has been speculated [16] that this fact might reflect the close association observed phylogenetically between the insulin and somatostatin cells (see above), and may indicate an important role for the somatostatin cells in controlling the function of the insulin cells during neonatal and early infantile periods of life [39; 41]. An anatomical substrate for such control - apparently in a paracrine mode - is offered by the long slender processes observed in somatostatin cells by means of three-dimensional reconstructions of electron micrographs [32].

Conclusions

It is self-evident that when the underlying structural lesions in disturbances of growth in the endocrine pancreas shall be quantitatively and qualitatively analyzed, it is imperative to perform this analysis against the background of the data about the evolution of the islet parenchyma and its postnatal maturation.

Aplasia/Hypoplasia of the Endocrine Pancreas

As mentioned in the Introduction, a genuine agenesis or a congenital hypoplasia of the endocrine pancreas seems to be exceedingly rare [45]. There are, to the best of our knowledge, only two reports claiming that a real agenesis had occurred of the whole pancreatic gland with its duct system and exocrine acinar pancreatic parenchyma [55; 60]. In the "lipomatous atrophy" (or "pseudohypertrophy") of the endocrine pancreas, associated with the Shwachman syndrome, the acinar cells are admittedly also more or less absent, but the duct system is said to be normal, as well as the islets of Langerhans [45]. These facts indicate that at least some kind of pancreas anlage has existed and that a complete agenesis is not present. Although familial clustering might indicate a genetic defect, the lipomatous atrophy has also been thought to be an effect of an intrauterine viral infection [45]. Neither does the so-called McQuarrie syndrome, where it has been claimed that a congenital absence of the glucagon cells in the islets of Langerhans occurs [33], fulfill the criteria of a genuine agenesis or congenital hypoplasia; with the advent of immunohistochemical and morphometric techniques it has been shown that no cases of PNHHN (to which McQuarrie's syndrome belongs) have had complete absence of glucagon cells [27; 28; 42].

The question to what extent congenital hypoplasia of the islet parenchyma is the cause of diabetes mellitus is dealt with in other chapters in this volume. In brief, it can be stated here that neither complete agenesis nor congenital hypoplasia of the endocrine pancreas is seriously considered to be involved in the etiology or pathogenesis of this disease apart from exceptional cases [60]. However, it is a well-known fact that an acquired hypoplasia of the islets of Langerhans is the structural basis of the hypoinsulinism that characterizes type 1 diabetes mellitus (see chapters by Lefèbvre, by Rahier, and by Hellerström et al. in this volume).

Hyperplasia of the Islet Parenchyma

Some Basic Concepts

In the endocrine pancreas, as in most other endocrine glands of classical type in the human body, it is sometimes difficult for the pathologist to distinguish between hyperplastic and genuinely neoplastic lesions. By definition, a neoplasm is an irreversible condition; a hyperplasia can be reversible. The fact that in the endocrine glands hyperplastic nodules and clear-cut neoplasms are closely linked to each other is well known to every pathologist who scrutinizes the endocrine organs at postmortem examinations; some hyperplastic nodules can usually be found in the thyroid, the adrenals, and the pituitary gland, at least microscopically. In the thyroid even so-called occult carcinomas can be found at surprisingly high incidence in both children and adults [4; 21]. Experimentally, it has recently been shown that also the second part of the neuroendocrine system, namely the disseminated endocrine cells in the gut mucosa (see above), can undergo a sequence of events similar to those in the solid endocrine glands when genuine neoplasms develop; typical examples are the carcinoid tumours of the gastrointestinal tract [24]. A schematic illustration of the proposed interrelationship between hyperplastic and neoplastic lesions in both endocrine glands and disseminated neuroendocrine cells is given in Fig. 3.

Nesidioblastosis

Differentiation from Genuine Neoplasms

Although PNHHN is a disease caused by a primarily hyperplastic growth of the endocrine pancreas (Fig. 3), it can sometimes be difficult to draw a sharp dividing line between the genuine hyperplasia ("nesidioblastosis") and such concepts as "diffuse microadenomatosis" [29] and "multi-focal adenomatosis" (Fig. 3) - in fact, the morphological spectrum of the lesions in PNHHN has been referred to as a "fascinating diversity" [27]. This is further illustrated by the great variety of additional synonyms that exist, such as "nesidiodysplasia" [23], "endocrine dysplasia"

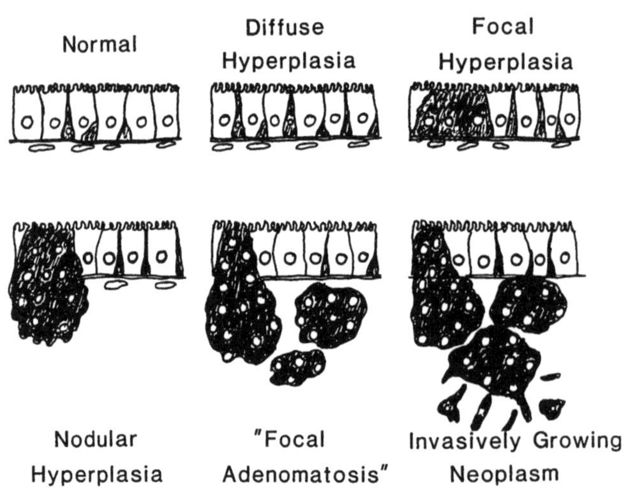

Fig. 3. Proposed development and interrelationship between various kinds of hyperplastic lesions in neuroendocrine cells of the mucosa in the alimentary tract (24) and in endocrine glands of classical type, including the islets of Langerhans

[26], "diffuse/multifocal abnormal distribution of endocrine cells" [28] and "diffuse and focal ductuloinsular proliferation" [27].

A persistent hypoglycemia with hyperinsulinism in early infancy can, however, also be caused by a genuine neoplasm, namely an insulin-producing islet-cell adenoma (insuloma) [27; 28; 42]. It is of utmost clinical importance to differentiate between hyperinsulinism evoked by a single neoplasm and that caused by diffuse-hyperplastic nesidioblastosis; in the former case, the patient can be cured by a simple excision of the focal lesion because the rest of the endocrine pancreas is normal. The diagnosis "nesidioblastosis" has far more severe clinical implications. When attempts to suppress (a) the hyperinsulinism by means of long-term treatment with diazoxide [46] or somatostatin [59], or (b) the hypoglycemia with long-acting glucagon [43] have failed, a subtotal or near-total pancreatectomy usually has to be carried out in order to avoid the threat of hypoglycemic damage to the brain [31; 34]. After such an operation the infants can become diabetic. In addition, the diagnosis "nesidioblastosis" also implies an "islet-cell dysmaturation syndrome" [22], not seldom of familial type [17] that may be associated with other malformations as well [35]. In exceptional cases there is even an association with "multiple endocrine neoplasia (MEN) type 1" [57], though mainly only when appearing as a "diffuse micro-adenomatosis", usually without a concomitant genuine islet hyperplasia [29].

Consequently, it is important to establish strict histopathological and immunohistochemical criteria for the underlying lesions in PNHHN; in the individual case the histopathological differential diagnosis can be rather dramatic. When the surgeon at operation cannot find any focal lesion by naked-eye inspection and palpation, a frozen-section diagnosis has to be made by the pathologist on a biopsy specimen. If the criteria for nesidioblastosis are fulfilled, the surgeon should continue with a near-total pancreatectomy; if not, efforts to find a focal lesion should be increased [42].

Histopathologic and Immunohistochemical Diagnostic Criteria

Macroscopically, the pancreatic gland in PNHHN is normal [27]. Microscopically, the most characteristic lesions are easily recognized (Fig. 4). The hallmarks are distinct hyperplasia and hypertrophy of the islets of LANGERHANS with loss of their sharp boundaries, widespread dissemination of individual islet parenchymal cells into the acinar exocrine pancreatic tissue, and clear-cut outbudding of islet cells from the epithelium of the small branches of the pancreatic duct system [8; 23; 26; 27; 28]. Since the advent of improved histochemical techniques [40; 58], it soon became evident that all these features could also be found in the pancreas of age-matched controls without any signs of hyperinsulinism [3; 16; 23; 26; 42]. Additional criteria were thus required for the histopathologic diagnosis of PNHHN. One such criterion was the presence of insulin cells with large nuclei [42]; another was a marked decrease in the relative incidence of somatostatin cells, as established by immunohistochemical morphometry, by radioimmuno assay [3; 16; 26] and by nonimmunological techniques [46]. A third criterion was the relative increase in the number of argyrophil (Grimelius' silver nitrate procedure) islet parenchymal

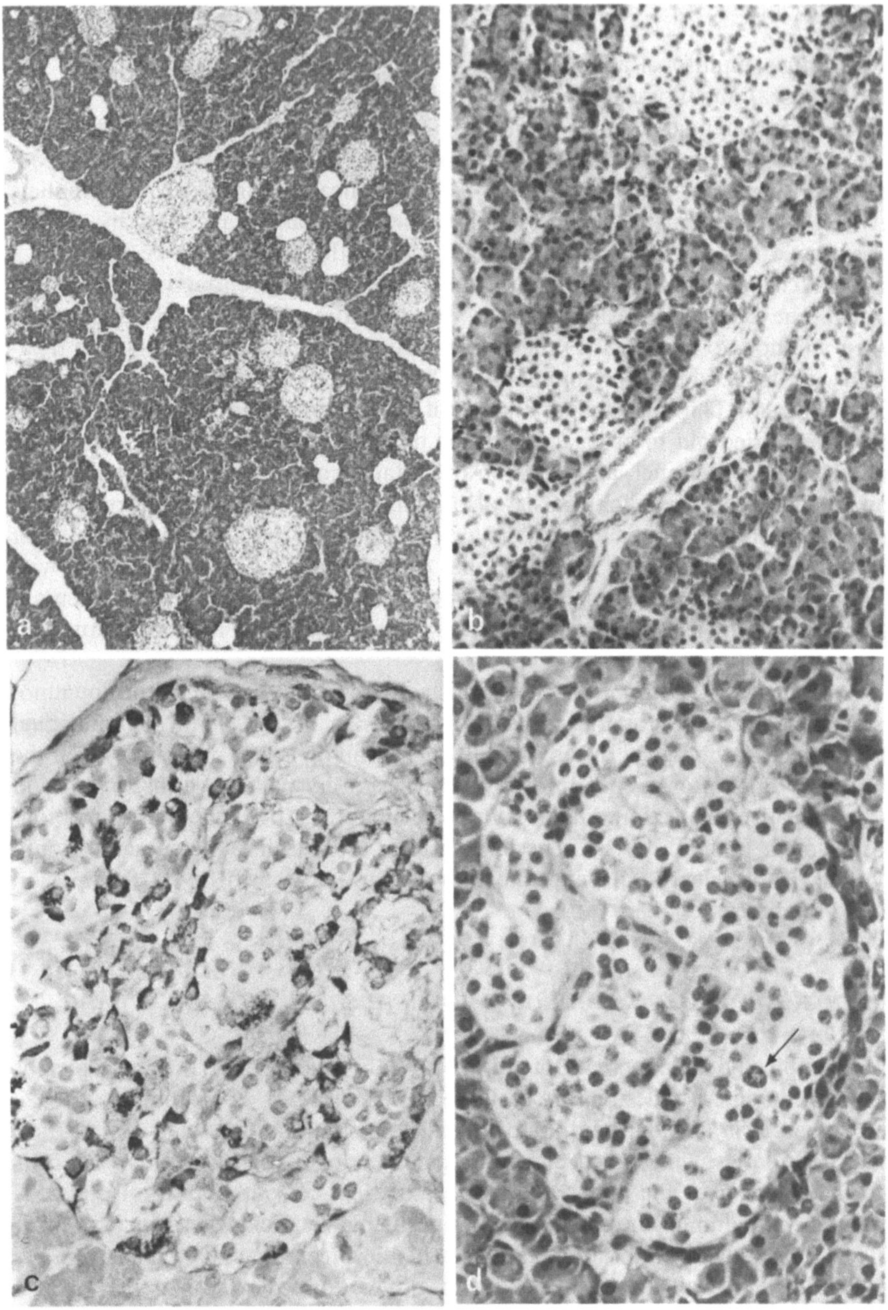

Fig. 4 a–d. A series of photomicrographs illustrating some of the major lesions in nesidioblastosis (adult, unpublished case). **a** Low-power survey picture showing the combined hypertrophy and hyperplasia of the islets of Langerhans *(pale)*. **b** Medium-power photomicrograph showing the outbudding of islet cells *(pale)* from the duct epithelium and their dissemination in the acinar, exocrine pancreatic parenchyma *(dark)*. The major part of the islet cells, however, form genuine islets of Langerhans of varying sizes and shapes. **c, d** Rather high-power photomicrographs showing two additional features of nesidioblastosis, i.e., the high incidence of argyrophil (Grimelius' procedure) cells (*black* in **c**) and the occurrence of insulin cells with large nuclei (*arrow* in **d**)

cells [17] despite a slight decrease in the relative incidence of the glucagon-immunoreactive cells [16].

Although the value of all these additional criteria for the histopathological assessment of the underlying lesion in PNHHN has been seriously questioned [27; 28; 42], they can all give information on some aspects of the pathogenesis of this mysterious disease. Thus, the large nuclei of the insulin cells may indicate that these cells show an increased activity, resulting in the ubiquitous hyperinsulinism seen in these patients. The relative loss of somatostatin cells may - together with a concomitant increase in insulin cells - give rise to impairment of the normal paracrine [32] control on the release of insulin by somatostatin cells in the islet parenchyma [3; 16; 22; 26] and thus also explain the hyperinsulinism. Lastly, the presence of increased numbers of argyrophil islet parenchymal cells may support the hypothesis that PNHHN is an islet cell dysmaturation syndrome with the appearance of immature argyrophil insulin cells of a kind similar to those occurring in the *Blutinseln* of the pancreas of lambs and calves (see above) and in the normal fetal mammalian pancreas (see above). Such argyrophil insulin cells may have deficient control of their insulin release, resulting in hyperinsulinism. The fact that peculiar types of islet parenchymal cells can be found in PNHHN has also been shown ultrastructurally, where both alpha- and beta-granules have been observed intermingled with each other in one and the same cell [36]. It may also be that the endocrine parenchyma in PNHHN contains other "polycrine" cells able to produce neurohormonal peptides with an insulin-releasing effect [27].

Of all these histopathological and immunohistochemical/morphometric criteria the large nuclei of the insulin cells is the feature that can be of greatest help to the practising pathologist in his differential diagnosis between the diffuse hyperplasia in PNHHN and the focal lesion in an insulin-producing islet cell adenoma [42]. This statement applies in particular to cases where a diagnosis has to be made on frozen sections (see above).

DNA Content of the Insulin Cells

For the above mentioned reason, we have made a pilot study on the DNA content of the insulin-immunoreactive cells in the islet parenchyma of patients with PNHHN. Such analysis, applying modern cytochemical techniques [2] and including also the islet parenchyma of age-matched controls, can show whether the insulin cells in PNHHN are diploid, "near-diploid" (as proliferating cells often are), polyploid (tetraploid or octaploid), or even aneuploid.

So far, only pilot studies have been made, using resection specimens of the whole pancreatic parenchyma from four young infants with typical PNHHN. The following procedure was used [2]. From formalin-fixed, paraffin-embedded specimens, sections about 50 μm thick were cut. These thick sections were deparaffinized, rehydrated, and enzymatically disintegrated by means of 30 min incubation (with regular Vortex mixing every 5 min) in 0.05% pronase at 37°. The density of the disintegrated cells on the microscope slides was adjusted by means of a cytospin technique. The nuclei of the disintegrated cells were stained by the Feulgen procedure for determination of the DNA content in a microspectrophotometer by means of their absorption at 546 nm wavelength [2]. On average about 100 nuclei of each of the four specimens were measured. Particular attention was paid to select those disintegrated cells that from their structural features could be assumed to be insulin cells with large nuclei.

The results obtained so far indicate that the DNA content of the nuclei of the hypertrophic insulin cells is of the pattern observed in tetraploid cells (Fig. 5). The rest of the cells, both endocrine and exocrine, show a nuclear DNA content distribution pattern which indicates that they are diploid cells (Fig. 5).

Concluding Remarks

There are several reasons for the widely diverging opinions about the pathogenesis of PNHHN; they have recently been rather comprehensively reviewed [27; 28]. The discrepancies are due to differences both of histotechnical and of more clinical nature. In conclusion, it can be stated that the available data definitely support the "islet dysmaturation" [22] and "nesidiodysplasia" [23] hypothesis, i.e., a maturation defect, resulting in a wide diversity of lesions (Fig. 3), where the overwhelming majority [27] are of diffuse hyperplastic nature, others are of focal hyperplastic character, and still others closely approach actual neoplasia [27; 28].

Beckwith-Wiedemann Syndrome

The BECKWITH-WIEDEMANN syndrome (BWS) is another example of how a hyperplastic lesion in the endocrine pancreas can be associated with a genuine neoplasia. Here, however, the genetic background is better known than in the case of PNHHN.

BWS is characterized by omphalocele, macroglossia, gigantism, hyperplastic visceromegaly, Leydig cell hyperplasia, dysplasia of the kidneys, and hypoglycemia caused by a hyperinsulinism. It is this hyperinsulinaemic hypoglycemia that is the major clinical problem in most newborns affected by BWS.

A comprehensive immunohistochemical/morphometric study of endocrine pancreas in two cases of BWS was recently made [50]. Both cases showed a massive islet cell proliferation ("islet-cell adenomatosis"); in particular the insulin- and glucagon-immunoreactive cells were increased, whereas the somatostatin cells were decreased. These observations, in addition to other alterations, showed that the pancreas in BWS had undergone abnormal development, in some respects similar to that seen in PNHHN [50].

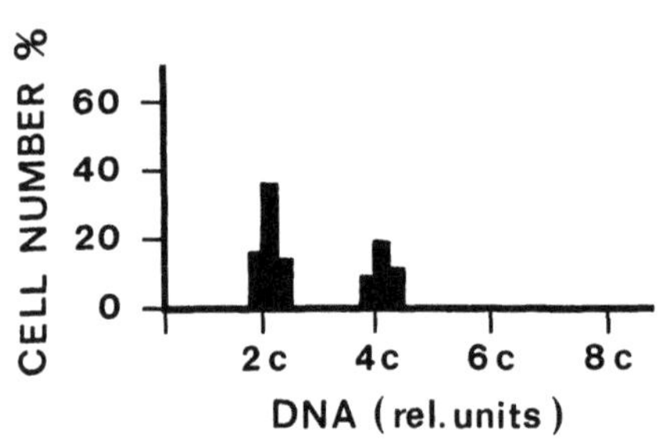

Fig. 5. DNA distribution pattern in a parenchyma, consisting only of diploid cells (2c) and tetraploid cells (4c) [2]. This DNA distribution pattern was found in the pancreas from four young infants with PNHHN, where the insulin cells with large nuclei correspond to the tetraploid cells. No aneuploid cells have been found, and no scattered values between 2c and 4c

Neonates with BWS may have a duplication of parts of chromosome 11, namely in its short arm (11p13-11p15 region). Such neonates have been shown to be predisposed to develop embryonal tumors, such as Wilms' tumor, hepatoblastoma, and rhabdomyosarcoma [30; 44].

As BWS is a rare disease, it is of rather limited clinical importance compared with PNHHN.

Islet Cell Neoplasia

One pattern that the development of a neoplastic disturbance of growth of the endocrine pancreas can follow has already been given in the preceding paragraphs (Fig. 3). The ensuing tumors comprise both benign adenomas and carcinomas with the ability to metastasize. They are also notorious for their ability to produce characteristic clinical syndromes due to hormone overproduction. As a matter of fact, the islet neurohormonal peptides and their precursors are so-called tumor markers. A comprehensive review of the islet cell neoplasms is given by SOMERS and DE VROEDE in this volume.

Acknowledgements. Thanks are due to the Director and the Staff of the Kristineberg Marine Biology Station at Fiskebäckskil, Sweden, for excellent working conditions (in the phylogenetical parts of this work).

References

1. Andrew A (1984) The development of the gastro-entero-pancreatic neuroendocrine system in birds. In: Falkmer S, Håkanson R, Sundler F (eds) Evolution and tumour pathology of the neuroendocrine system. Elsevier, Amsterdam, pp 91-110
2. Auer GU, Askensten UG, Zetterberg A (1987) Microspectrophotometric nuclear DNA analysis in clinical tumour material. Adv Clin Cytol (to be published)
3. Bishop AE, Polak JM, Chesa PG, Timson CM, Bryant MG, Bloom SR (1981) Decrease of pancreatic somatostatin in neonatal nesidioblastosis. Diabetes 30: 122-126
4. Bondeson L, Ljungberg O (1984) Occult papillary thyroid carcinoma in the young and the aged. Cancer 53: 1790-1792
5. Bonner-Weir S, Like AA (1980) A dual population of islets of Langerhans in bovine pancreas. Cell Tissue Res 206: 157-170
6. Conlon JM, Dafgård E, Falkmer S, Thim L (1987) The primary structure of ratfish insulin reveals an unusual mode of proinsulin processing. FEBS Lett 208: 445-450
7. Chejfec G, Falkmer S, Grimelius L, Jacobsson B, Rodensjö M, Wiedenmann B, Franke WW, Lee I, Gould VE (1987) Synaptophysin: a new marker for pancreatic neuroendocrine tumors. Am J Surg Pathol 11: 241-247
8. Dahms BB, Landing BH, Blaskovics M, Roe TF (1980) Nesidioblastosis and other islet cell abnormalities in hyperinsulinemic hypoglycemia of childhood. Hum Pathol 11: 641-649
9. Edström C (1973) Course of alloxan diabetes in duct-ligated rats. A functional and morphological study. Acta Path Microbiol Scand 81A: 21-36
10. El-Salhy M, Falkmer S, Kramer KJ, Speirs RD (1983) Immunohistochemical investigations of neuropeptides in the brain, corpora cardiaca, and corpora allata of an adult lepidopteran insect, *Manduca sexta* (L). Cell Tissue Res 232: 295-317

11. Falkmer S (1985) Comparative morphology of pancreatic islets in animals. In: Volk BW, Arquilla ER (eds) The diabetic pancreas, 2nd edn. Plenum, New York, pp 17-52
12. Falkmer S (1985) Phylogenetical aspects of the brain-gut axis, with special reference to islet hormones in invertebrates and lower vertebrates. In: Kobayashi H, Bern HA, Akihisa U (eds) Neurosecretion and the biology of neuropeptides. Jpn Sci Soc Press, Tokyo, pp 317-325
13. Falkmer S, Boquist L (1976) Onto- and phylogenetical aspects on insulin-producing islet cell tumors. Horm Metab Res 6 [Suppl]: 55-62
14. Falkmer S, Emdin SO (1981) Insulin evolution. In: Dodson G, Glusker JP, Sayre D (eds) Structural studies of molecules of biological interest. Oxford University Press, Oxford, pp 420-440
15. Falkmer S, Van Noorden S (1983) Ontogeny and phylogeny of the glucagon cell. Handb Exp Pharmacol 66/I: 81-119
16. Falkmer S, Søvik O, Vidnes J (1981 a) Immunohistochemical, morphometric, and clinical studies of the pancreatic islets in infants with persistent neonatal hypoglycemia of familial type with hyperinsulinism and nesidioblastosis. Acta Biol Med Germ 40: 39-54
17. Falkmer S, Rahier J, Søvik O, Vidnes J (1981 b) Significance of argyrophil parenchymal cells in the pancreatic islets in persistent neonatal hypoglycemia with hyperinsulinism of familial type. Ups J Med Sci 86: 111-117
18. Falkmer S, El-Salhy M, Titlbach M (1984) Evolution of the neuroendocrine system in vertebrates. A review with particular reference to the phylogeny and postnatal maturation of the islet parenchyma. In: Falkmer S, Håkanson R, Sundler F (eds) Evolution and tumour pathology of the neuroendocrine system. Elsevier, Amsterdam, pp 59-87
19. Falkmer S, Gustafsson MKS, Sundler F (1985) Phylogenetic aspects of the neuroendocrine system. A minireview with particular reference to cells storing neurohormonal peptides in some primitive protostomian invertebrates (flatworms, annelids). Nord Psykiatr Tidsskr 39 [Suppl 11]: 21-30
20. Falkmer S, Conlon JM, Dafgård E, Thim L (1986) Phylogenetic aspects on regulatory peptides, in particular islet hormones in some lower vertebrates. Exp Brain Res 16: 195-200
21. Franssila KO, Harach HR (1986) Occult papillary carcinoma of the thyroid in children and young adults. A systemic autopsy study in Finland. Cancer 58: 715-719
22. Gabbay KH, Gang DL (1978) Hypoglycemia in a three-months-old girl. N Engl J Med 299: 241-248
23. Gould VE, Memoli VA, Dardi LE, Gould NS (1983) Nesidiodysplasia and nesidioblastosis of infancy: structural and functional correlations with the syndrome of hyperinsulinemic hypoglycemia. Pediatr Pathol 1: 7-31
24. Havu N (1986) Enterochromaffin-like (ECL) cell carcinoids of gastric mucosa in rats after lifelong inhibition of gastric secretion. Digestion 35 [Suppl 1]: 42-56
25. Heitz PU, Klöppel G (1984) Pancreatic endocrine tumours. In: Falkmer S, Håkanson R, Sundler F (eds) Evolution and tumour pathology of the neuroendocrine system. Elsevier, Amsterdam, pp 481-496
26. Jaffe R, Hashida Y, Yunis EJ (1980) Pancreatic pathology in hyperinsulinemic hypoglycemia of infancy. Lab Invest 42: 356-365
27. Klöppel G, Heitz PU (1984) Nesidioblastosis: A clinical entity with heterogenous lesions of the pancreas. In: Falkmer S, Håkanson R, Sundler F (eds) Evolution and tumour pathology of the neuroendocrine system. Elsevier, Amsterdam, pp 340-379
28. Klöppel G, Heitz PU (eds) (1984) Pancreatic pathology. Edinburgh, Livingstone, pp 1-240
29. Klöppel G, Willemer S, Stamm B, Häcki WH, Heitz PU (1986) Pancreatic lesions and hormonal profile of pancreatic tumors in multiple endocrine neoplasia type I. An immunocytochemical study of nine patients. Cancer 57: 1824-1832
30. Koufos A, Hansen MF, Copeland NG, Jenkins HA, Lampkin BC, Cavenee K (1985) Loss of heterozygosity in three embryonal tumours suggests a common pathogenetic mechanism. Nature 316: 330-334
31. Kramer JL, Bell MJ, De Schryver K, Bower RJ, Ternberg JL, White NH (1982) Clinical and histologic indications for extensive pancreatic resection in nesidioblastosis. Am J Surg 143: 116-119
32. Larsson L-I, Goltermann NR, de Magistris L, Rehfeld JF, Schwartz TW (1979) Somatostatin cell processes as pathways for paracrine secretion. Science 205: 1393-1394

33. McQuarrie I (1954) Idiopathic spontaneously occurring hypoglycemia in infants. Clinical significance of problem and treatment. Am J Dis Child 87: 399-428
34. Moazam F, Rodgers BM, Talbert JL, Rosenbloom AL (1982) Near-total pancreatectomy in persistent infantile hypoglycemia. Arch Surg 117: 1151-1154
35. de Morais CF, Lopes EA, Bisi H, Alves VAF, de Marcede Santos RT (1986) Nesidioblastosis associated with congenital malformations of the heart. Morphological and immunohistochemical study of 5 necropsy cases. Pathol Res Pract 181: 175-179
36. Newman GR, Jasani B, Williams ED (1986) Multiple hormone storage by polycrine cells in the pancreas (from a case of nesidioblastosis). Histochem J 18: 67-79
37. O'Neill GS, Falkmer S, Thorndyke MC (1986) Insulin-like immunoreactivity in the neural ganglion of the ascidian *Ciona intestinalis*. Acta Zool 67: 147-153
38. Orci L (1984) Patterns of cellular and subcellular organization in the endocrine pancreas. J Endocrinol 102: 2-11
39. Orci L, Stefan Y, Malaisse-Lagae F, Perrelet A (1979) Instability of pancreatic endocrine cell population throughout life. Lancet I: 615-616
40. Polak JM, Van Noorden S (eds) (1986) Immunocytochemistry. Modern methods and applications, 2nd edn. Wright, Bristol, pp 1-736
41. Rahier J, Wallon J, Henquin JC (1981) Cell populations in the endocrine pancreas of human neonates and infants. Diabetologia 20: 540-546
42. Rahier J, Fält K, Müntefering H, Becker K, Gepts W, Falkmer S (1984) The basic structural lesion of persistent neonatal hypoglycaemia with hyperinsulinism: deficiency of pancreatic D-cells or hyperactivity of B-cells? Diabetologia 26: 282-289
43. Rose SR, Chrousos G, Cornblath M, Sidbury J (1986) Management of post-operative nesidioblastosis with zinc protamine glucagon and oral starch. J Pediatr 108: 97-100
44. Scott J, Cowell J, Robertson ME, Priestley LM, Wadey R, Hopkins B, Pritchard J, Bell GI, Rall LB, Graham CF, Knott TJ (1985) Insulin-like growth factor-II gene-expression in Wilms' tumour and embryonic tissues. Nature 317: 260-362
45. Seifert G (1984) Congenital anomalies. Lipomatous atrophy and other forms. In: Klöppel G, Heitz PU (eds) Pancreatic pathology. Livingstone, Edinburgh, pp 22-31
46. Søvik O, Vidnes J, Falkmer S (1975) Persistent neonatal hypoglycemia. Acta Pathol Microbiol Scand (A) 83: 155-166
47. Stefan Y, Falkmer S (1980) Identification of four endocrine cells types in the pancreas of *Cottus scorpius* (Teleostei) by immunofluorescence and electron microscopy. Gen Comp Endocrinol 42: 171-178
48. Stefan Y, Ravazzola M, Orci L (1981) Primitive islets contain two populations of cells with differing glucagon immunoreactivity. Diabetes 30: 192-195
49. Stefan Y, Grasso S, Perrelet A, Orci L (1983) Quantitative immunofluorescent study of the endocrine cell population in the developing human pancreas. Diabetes 32: 293-307
50. Stefan Y, Bordi C, Grasso S, Orci L (1985) Beckwith-Wiedemann syndrome: A quantitative, immunohistochemical study of pancreatic islet cell populations. Diabetologia 28: 914-919
51. Thorndyke MC, Falkmer S (1985) Evolution of gastro-entero-pancreatic endocrine systems in lower vertebrates. In: Foreman RE, Gorbman A, Dodd JM, Olsson R (eds) Evolutionary biology of primitive fishes. Plenum, New York, pp 379-400
52. Titlbach M, Fält K, Falkmer S (1987) Ontogeny of the pancreatic islet parenchymal cells in the rabbit. An immunohistochemical and ultrastructural study with particular regard to the earliest appearance of argyrophil insulin-immunoreactive cells. Diabetes Res 5: 105-117
53. Titlbach M, Fält K, Falkmer S (1985) Postnatal maturation of the islets of Langerhans in sheep. Light microscopic, immunohistochemical, morphometric, and ultrastructural investigations with particular reference to the transient appearance of argyrophil insulin immunoreactive cells. Diabetes Res 2: 5-15
54. Titlbach M, Chejfec G, Grimelius L, Falkmer S (1986) Neuroendocrine background of the pathology of the islets of Langerhans: A minireview with particular reference to synaptophysin and chromogranin A as neuroendocrine markers and to the ontogeny of argyrophil insulin immunoreactive cells in the rabbit. Exp Clin Endocrinol 89: 242-250
55. Töpke B, Menzel K (1976) Die Pankreasagenesie des Neugeborenen, ein seltenes, klinisch aber charakteristisches Krankheitsbild. Acta Paediatr Acad Sci Hung 17: 147-151
56. Van Noorden S (1984) The neuroendocrine system in protostomian and deuterostomian in-

vertebrates and lower vertebrates. In: Falkmer S, Håkanson R, Sundler F (eds) Evolution and tumour pathology of the neuroendocrine system. Elsevier, Amsterdam, pp 7-38
57. Vance J, Stoll RW, Kitabchi AE, Williams RG, Wood FC (1969) Nesidioblastosis in familial endocrine adenomatosis. JAMA 207: 1679-1682
58. Weibel ER (1973) Sterological techniques for electron microscopic morphometry. In: Hayat MA (ed) Principles and techniques of electron microscopy. Van Nostrand Reinhold, New York, pp 239-296
59. Wendel U, Kardorff C, Dorittke P, Bremer HJ (1985) Somatostatin in the treatment of neonatal persistent hypoglycemia due to hyper-insulinism (nesidioblastosis). Mschr Kinderhk 133: 527-531
60. Wöckel W, Scheibner K (1977) Aplasie des Pancreas mit Diabetes mellitus, intrahepatische Gallengangsaplasie und weitere Mißbildungen bei einem hypotrophen Neugeborenen. Z Pathol 121: 186-194

Islet Cell Replication and Diabetes*

C. Hellerström, I. Swenne and A. Andersson

Introduction

The maintenance of appropriate plasma insulin levels is the result of two major mechanisms, namely minute-to-minute regulation of the insulin release from individual B-cells and long-term adaptation of the total B-cell mass to the peripheral demand for insulin. Diabetes mellitus is characterized by an inadequate supply of insulin resulting in severe hyperglycemia and disastrous vascular complications. In the case of insulin-dependent diabetes mellitus (IDDM), this inadequacy clearly reflects B-cell destruction, most probably caused by autoimmune aggression [57, 45]. In the case of non-insulin-dependent diabetes mellitus (NIDDM), the pathogenesis is less obvious, although there is evidence to suggest that in patients with NIDDM an increased peripheral insulin requirement is combined with a genetic deficiency in the ability of the B-cell to replicate [24, 68–70, 85] and a reduced insulin response to glucose [44]. It has furthermore been proposed that B-cell regeneration may also be of some significance in the course of IDDM, since in the early stages of the disease some patients exhibit both morphological and functional signs of a returning insulin production ("the honeymoon period") possibly reflecting an effort of the reduced B-cell mass to meet the insulin demand.

It is the purpose of this chapter to present a discussion of the mechanism of islet cell replication and the growth pattern of the islet organ in the light of recent observations. Both basic and clinical data have been reviewed, with particular attention to the ability of the islet organ for adaptive B-cell growth and to changes in replication and in the number of other islet cell types. During the course of this work, it was the strong feeling of the authors that more research on the regulation of islet cell replication would be instrumental for a better understanding of the cause and the natural history of any form of diabetes mellitus.

* The work by the authors included in this review was supported by the Swedish Medical Research Council (12X-109, 17X-07501, 12P-6947), the Swedish Diabetes Association, the Nordic Insulin Fund, the Novo Company, the Expressen Prenatal Research Foundation, the Edla Johansson Fund, the Åke Wiberg Fund, the Ernfors Diabetes Foundation, the Juvenile Diabetes Foundation International, and the Kroc Foundation.

Regulation of Islet Cell Replication

Islet Cell Cycle Kinetics

A large number of studies on effects of various substances on the B-cell proliferation have employed the incorporation of ^{3}H-thymidine into DNA as an index of proliferation [70]. These methods, however, have the inherent limitation of yielding only relative values for different rates of proliferation. Moreover, changes in the duration of the DNA-synthesizing S phase of the cell cycle may, in the absence of parallel changes in the rate of mitotic division, alter the incorporation of ^{3}H-thymidine. A cell cycle analysis of proliferating islet cells should overcome this problem and also yield estimates, expressed in absolute numbers, of the rate of formation of new cells.

It has been possible to perform cell cycle analyses in vitro using isolated fetal rat islets which have a high proportion of proliferating cells [150, 151]. In these studies, the cell cycles of the proliferating cells were synchronized by the addition of hydroxyurea to the culture medium. This drug reversibly inhibits DNA synthesis, and cells progressing through the cell cycle were collected at the boundary between the G_1 and the S phase [141]. When the drug was removed, the synchronized cells entered the S phase simultanously, and their progress through the cell cycle could be monitored by pulse-labeling with ^{3}H-thymidine [152]. As seen in Fig. 1, the S phase duration of the islet cells could be measured as the width of the first DNA-synthesizing wave, and the generation time (i.e., the duration of a full cell cycle), as the distance between the two DNA-synthesizing waves. Furthermore, when histological sections of the synchronized islets were examined for mitotic figures, it was possible to measure the duration of the G_2 phase as the distance between the DNA-synthesizing and mitotic waves [150]. On the basis of this combined information, the generation time of fetal rat islet cells was estimated to be 14.9 h. Assuming that the mitotic duration is 0.5 h, the cell cycle could be further subdivided into a G_1 phase of 2.5 h, an S phase of 6.4 h, and a G_2 phase of 5.5 h (150). It was also of interest to note that the islet cell cycle proceeded similarly at different glucose concentrations. This observation suggests that glucose stimulates islet cell proliferation by regulating the number of cells entering an active cell cycle. Furthermore, this finding lends support to the rationale for using the incorporation of ^{3}H-thymidine as an index of proliferation, since such estimates are not confounded by variations in S phase duration. It was also possible, from the cell cycle data and the autoradiographic labeling indices of unsynchronized cultured islets, to calculate the proportion of islet cells in the active cell cycle at a given moment, i.e., the proliferative compartment. This was found to be about 3% in 2.7 m*M* glucose and increased to about 7% in 16.7 m*M* glucose. Using these figures, the cell birth rate (i.e., the production of new cells per 24 h) was calculated to be approximately 4% and 10% in 2.7 m*M* and 16.7 m*M* glucose respectively [150].

It can be seen in the cell cycle curve of Fig. 1 that the ^{3}H-thymidine incorporation sank to very low levels between the two DNA synthetic waves, suggesting that very few, if any, islet cells entered the S phase during this interval. A similar observation has been made in an islet cell cycle analysis performed in vivo in mice [22]. These observations suggest that only a limited fraction of the islet cells are capable

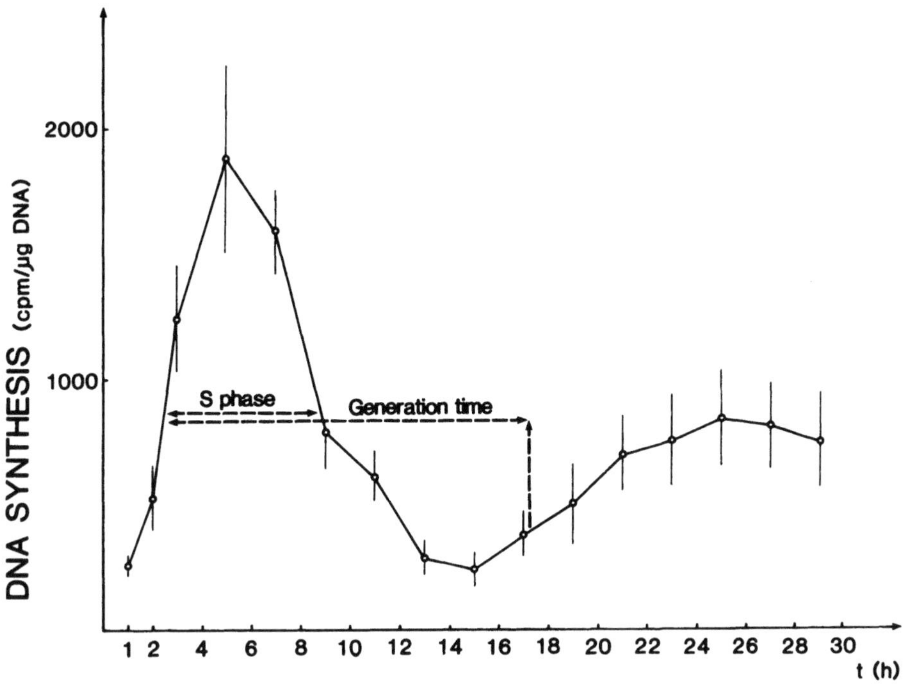

Fig. 1. DNA synthesis in fetal rat islets after synchronization of the cell cycle in tissue culture medium containing hydroxyurea. This drug synchronizes proliferating cells by collecting them at the G_1/S boundary. When the hydroxyurea was removed, proliferating cells entered the S phase as a synchronized population and their progress through the cell cycle was monitored by labeling with ^3H-thymidine in 1-h pulses. The duration of the S phase was measured as the width of the DNA synthetic wave occurring immediately after removal of the hydroxyurea. The generation time, i.e. the duration of a full cell cycle, was measured as the distance between the first and second DNA synthetic waves. (Modified from ref. 150)

of entering the cell cycle. The hypothesis that only a small fraction of the islet cells can be stimulated to proliferate and that the majority have entered an irreversible G_0 phase introduces a new concept of how B-cell proliferation is controlled. The ability of the B-cell mass to expand would then depend not only on the proliferative stimulus, but also on the number of B-cells able to respond. It has been possible to estimate the maximal proliferative compartment, i.e., the fraction of cells capable of entering an active cell cycle, as roughly 10% in cultured fetal rat islet cells [153].

As an animal's age increases, the rate of DNA replication in cultured islets decreases [151, 154, 156]. Cell cycle analysis revealed that the proliferative response to glucose does not change with age, but that the number of cells capable of responding diminishes [151]. Thus, in 3-month-old rats the maximal proliferative compartment has decreased to less than 3%. It is, moreover, of interest to note that not only age, but also genetic factors, may set a limit to the maximal proliferative compartment [154]. Further discussion of the effect of age on islet growth and function will be found below.

Against the background outlined above, a model for the regulation of glucose-stimulated B-cell replication would be based on the assumption that the majority of the B-cells have entered an irreversible G_0 phase and are incapable of proliferation. The size of the small fraction of B-cells with proliferative capacity is probably set by genetic factors, but may also be subject to environmental influences early in the organism's development. Proliferating B-cells respond to glucose by leaving a reversible G_0 phase, entering an active cell cycle, and subsequently undergoing mitosis (Fig. 2). With increasing age, there is a gradual loss of proliferating B-cells into the irreversible G_0 compartment, but the B-cells which retain the ability to proliferate respond similarly to glucose at different ages. It thus appears that it is the number of cells able to respond to glucose, rather than the quality of their response, which limits the glucose-stimulated expansion of the B-cell mass.

Role of Substrates and Growth Factors in the Regulation of Islet Cell Proliferation

There is ample documentation of the stimulatory effect of glucose on B-cell proliferation [70], but the mechanism by which glucose stimulates the individual B-cells to enter an active cell cycle remains unclear. Of the sugars tested apart from D-glucose, only D-mannose stimulates B-cell replication, whereas L-glucose, D-fructose, and 3-*O*-methylglucose are nonstimulatory [80, 81]. Mannoheptulose, on the other

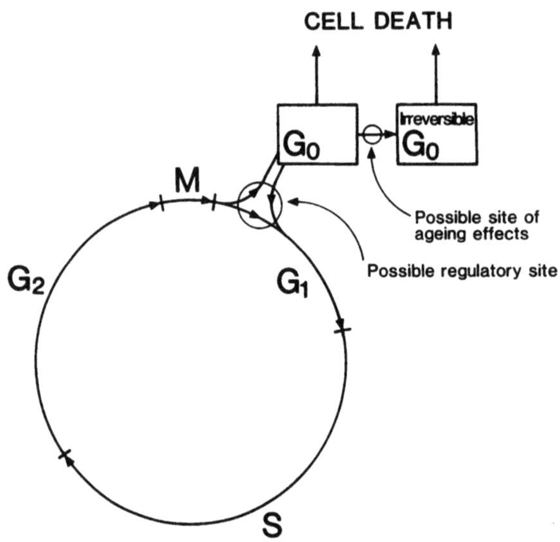

Fig. 2. Hypothetical model of the cell cycle of the pancreatic B-cell. The figure shows that after completing a cell cycle the daughter cells can either continue into new proliferative cycles or enter a resting G_0 state. From the G_0 state the B-cells can be recruited back into an active cell cycle provided appropriate proliferative stimuli are applied. This transition from a resting to a proliferative state appears to be a site of regulation of B-cell proliferation. According to this model the loss of proliferative capacity with age would be explained by an increasing number of B-cells entering an irreversible G_0 state from which they cannot reenter the cell cycle and resume proliferation

hand, inhibits glucose-stimulated replication [82]. In contrast to the other carbohydrates, D-glucose and D-mannose are metabolized by the B-cell, while mannoheptulose acts by blocking hexose metabolism at the level of the initial phosphorylation [6]. It thus appears that glucose stimulation of B-cell replication, in concert with glucose stimulation of insulin biosynthesis and secretion [7, 66], is linked to a substrate site and requires metabolic processing of the sugar.

Other metabolic substrates, such as a mixture of essential amino acids, also stimulate islet cell replication [36, 153, 156]. Individual amino acids have as yet not been tested, but α-ketoisocaproic acid, the deamination product of leucine, has been shown to stimulate islet cell replication in vitro [99]. In studies performed on fetal rat islets, growth stimulation by essential amino acids could be demonstrated, while there were only small effects on insulin biosynthesis and secretion by these compounds [153, 156]. It thus seems that the substrate site regulating entry into an active cell cycle is different from the one regulating insulin production. It should be emphasized in this context that only a small proportion of the islet cells take part in proliferation (see above) and that these cells may have regulatory mechanisms different from those of cells which have entered an irreversible G_0 phase. B-cells in S phase and mitosis are well granulated [94, 95, 156, 163] but it is unknown whether the proliferating cells respond to insulin secretagogues in the same manner as nonproliferating cells. Due to their low number, they would hardly cause detectable changes of the insulin output from isolated islets. When ^{3}H-thymidine incorporation into DNA during the S phase is used as an index of proliferation, there is no detectable uptake into DNA either during the other phases of the cell cycle in proliferating cells or in nonproliferating cells [135]. Findings of apparently qualitatively or quantitatively differing effects of a growth factor on insulin production on the one hand and cell proliferation on the other may thus reflect the fact that different sub-populations of one and the same islet cell type are being studied.

As indicated above, proliferating islet cells maintain a similar response to glucose during aging from late fetal to adult life. However, up to day 20 of gestation, the fetal rat islet cells do not respond to a high glucose concentration with an increased proliferation [36, 153]. In this respect, the regulation of islet cell replication forms a parallel with the development of insulin biosynthesis and secretion in that both attain adult characteristics during the perinatal period [9, 47]. The factors governing these processes are unknown, but it is noteworthy that glucose, which in itself is able to induce the development of a glucose-sensitive insulin secretory response [10, 51], does not have such an effect on islet cell replication [153]. The possibility that hormones may influence the sensitivity of islet cell replication to glucose has also been put to a test, but neither growth hormone (GH) nor thyroid hormone had any effect in this respect [153]. Thus, while the rat fetal B-cell responds poorly to glucose until the end of gestation, a mixture of essential amino acids strongly stimulates islet cell proliferation prior to this period [36, 153]. The degree of stimulation diminishes towards the end of gestation [153], but a modest capacity to stimulate replication by amino acids is retained in adult rat islets (SWENNE, unpublished). Indeed, the amino-acid-enriched medium resembles the physiological condition for the rat foetus late in gestation when the serum level of glucose is low [46] and that of amino acids high [61]. It may be that during fetal development an ample supply of amino acids is necessary both as a source of energy and as a source of building blocks for constructing peptides.

Although nutrients seem to be the most important regulators of B-cell proliferation, macromolecular growth factors may be necessary to modulate, or even maintain, the proliferative response to sugars and amino acids. This notion is supported by the stimulatory effect of serum on islet cell proliferation [119, 120, 156] and by the lack of a replicatory response to glucose in islets cultured in the absence of serum [155, 157]. Interestingly, fetal rat islets can be maintained in a serum-free, chemically defined medium provided it is supplemented with, among other substances: transferrin, insulin, prolactin, growth hormone, and epidermal growth factor [103].

The stimulatory effect of GH on islet cell replication and insulin production is well documented [70]. In a number of other tissues, GH stimulates proliferation by inducing the local production of somatomedins/insulin-like growth factors (SM-C/IGF I) which act by promoting the entry of cells into an active cell cycle [37, 106]. When added to the tissue culture medium, multiplication-stimulating activity (MSA or rat IGF II) stimulated B-cell replication [119, 120], indicating a possible physiological role for this group of substances in the regulation of islet growth. Moreover, using immunocytochemistry, somatomedins have recently been demonstrated in adult rat [5] and fetal human islets of Langerhans (D. J. Hill, personal communication), suggesting a local production of these peptides. Finally, the production of somatomedins by islet cells in monolayer culture has been demonstrated [133]. Careful biochemical characterization of the secreted peptides revealed that the islet cell somatomedin was of the SM-C/IGF I type and that no MSA could be detected [133].

In a study of the regulation of the SM-C/IGF I production in cultured fetal rat islets, it was observed that GH stimulated the secretion of this peptide into the medium [157]. This effect on replication of GH could be partially blocked by an antibody against SM-C/IGF I known to neutralize the biological effects of somatomedins in vitro. The above finding supports the view that GH can stimulate islet cell replication via an autocrine or a paracrine mechanism, i.e., by increasing the local production of growth factors. It is, however, noteworthy that the antibody did not bring GH-stimulated islet cell replication back to basal levels, but rather that some somatomedin-independent stimulation persisted. This suggests that GH also exerts a direct effect on the B-cell. Glucose itself did not stimulate SM-C/IGF I production. However, a high glucose concentration was necessary to achieve a substantial GH stimulation of replication and SM-C/IGF I production. It would thus appear that GH and GH-induced somatomedin production can modulate the islet growth response to glucose and perhaps to other nutrients.

GH was able to substitute for serum and restored a glucose-stimulated islet cell replication in serum-free medium, whereas the very low insulin secretion into such medium was not affected [157]. It is of interest in this context to scrutinize the composition of the chemically defined medium intended for islet culture which was referred to above [103]. In addition to GH, prolactin stimulates islet cell replication [107]. The latter may exert its action by cross-reacting with the receptor mediating the effects of GH [62]. Insulin is included in the medium at a very high concentration (5 μg/ml) and may under such conditions act as a somatomedin analogue and stimulate islet cell replication via a somatomedin receptor [119]. This group of substances is apparently of great importance for the maintenance of islet cell proliferation. It is noteworthy, though, that the addition of small amounts of serum to the culture medium is necessary for GH to have its full effect and that GH has little effect on insulin secretion in a serum-free medium [157]. This would suggest that other, hitherto unknown, serum factors are needed for the maintenance and growth of the B-cell in vitro.

Islet Cell Differentiation and Islet Growth at Different Ages

Differentiation and Proliferation of Islet Cells During Intrauterine Life

Basically, the process of differentiation of the islet cells is a reflection of the activation of genes coding for the various islet hormones. With regard to the B-cell, the nucleotide sequence of the insulin gene has been known for several years [13, 32, 100]. Recent studies have aimed at clarifying the mechanism that governs the expression of this gene and the control of its phenotypic activity. In several experiments using mice, a DNA fragment including the human insulin gene was microinjected into fertilized mouse eggs. These experiments resulted in transgenic progeny containing the human insulin gene in its genomic DNA [21, 138]. Transcripts of the human insulin gene were found in the pancreas but not in other tissues, and production of human insulin was revealed by the detection of human C-peptide in the plasma and urine of the transgenic mice. Immunocytochemical studies clearly showed that human insulin, identified by an anti-human C-peptide antibody, was present only in pancreatic islet cells [138]. It was also found that the serum levels of human insulin were properly regulated by glucose, amino acids, and tolbutamide. These combined observations indicate that the human DNA fragments present in the genomic DNA of the transgenic mice carried, in addition to the insulin gene, the sequences necessary for the tissue-specific expression of this gene and that these regulatory sequences reacted to homologous signals in the mouse.

Further studies of the molecular biology of the insulin gene have indicated a tight regulation of its cellular transcription. EDLUND et al. [42] have presented evidence for the existence, in the 5′ flanking DNA of the rat insulin I gene, of sequences controlling its cell-specific expression. Analyses of this region suggested that a transcriptional enhancer might be located in the distal position of the 5′ flanking DNA. They also presented evidence for the existence of another controlling element located more proximally to the transcription start site and for the view that the activity of both these controlling sequences is restricted to pancreatic B-cells. Recent studies have also demonstrated the existence of nuclear factors derived from an insulin-producing tumor cell line which interact with three distinct regions within the insulin enhancer [109]. Further data suggest that the insulin enhancer is controlled by both positive and negative regulators and that the negative regulators may repress the enhancer in non-islet cells [108]. Taken together, these studies suggest that the cell-specific regulation of insulin gene transcription involves a complicated pattern of molecules which can act upon a relatively small DNA domain.

The genes for both glucagon and somatostatin have been cloned and sequenced, but to this date virtually nothing is known of their regulation [14, 140]. Therefore, the molecular biology of the differentiation of the A-, D-, and PP-cells is still virgin territory.

While it is only in the last five years or so that it has been possible to analyze the molecular biology of islet cell gene expression, the morphology of this process, as reflected in islet cell differentiation, has been a matter of study for decades. Such studies have been focused on the development of islet cells and on their embryonic location and growth. Earlier observations in this field have been reviewed by PICTET and RUTTER [113], HELLERSTRÖM [68], and HELLERSTRÖM and SWENNE [70]. The introduction of sensitive and highly specific immunocytochemical methods has greatly contributed to the precise definition of the developmental stage when the islet cells first appear. FUJI [52] and YOSHINARI et al. [167], have exploited such methods in a light-microscopic study of the sequential appearance of endocrine cells in the rat pancreas. The first cell to be identified was the A-cell. It appeared in the embryonic pancreas on day 11 of gestation (the day of the vaginal plug was denoted as day 0), which is just before the fusion of the ventral and dorsal rudiments of the embryonic rat pancreas. At this stage glucagon-reactive cells were found in the epithelium of the foregut and in cap-like pancreatic primordia on both the ventral and the dorsal intestinal walls. The next endocrine cells to appear in the embryonic rat were the B-cells on day 12.5–13.5 and the PP-cells on day 14. These cells seemed to be located entirely within the pancreatic bud, in which islet-like structures could be seen as early as day 13. D-cells appeared 3 days after the B-cells and were located within the primitive islets. The typical adult arrangement of the islet cells in the rat, which consists of a B-cell core surrounded by the other cell types, was attained on gestational day 18. Moreover, it was notable that the intrauterine decapitation of the fetuses on gestational day 16 did not influence the development of the islet cells until day 20 [167].

The ontogeny of islet cells in the porcine pancreas has been reported by ALUMETS et al. [2]. At a fetal age of 4 weeks, A-, B-, and D-cells were present in the dorsal pancreatic primordium. PP-cells were identified at the same developmental stage, but only in the ventral primordium. It was noteworthy that at this early stage the two pancreatic primordia were entirely made up of strains of endocrine cells with a total lack of ducts or acini. The duodenal pancreatic portion (derived from the ventral bud) became populated with A-, B-, and D-cells around the 10th week of gestation, although the PP-cells maintained predominance in this area until birth. There were few PP-cells in the splenic part of the pancreas throughout the period of intrauterine development. Typical islets, with a core of B-cells surrounded by the other islet cell types, did not form until the time of birth. Recently, corresponding ontogenetic studies of the four islet cell types have also been performed in ruminants [129, 130].

Of particular interest in this context is the qualitative and quantitative development of the human fetal endocrine pancreas. Immunocytochemical staining has been used for both identification and quantitation of the various islet cells at very early stages of fetal life. With this technique, the first light-microscopic appearance of endocrine cells has been demonstrated as early as the 8th fetal week, when A-, B-, D-, and PP-cells were found either in primitive islets or as isolated cells adjacent to duct cells [27, 144]. No immunoreactive cells could, however, be traced at 7 weeks of intrauterine age [27]. It was noteworthy that in the 8-week-old fetal pancreas there was a sizable population of endocrine cells reacting only with antiglicentin antiserum, while the A-cells reacting with both antiglucagon and antiglicentin antisera appeared at 12-13 weeks of gestational age [144].

The morphological observations on the differentiation of human islet cells indicate that the four cell types appear earlier than was hitherto believed. It also seems that the different human endocrine islet cells begin their intrauterine hormone production more simultaneously than is the case with the fetal rat, in which a distinct sequential appearance of the islet cells seems to occur. It should be pointed out in this context that by definition, the process of islet cell differentiation involves several steps in addition to the mere transcription and translation of the gene for a specific hormone. Thus the mechanisms of hormone processing and of intracellular transport, storage, and release are intimately involved in the differentiation process and require the expression of numerous genes for their maturation. Examples which support this conclusion include: the above-mentioned observations showing that only glicentin has immunoreactivity in the immature A-cells [144], an unequal expression of the two nonallelic genes for rat insulin I and II in the fetal rat [35], and the deficient glucose regulation of insulin release in the fetal stage of several different species, including man [11, 51, 136, 159].

The growth of the human islet organ during fetal and neonatal life has been the subject of a careful quantitative study by Stefan et al. [144]. In their report, the total volumes of the different islet cell types were measured in fetuses from the 12th intrauterine week up to 5 months postnatally. The collected data were subdivided into five different age groups, and the volume densities of islet cells, as measured in immunocytochemically stained sections, were transformed to absolute volumes on the basis of estimates of the total volume of fresh and nonfixed pancreatic samples. Thus, the observations provide substantial information on both relative and absolute growth of islets early in human life. The volume density of endocrine tissue was high in the younger fetuses, but decreased by 50% in the neonates. In the fetus the proportion of islet tissue in both the PP-rich and the glucagon-rich pancreatic regions differed from the corresponding regions of the adult pancreas. In the former region the fetal pancreas contained about twice as much islet tissue as in the adult, while in the latter region there was up to ten times more islet tissue in the fetus than in the adult. In the whole fetal pancreas there was a parallelism between the increase in B-cell volume and in total glandular tissue, while the relative A-cell volume reached a peak at a fetal age of 17-19 weeks and was followed by a marked decrease until the start of neonatal life. The B-cell/A-cell ratio therefore increased from approximately 1.5 in the 20- to 24-week fetuses to approximately 5 in the infants. It was also observed that the D-cells reached their highest volume density in the neonatal period, which confirms several previous observations [27, 121, 122, 164].

Volumetric measurements of the growth of the different endocrine cells showed that the B-cell mass increased more than 130-fold (from 0.43 μl to 59 μl) between the 12th intrauterine week and the 5th postnatal month. The corresponding growth rate for the A-cells was only about half that of the B-cells, while that of the D-cells was over 150-fold. The increase in PP-cells was about 100-fold during the same period. By comparison, the increase in total glandular tissue (endocrine + exocrine) was on the order of 130-fold. These data clearly illustrate the dynamic islet growth in the human fetus and neonate and the gradual change in islet cellular composition which takes place both before and after birth. They also provide practical information on quantities of B-cells which may be obtained from human fetal pancreatic glands intended for transplantation.

Islet Growth in Postnatal Life

It is conceivable that both islet cell replication and islet growth in postnatal life are under the influence of numerous complex factors related both to genetic background and environment. Among the obvious environmental influences are nutritional state and physical activity. More subtle influences may be effected through the central nervous system and the hormonal balance. Presumably age in itself is highly significant. It may also be that age acts in concert with other factors such as eating and exercise habits. Glucose homeostasis is intimately related to the growth responses of the islet organ, and any inadequacy in islet hormone production may lead to aberrations in glucose tolerance. This section summarizes some recent observations on the normal postnatal growth pattern of the islets and the changes in islet growth and function which may be observed with advancing age. It follows from the complexity of this subject that most of the studies have been carried out in animals.

A comprehensive volumetric study of the postnatal development of A-, B-, and D-cell populations in the rat pancreas up to 210 days of age has been presented by McEvoy [101]. The percentage volume contribution of islet cells to the total pancreatic volume diminished from just over 4% on the 10th day after birth to about 1,5% at day 210. The total islet volume continued to expand throughout this period, though there were marked differences between the different islet cell types. The B-cell volume was relatively constant between days 10 and 20 and subsequently increased 10-fold up to day 210. In contrast, the A-cell volume observed on day 50 was not significantly different from that observed on day 210. The D-cell population had already reached its adult volume on day 35. The pancreatic contents of insulin and glucagon closely reflected the growth of the B- and A-cell volumes respectively. The plasma concentration of insulin, on the other hand, was constant over the whole observation period, while that of glucagon showed a significant decrease with age. These data suggest that in the rat the B-cell volume shows a continuous increase with age, while the A- and D-cell volumes reach a maximum value relatively early in life. The growth of the B-cell volume during the adult life of the rat conforms to previous observations by Hellman [73] and Remacle [131] which indicate that the rat islet volume continues to increase up to 700 days of age. Although body weight also continues to increase, the islet organ grows at a faster rate, leading to a gradual increase in the islet volume/body weight ratio.

The capacity of the islet organ to respond with cell proliferation and growth during old age is of particular interest, since glucose intolerance is a common feature in aging individuals. To what extent this reflects a deficiency in the adaptability of the islet cells is still controversial, and clinical knowledge on this issue is scarce. In the rat, however, a series of observations have been reported on the effects of age on both the structure and the function of the islet organ. Several studies [34, 132, 151] demonstrated, on the whole, slight pathological islet changes with advancing age, though a certain decrease in proliferative capacity could be shown. In isolated islets obtained from rats aged 2–18 months, however, REAVEN et al. [126] demonstrated the existence of an insulin response to glucose and leucine which progressively decreased with age. This deficient insulin response to glucose has since been confirmed in other studies using rats up to 24 months of age [40, 137]. In contrast, the islet size, total islet mass, the number of B-cells per islet, and the volume of mature B-cell granules per B-cell steadily increased with age. As a result, there was a profound decrease in the amount of insulin release per B-cell. Attempts to affect the aging process by exercise or caloric restriction did not stop the decline in B-cell function with age, despite the fact that each of these experimental situations decreased the blood sugar levels and prevented the age-dependent pathological changes of islet morphology [125]. In further studies, the maximal insulin response to glucose in 12-month-old rats was measured in a pancreas perfusion system and compared to that of 2-month-old rats [127]. The animals were fed standard laboratory chow, a sucrose-rich diet, or a calorie-restricted diet. The results indicated that the maximal insulin response per unit of endocrine pancreas was markedly reduced in all three groups of 12-month-old animals: it was only 25%–33% of that in the corresponding younger groups. The islet mass of the 12-month-old animals fed either the sucrose rich diet or standard chow was, however, 3–4 times larger than that of the young rats, and these older rats were able to secrete as much insulin per unit of pancreas volume as the younger rats. The above observations were interpreted as suggesting that aging animals, which have a deficient insulin response to glucose, can overcome this deficiency of response by expanding the pancreatic pool of B-cells. These observations also suggest that the decline in insulin secretion of the individual B-cell is a function of age per se and is not influenced by variations in the amount and kind of calories ingested.

The notion that aging rats are able to compensate for the decreased insulin response of the individual B-cell to glucose is supported by observations concerning the oral glucose tolerance of old rats. In the same dietary groups referred to above, REAVEN et al. [128] found virtually normal plasma glucose levels after oral glucose tolerance tests. However, plasma insulin values were different between the groups, and the in vitro insulin response to glucose of isolated islets diminished, which was shown to reflect marked variations in insulin sensitivity. These observations also confirm a previous report by YOSHINO et al. [168] showing a normal oral glucose tolerance in rats up to 18 months of age. It is worthy of note, however, that the repeated observation of an insulin secretory defect in the B-cells of old rats [40, 126, 137] has not remained undisputed. A recent paper by BURCH et al. [23], which employed a more careful islet isolation technique presented evidence for an activated, rather than reduced, insulin release in vitro from islets of 12- to 18-month-old rats. Therefore, the possibility that diabetogenic factors which act in old age may lead to both B-cell hyperplasia and hyperfunction cannot be entirely excluded.

Nutrition and Islet Cell Proliferation

As indicated above, metabolic substrates - notably glucose - may be among the physiologically most important stimuli of islet cell proliferation. In vivo studies of islet growth employing diets of different nutritional compositions would therefore form interesting parallels with in vitro experiments performed on isolated islets. Force-feeding rats with diets rich in complex or refined carbohydrates in amounts sufficient to cause glycosuria resulted in considerable islet hyperplasia without signs of B-cell degeneration [165]. Likewise, parenteral administration of glucose caused islet hyperplasia and increased replicatory activity in islet cells [63, 99, 166]. When the animals have been fed carbohydrate-rich diets ad libitum, the effects on the islets have been divergent. In one report there was an enhanced growth of the islets in rats receiving a high carbohydrate diet compared to those fed diets rich in fat or proteins [158]. However, this observation was not confirmed by other investigators [74, 91]. In this context it should be noted that laboratory rodents often change the amount of food they take in, and consequently their rate of body weight gain, if the composition of their diet is changed [26, 77, 92]. It may therefore be difficult to separate the effects of dietary components from those caused by an altered caloric intake. Nevertheless, the weight of evidence suggests that carbohydrates have a stimulatory effect on islet cell growth, though the effect of carbohydrates per se is difficult to separate from that of an increased caloric intake.

Complete withdrawal of food from laboratory rodents resulted in a weight loss of about 25% over 48 h, but the total islet volume did not change [64, 149]. A period of 2 days is probably too short for the development of significant changes in islet volume. This would emphasize the hypothesis that changes in islet mass occur as part of the long-term regulation of insulin production. Restricting the amounts of an adequately composed diet fed to animals allows longer periods of observation under conditions of caloric deficiency. In such conditions growth is retarded and total islet volume is decreased [8, 39, 111]. However, if the islet volume is expressed per unit of body weight, there is either no change or possibly a slight increase in relative volume, which suggests that the islet cells adapt to the nutritional conditions.

Rats fed a diet with inadequate protein content reduce their food intake spontaneously and develop a state of protein-calorie malnutrition [77]. Body weight gain is severely retarded or even completely arrested, and the animals show several signs of malnutrition [142]. Morphological examinations of the pancreas indicated atrophy, decreased islet size, diminution of B-cell cytoplasm and cell size, and an increased A-cell/B-cell ratio in the islets. There was, however, no evidence of B-cell necrosis at either the light- or the electron-microscopic level [65, 114, 146,

160]. In one quantitative study, the islet volume relative to body weight was reduced by one-third [160]. Another study failed to demonstrate that protein-calorie malnutrition had a similar effect [39]. However, the latter study included an additional experimental group which received a nutritionally adequate diet restricted to amounts equal to those consumed by the rats on low-protein diet. The growth of rats on such a calorically restricted diet was retarded, but not to the same degree as was the growth of animals suffering from protein-calorie malnutrition. The calorie-restricted rats had a B-cell volume per kilogram body weight which was 30% larger than that of rats on the low-protein diet. Taken together, these findings suggest that protein-calorie malnutrition reduces the growth of the islet organ, presumably by inhibiting both proliferation and increase in the size of individual cells.

The effects of protein-calorie malnutrition on the endocrine pancreas are of special interest in view of their hypothesized role in the pathogenesis of tropical or malnutrition-related diabetes [38]. During protein-calorie malnutrition there is in addition to the changes in endocrine pancreatic morphology described above, a severe impairment both of the insulin secretory response to glucose and of glucose tolerance. Epidemiological data suggest the possibility that despite nutritional rehabilitation, structural and/or functional abnormalities persist later in life and predispose for diabetes [1, 124]. This hypothesis has now been approached experimentally by feeding weanling rats a low protein diet for a limited period and subsequently refeeding them with an adequate diet. Upon refeeding, growth was resumed and glucose tolerance improved, but a blunted insulin secretory response to glucose persisted [33]. This experimental model may prove valuable for studies of the effects of an early nutritional insult on the growth and function of the B-cell in adult life.

Islet Growth in Diabetes

Experimental Diabetes in Animals

The literature abounds with papers dealing with experimentally induced diabetes in animals, but relatively few of them directly address the subjects of islet growth and islet cell replication in these models. Perhaps this omission reflects a hesitation to apply the relatively cumbersome techniques for the morphometric assay of islet volumes and for obtaining autoradiographic estimates of the number of islet cells in S phase. It is an omission which might also be due to a legitimate suspicion that experimental animal models presently available for this purpose may not be ideal. No doubt, caution should be exercised in the interpretation of data on islet cell regeneration obtained in experiments in which the B-cells have been directly exposed to the cytotoxic action of, for example, alloxan or streptozotocin (STZ). This is also true, although to a lesser extent, for studies of regeneration after partial pancreatectomy, since in these cases not only the B-cells but also some of the other endocrine cells and part of the exocrine parenchyma have been removed. Indeed, almost all studies of islet cell regeneration in animal models of experimental diabetes can be criticized for not exactly fulfilling the criteria for human diabetes. Nevertheless, as exemplified below, such studies may provide valuable information on various aspects of adaptive islet growth.

Although there are previous reports on the regeneration of islet cells in alloxan diabetic animals [19, 43, 48, 79, 86, 87], the weight of evidence suggests that at least in the rat this is a transient phenomenon which does not result in complete amelioration of diabetes. Indeed, McEvoy and Hegre [102] reported a lasting reduction in B-cell mass down to less than 6% of the normal during an observation period of over 14 months in rats made severely diabetic with alloxan. However, when the pancreatic duct was ligated in rats before alloxan administration, Edström [43] was able to demonstrate considerable B-cell regeneration and the return of fasting hyperglycemia to normal levels after 5 months. The alloxan-treated, duct-ligated rats nevertheless continued to have grossly abnormal glucose tolerance tests 8 months after alloxan administration. While the A-cell volume of alloxan-diabetic animals does not seem to differ from normal [102], there are several reports that indicate significant hyperplastic changes in the D-cells in both alloxan- and STZ-diabetic rats [75, 102, 110]. To what extent this reaction is a sign of adaptation to a state of insulin deficiency and hyperglycemia remains unclear. Indeed, both the D-cell mass and the pancreatic somatostatin content are decreased in the diabetic Chinese hamster [112]. It is worthy of note, however, that a deficiency of D-cells may also exist in the opposite metabolic state - namely, hyperinsulinemic hypoglycemia in infancy [83].

Regeneration of the islet cells in severe STZ-diabetes in the adult rat seems to be as rare as in alloxan diabetes [98, 145]. This, however, contrasts with the situation in the newborn rat, in which administration of STZ is followed, after an initial B-cell necrosis, by a marked regeneration of B-cells. This interesting model for the study of B-cell regeneration after chemical destruction was described first by Portha et al. [117] in newborn rats and later by Bonner-Weir et al. [15] in 2-day-old rats. In the model of Portha et al. [117], an intravenous injection of 100 μg STZ on the day of birth was rapidly followed by hyperglycemia which reverted to normal values within a week. The initial diabetic phase was accompanied by a marked destruction and loss of B-cells [25]. From postnatal day 4 onward, signs of regeneration became apparent in that numerous insulin-positive cells were found throughout the acinar parenchyma and within the duct epithelium. The apparent budding of islets from the ducts was a common feature. A study of the mitotic rate in colchicin-treated animals by Dutrillaux et al. [41] suggested that most B-cells were formed by mitoses of undifferentiated cells. The long-term study of blood glucose homeostasis, however, indicated that the regeneration process was incomplete, since in adult life the rats remained glucose-intolerant [116]. Notably, this study concludes that insulin therapy during the initial, hyperglycemic phase leads to a significantly improved glucose tolerance in adult life [116].

In the model developed by Bonner-Weir et al. [15], 2-day-old rats were given an i.p. injection of 90 mg/kg STZ. This treatment caused a peak of hyperglycemia at 4 days of age, followed by nearly normal blood glucose values at 1 week of age and a recurrence of overt hyperglycemia by 6 weeks of age. Morphometric evaluation of the B-cells in these animals showed a dramatic decrease at 48 h of age, when the fraction of B-cells per islet was not more than 27%. This fraction had increased to 40% by 10 days of age, when the animals showed a near normal blood glucose concentration. This was accompanied by the more frequent appearance of mitotic figures in the B-cells of STZ-treated animals than in the controls. From 4 days until 6 weeks of age, the non-B-cell mass increased fourfold in both the control and the experimental animals. During the same time period, the B-cell mass increased 2.5-fold in the control, and 4.6-fold in the experimental animals. At variance with DUTRILLAUX et al. [41], the authors interpreted their observations on B-cell regeneration as being due to the replication of preexisting B-cells, rather than neogenesis from undifferentiated precursors. It was also noteworthy that when 2-day-old rats received STZ, they relapsed into hyperglycemia at 6 weeks of age despite a proportion of islet B-cells which was similar to that at 10 days of age when they were normoglycemic. This hyperglycemia persisted up to at least 13 weeks of age. This obvious insufficiency of regeneration could not be corrected by injections of dexamethasone which significantly increased the number of B-cells per islet, the islet size, and the pancreatic insulin content of the control animals [16]. The question therefore remains: Why, in both these models of neonatally STZ-injected pups, did the B-cells show a deficient regeneration in response to the peripheral insulin demand? Although the possibility that STZ has a toxic effect cannot be excluded from consideration, it appears more likely either that the growth capacity of the B-cells has a genetically determined limit or that a chronic functional load causes an arrest in their progress through the cell cycle. Indeed, an increased nuclear volume compatible with polyploidy was found in the B-cells of the neonatally STZ-injected rats [161].

In addition to the observations referred to above, BONNER-WEIR et al. have evaluated the effects of partial pancreatectomy on islet cell replication and B-cell function in the adult rat [17]. During the 6 weeks following 90% partial pancreatectomy, the animals showed moderate nonfasting hyperglycemia, but plasma insulin concentrations were comparable to those of the controls. Morphometric studies of the islet volume 8-10 weeks after surgery, indicated a considerable regeneration of both B-cells and non-B-cells, with remnant weight being 26%, B-cell mass 42%, and non-B-cell mass 47% of the values found in control whole pancreas. Islet morphology was variable: both normal-looking islets and abnormal islets having either marked hyperplasia or fibrosis were observed. The insulin response to intravenous glucose or to a glucose challenge of the perfused remnant was severely blunted, but responses following meals or arginine were normal. Taken together, the above observations demonstrate that during the 10-week period after surgery there was a considerable regeneration of islet cells, which, however, failed to fully normalize the glucose homeostasis. In addition, the chronic functional demand also seemed to lead to a selective defect in the glucose-induced insulin release. It is of interest in this context that CLARK et al. [28] observed that islet cells did not regenerate when rats were subjected to 95% partial pancreatectomy. Their observations indicated that neither the acinar nor the islet cells regenerated, possibly reflecting the more severe diabetic state induced by the almost complete pancreatectomy.

Another model of severe, experimental diabetes involving a major loss of B-cells can be induced in certain strains of mice by the administration of multiple low doses of STZ [96]. The pathogenesis is more complex than after a single dose of STZ and seems to involve both a direct, B-cytotoxic effect from the drug and an autoimmune component [18]. As in the adult rat treated with a single dose of STZ, little or no regeneration of B-cells has been observed in the course of diabetes in these animals [18, 104]. The possibility that regenerating B-cells in these animals are rapidly damaged and removed by the autoimmune process should be considered.

Genetic Diabetes in Animals

Animals with hereditary traits for glucose intolerance or overt diabetes remain invaluable models in diabetes research. Such animals allow detailed study not only of the phenotypic expression of the diabetic syndrome, but also of the role played by the genetic background. The exploration of these animals has, indeed, underlined the marked pathogenetic heterogeneity of diabetes, a characteristic which probably occurs in the human syndrome as well. Excellent overviews of this field of research have recently been published [134, 139].

When it comes to the issue of islet growth in relation to genetic diabetes in animals, the most extensively studied species is the mouse. Among these models there are strains which are both genetically well defined and extensively characterized with respect to their syndromes. Mouse strains with obesity and hyperglycemia are of particular interest in the context of islet growth, since a prominent feature of these animals is a marked islet cell hyperplasia. The obese mouse (gene symbol *ob*) and the diabetic mouse (gene symbol *db*) are the two most studied diabetes-obesity syndromes in mice. Both varieties carry mutant genes with a recessive inheritance. At least in the early development of the syndromes, the homozygous mice carrying either gene exhibit hyperphagia, marked obesity, insulin resistance, hyperglycemia, and hyperinsulinemia. The islets of Langerhans are characterized by pronounced hyperplasia leading to a six- to tenfold increase in islet volume in the *ob* mouse [59, 76]. When placed on the genetic background of C57BL/6J, both the *ob* and *db* genes produce a sustained B-cell hyperplasia associated with relatively mild hyperglycemia and hyperinsulinemia. It is of considerable interest, however, that when either of the genes is maintained on a background of C57BL/KsJ, the initial islet hyperplasia is rapidly followed by islet degeneration and atrophy, and severe life-threatening diabetes. The exact definition of the genetic modifiers responsible for these important phenotypic differences remain to be established [29]. Contrary to a previous contention [91], however, there seems to be little association between the severity of the diabetes syndrome and the major histocompatibility complex (H-2) [89, 90]. In this, as in several other respects, this mouse model is compatible with human NIDDM. It is also interesting that the phenotypic expression of the *db* gene has been found to be modified by a number of environmental factors such as diet and treatment with various drugs. Thus in the C57BL/KsJ *(db/db)* mouse, islet growth was greatly stimulated by a protein-rich diet, while a high dietary content of refined carbohydrates predisposed the B-cells to degenerative changes [92]. When dietary carbohydrates were low, on the other hand, there was no B-cell atrophy [92]. In the same strain of mice there was a marked amelioration of the syndrome when animals were given either dehydroepiandrosterone or 17β-estriol, both of which prevented B-cell atrophy [30, 31]. In a recent study, PRICHAZKA et al. [118] showed that treatment with estrone was able to prevent hyperphagia, hyperinsulinemia, and B-cell degeneration, while insulin resistance and a modest obesity persisted. These interesting results were interpreted as indicating that insulin resistance plays a primary role in the development of the syndrome. Accordingly, the B-cell hyperplasia in the mouse strain may be an adaptive response to an increased functional demand. If this is so, the failure to meet this sustained demand would then be a reflection of atrophy and reduction of the B-cell mass and would eventually result in marked insulin deficiency and diabetes. It is notable in this context that SWENNE and ANDERSSON [154] found a diminished capacity for B-cell proliferation when isolated islets, which were also taken from lean KsJ mice, were exposed to glucose stimulation in vitro.

Studies of temporal changes in non-B-cell populations in spontaneously diabetic mice have been mainly confined to the *db* mouse. GAPP et al. [53] showed that the total islet volume in C57BL/6J *(db/db)* mice was three- and tenfold elevated above that of the normal controls by 8 and 10 weeks of age respectively. During the initial phase of B-cell hyperplasia, the D-cell volume density showed a transient increase followed by a gradual reduction. By 10 weeks of age and onwards, the absolute D-cell volume was similar in the *db/db* mice and their controls. The volume density of PP-cells remained stable over the period of observation, while the A-cell volume density was lower in the *db/db* mice than in their lean littermates. Thus there was no consistent hyperplasia of the non-B-cells, a result which supports the notion that the hyperplasia of the B-cells in this syndrome is indeed an adaptive response to functional demands rather than to a more general mitogenic stimulus.

Other spontaneously diabetic animals in which extensive islet studies have been performed include the Chinese hamster, the BB rat, and the NOD mouse. Of these models, the BB rat and the NOD mouse show marked signs of autoimmune aggression against the B-cell along with intense insulitis and B-cell degeneration but no signs of regeneration [93]. While the pathogenesis of the diabetic state in the Chinese hamster is more obscure, it seems to be related to factors such as genetic background and nutrition [60]. During the initial stage of the diabetic syndrome, there are some hyperplastic changes of the pancreatic islets associated with mild hyperinsulinemia. During the progress of the disease, the B-cells degranulate, the B-cell number declines, and the DNA synthesis of these cells decreases [97]. However, some animals show spontaneous remission from diabetes associated with hyperplastic changes of the B-cells. LIKE et al. [97] also found that administration of glucocorticoids to normal hamsters induced B-cell hyperplasia and increased ^{3}H-thymidine incorporation. A similar treatment of diabetic hamsters failed, however, to induce corresponding changes in their B-cells. On the basis of these observations it was suggested that the diabetic Chinese hamster may have a genetic defect that affects B-cell replication and is in part responsible for the declining number of B-cells and the deficiency in insulin-synthesizing capacity.

Human Diabetes

In contrast to the situation in experimental animals, a discussion of islet cell replication in humans having diabetes must be based mainly on observations of pancreatic autopsy material and must proceed with only limited quantitative information available. Furthermore, it is not surprising that in those few reports in which measurements of islet and B-cell volumes have been performed in humans with diabetes, the destructive, rather than regenerative, processes have attracted most attention, particularly in the context of IDDM [55, 57, 58]. The combined information available on both IDDM and NIDDM is nevertheless sufficient to form a point of departure for a discussion of islet cell regeneration in human diabetes.

There is now strong evidence suggesting that IDDM represents the end-point in a long process of autoimmune islet B-cell destruction which results in a dramatic reduction of the B-cell mass [45]. However, in concert with the predominant destruction of the B-cells unequivocal signs of regeneration and repair may be observed. In a recent review of this topic, GEPTS and LECOMPTE [58] pointed out that the regenerative activity in patients with IDDM seems to originate in centroacinar and duct cells. Proliferation of such cells may lead to the formation of islets composed largely of B-cells with a clear cytoplasm and often containing a fine granulation *(Körnchen)*. The distribution of newly formed islets in the pancreas is quite irregular and may be confined to a few lobules. A notable observation was that apparently neoformed islets were occasionally heavily infiltrated with lymphocytes, suggesting that newly formed B-cells may also be targets for a destructive autoimmune attack. In an earlier report, GEPTS [56] observed mitotic division among islet B-cells in only one of 23 cases of IDDM, which supports the view that regeneration of B-cells in the human diabetic's pancreas is largely a result of neoformation of these cells from undifferentiated precursors. In agreement with this hypothesis, POHL et al. [115] reported the occurrence of polyploid B-cells in the human diabetic's pancreas. Even though occasional enlarged islets have been observed in early cases of IDDM [49, 58, 84], the weight of evidence nevertheless indicates that signs of regeneration of B-cells in IDDM are relatively rare and that regeneration, if it occurs, is always outweighed by the destructive processes. The volumes of non-B-cells, on the other hand, do not seem to be affected at all in IDDM [84, 123, 143].

NIDDM is characterized by peripheral insulin resistance and glucose intolerance and is often associated with obesity. In addition, there is a strong genetic component, although the mode of inheritance remains unclear. While in IDDM the islet pathology is uniformly characterized by a strong reduction in B-cell mass, the alterations in NIDDM are more variable and controversial. In this latter condition islets may show hydropic degeneration, amyloid deposits, fibrosis, and hypertrophy, but neither insulitis nor B-cell destruction [57, 85]. The insulin release is low, at least in relation to the hyperglycemia, and shows a characteristic delay in its initial response to glucose [44].

While there is no doubt that B-cells are always present in the islets of patients with NIDDM, it is less clear to what extent the total B-cell mass is changed. Although a compensatory hyperplasia of the B-cells might be expected in a condition of sustained hyperglycemia, quantitative studies suggest that there is either no change in or, indeed, a reduction of this cell type in comparison with nondiabetic controls. STEFAN et al.[144] and RAHIER et al. [123], on the whole, found a normal mass of B-cells in their materials, while WESTERMARK and WILANDER [162] and KLÖPPEL et al. [85] found a marked decrease. The study by KLÖPPEL et al. is of particular significance, since comparisons were made between the B-cell mass in nonobese and obese patients with NIDDM on the one hand and weight-matched, healthy controls on the other. The results indicate that the obese, but otherwise healthy, controls had a significant enlargement of their B-cell mass in comparison with the normal-weight controls. Overweight patients with NIDDM showed a marked reduction of their B-cell mass in comparison with the overweight controls. By the same token, normal-weight patients with NIDDM had a much smaller B-cell volume than their normal-weight controls. These results suggest that there is, indeed, a hyperplasia of the B-cells in obese, but otherwise healthy, individuals and that this hyperplastic islet change is absent in patients with NIDDM. The possible significance of this finding for our understanding of the pathogenesis of NIDDM will be discussed below.

Growth of Transplanted Islets

It has long been known that a wide variety of tissues or organ slices have the capability to survive and sometimes even grow when grafted into different sites of isogeneic or immunosuppressed recipients. It is also well known that the graft survival and growth is improved when tissue from younger donors is utilized. With regard to the endocrine pancreas it has been observed that when fetal rat pancreatic glands were transplanted beneath the kidney capsule of isogeneic adult recipients the total islet mass increased over 20-fold during the 21 days following transplantation [20]. This islet growth in fetal rat pancreas grafts quantitatively seems to mirror mainly the natural development of the islet organ during fetal and neonatal life. In order to investigate which factors possibly influence the growth of mature islets we implanted islets at different sites into mice suffering from either spontaneous diabetes or diabetes induced by chemical compounds. By varying the number of islets implanted, the degree of diabetic milieu in the recipient could be modulated. The following presentation will briefly summarize the results of our previous studies on the capability of transplanted islets to grow. For reviews on different aspects of transplantation of the endocrine pancreas reference should be made to LAZAROW et al. [88], SUTHERLAND [148], and HEGRE [67].

Methodological Considerations

The ideal measurement of transplanted islet growth would be a volume or mass estimation before and after grafting. However, it is technically difficult to determine the isolated islet mass first before transplantation and then after the islets have grown at the site of transplantation. Islets may also be lost during the grafting procedure, or they may be difficult to find in, for instance, the liver [12]. We have circumvented some of these problems by studying transplanted islets after syngeneically grafting them to the spleen, where they could be easily located after histological processing. The mean islet volume was measured by conventional morphometric techniques, and corrections were made for overrepresentation of sections from larger islets. Relevant comparisons were made between groups of animals with experimental or spontaneous diabetes and their normal controls.

Transplanted islet cells in the S phase were identified by autoradiography after the recipient was intraperitoneally injected with ^{3}H-thymidine 1-2 h before being sacrificed. In these experiments, islets were grafted not only to the spleen, but also to the liver, and to a subcapsular site in one of the kidneys. These organs were subsequently removed, fixed in Bouin solution, and prepared for autoradiography. After identification of islets in hematoxylin-eosin (HE)-stained sections, B-cells were recognized by their typical location in the islets and a labeling index was determined. In more recent studies, specific B-cell staining was employed along with immunocytochemical staining for insulin before the autoradiographic processing.

In studies of proliferation of transplanted islet cells, certain inherent limitations of the technique should be kept in mind. Grafts consisting of isolated islets are devoid of acinar cells and, at least initially, of nerves and blood vessels. Corresponding conditions pertain to pancreatic fragments. In addition, such fragments pass through an initial phase of exocrine cell degeneration. Additional problems can be posed by conditions at the site of islet transplantation and immune incompatibility. The latter problem has been eliminated by the use of inbred animals, but little is known about the significance of several of the other factors for the proliferation of transplanted islet cells.

Growth of Transplanted Islets in Animals with Experimental and Spontaneous Diabetes

Our initial studies indicated that syngeneic islets isolated from lean mice grew quite extensively when implanted intrasplenically into obese-hyperglycemic mice [4]. The aim of this study was to reevaluate previous reports [54, 147] suggesting that implantation of islets isolated from lean mice into obese mice ameliorated the obese-hyperglycemic syndrome of the recipients. It was, however, not possible to confirm this observation, since islet transplantation failed to affect either the weight gain or the hyperglycemia of the obese-hyperglycemic mice. Morphometric examination of the grafted islets showed that 8 weeks after transplantation the mean islet volume had increased more than fivefold. When islets were implanted into lean alloxan-diabetic mice in numbers sufficient to revert hyperglycemia, there was a doubling of the mean islet volume [4]. In contrast, when islets were implanted into old (>1 year) obese-hyperglycemic mice which were still hyperinsulinemic but normo- or even hypoglycemic before transplantation, they did not grow at all [3]. These combined observations suggest that in addition to hyperglycemia, hyperinsulinemia might be required to induce the enhanced growth found in the obese-hyperglycemic mice. These studies also indicate that not only fetal, but also adult islets are able to respond with a remarkable hyperplasia when transferred to a diabetic environment.

Volumetric estimates of transplanted islets were also used to evaluate the significance of genetic background for the growth of intrasplenically implanted islets. In these studies, the growth of transplanted islets originating in C57BL/6J mice was compared with that of islets from C57BL/KsJ mice [3]. As discussed above there is strong evidence to suggest a difference in islet growth capacity between these strains of mice [29]. To what extent this difference can be attributed to differences in the islet cell capacities to increase replication in a diabetic environment was elucidated by implanting, into alloxan-diabetic mice, a number of islets that was insufficient to revert the animals to normoglycemia. The volume of the C57BL/6J islets remained unchanged during these circumstances, while that of the C57BL/KsJ islets decreased. When, however, KsJ islets were implanted in numbers sufficient to completely normalize the serum glucose, there was an increase in the islet volume, indicating that a diabetic environment may be detrimental for KsJ islets. That this observation could reflect a reduced islet cell replicatory capacity was demonstrated in a more recent study [154] by means of autoradiographic techniques. It was found that after exposure to high glucose concentrations, both transplanted islets and cultured islets from C57BL/KsJ mice had ^{3}H-thymidine labeling indices that were only about half that of the 6J islets. It is worthy of note that a corresponding difference between the strains could not be demonstrated for glucose-stimulated (pro)insulin biosynthesis [154].

Islets have been implanted into many different organs, but little is known of the relationship between islet growth and the transplantation site. In a recent study [105] we compared the labeling indices of islets implanted into either the spleen or the liver, or under the kidney capsule. The highest labeling index was consistently found in the kidney grafts, followed by that found in the islets implanted into the liver, which had an index about half as high. The intrasplenically implanted islets had an index only about one-third of those implanted in the liver. The reason for these differences remains obscure, since all three organs are well vascularized.

Growth of Human Fetal Pancreas Transplanted into Nude Mice

As mentioned above, experimental diabetes in animals can be cured by syngeneic transplantation of fetal pancreas. These promising results have prompted investigations exploring the usefulness of human fetal pancreas for transplantation to diabetic patients. Since isolation of islets from the human fetal pancreas is not feasible, a suitable preparation of endocrine cells could be obtained only after a suspension of pancreatic fragments obtained from 10- to 24-week-old fetuses were tissue-cultured [71, 136]. The resulting islet-like cell clusters (ICC) were characterized by morphological and functional techniques, and samples of about 50 each were xenotransplanted beneath the kidney capsule of athymic nude mice [136]. At the time of implantation these ICC were composed of a majority of nondifferentiated cells, sometimes arranged in duct-like structures, and a few insulin-positive B-cells. The recipient mice were killed 8 weeks later after being injected with ^{3}H-thymidine. The transplantation site was then identified and processed for histology and autoradiography. In seven of nine animals receiving transplants, histological sections from the graft stained for insulin or glucagon showed groups of cells composed of B- or A-cells arranged in an islet-like pattern and surrounded by nonstained epitheloid cells. There were also duct-like structures composed of occasional hormone-containing cells. The number and proportion of B-cells had increased dramatically in the grafted ICC as compared to the nongrafted ones. In four mice estimates of ^{3}H-thymidine labeling indices were performed on HE-stained sections of ICC grafts. The labeling index for the entire cell population in the grafts was found to be about fivefold higher than the corresponding values for islets prepared from adult mice.

This study clearly demonstrates that viable explants suitable for transplantation can be prepared from the human fetal pancreas obtained after prostaglandin-induced abortions. The ICC are well suited for the study of growth and differentiation of the endocrine human fetal pancreas. The high labeling index and proportion of insulin-containing B-cells demonstrated in vivo suggests that fetal human islet cells are able to both differentiate and replicate after transplantation. It is conceivable that the nude mouse will become a valuable tool in the further detailed exploration of the optimal conditions for growth of B-cells obtained from the human fetal pancreas.

Failure of Adaptive B-Cell Growth as a Cause of Diabetes

The concept of adaptive cell proliferation implies that the functional demand imposed on a given cell population represents a basic element in the control of its DNA replication. This notion may be exemplified by the growth of the liver after partial hepatectomy or of the mammary gland during pregnancy and lactation. Such adaptive growth processes are initiated and maintained by signal molecules of high specificity which bind to receptors on, or inside, the target cells. Many of these molecular species have been identified and the nature of their signals characterized.

In the previous sections of this chapter several examples of adaptive proliferation also of the islet B-cells have been put forward. Perhaps the most impressive is the almost tenfold increase in B-cell mass in the obese C57BL *ob* or *db* mice. Observations of the growth of islets in glucose-infused rats or of islets transplanted into alloxan-diabetic mice also clearly demonstrate the ability of the B-cell to respond to an increased functional demand with replication in both hereditary and experimental diabetes. Still other examples, which have not been referred to above, are islet growth in pregnancy and in the offspring of the diabetic mother [72, 78]. Although hyperglycemia seems to be the common denominator in most, if not all, of these conditions, glucose is by no means the only factor of regulatory significance for B-cell growth. As indicated above, there are a number of other molecules, including both metabolic substrates and receptor-specific peptides, which affect the DNA replication of the B-cell. To what extent the growth-stimulating effect of glucose is maintained and/or mediated by such factors is at present unclear, but it is notable that serum is required in vitro for this stimulating effect of glucose to become manifest.

Despite the obvious ability of even adult islet B-cells to respond with DNA replication to a sustained functional stimulation, there are several well-documented situations in which regeneration of B-cells is absent or insufficient. This is the case in severe alloxan- or STZ-diabetes, after subtotal (i.e., $>95\%$) pancreatectomy, and in diabetes induced by multiple low doses of STZ. In all these situations a small number of B-cells is still present in the pancreas but functional amelioration of the diabetic state is rare and significant morphological signs of regeneration are absent. There is so far no explanation for this almost complete lack of recovery but the possibility of B-cell "exhaustion" has been repeatedly put forward. With regard to mice injected with multiple low doses of STZ an autoimmune destructive process could also be involved [104].

The capacity for adaptive proliferation of the islet B-cells is obviously under genetic control. In support of this, the phenotypic expression of both the *db* and *ob* genes is quite different depending on the genetic background. With respect to the islets there is a sustained proliferation of the B-cells in the 6J mice, whereas this process seems to become arrested at a relatively young age in the KsJ mice. The latter animals develop a severe insulin lack and ketotic diabetes. By the same token, only those Chinese hamsters which develop the most severe form of diabetes show a grossly deficient B-cell replication. The possibility that the B-cells of both the KsJ mice and the diabetic Chinese hamster have a genetic restriction on the number of mitotic cycles through which they can pass should be considered.

The role of B-cell regeneration in the natural history of human diabetes is still largely unknown. It seems nevertheless possible to consider some fundamental aspects in this context based on observations in both animals and man. The lack of lasting regeneration of the B-cell volume in IDDM may thus indicate that newly formed B-cells remain targets of autoimmune attack. It is, furthermore, possible that NIDDM is a reflection of the combined effects of peripheral insulin resistance and a genetic deficiency in the capacity for B-cell regeneration. In support of this notion, obese and insulin-resistant individuals with normal glucose tolerance have a much larger B-cell mass than those with NIDDM. Insulin resistance is also a characteristic of normal pregnancy, and animal studies have shown that the B-cell mass increases during pregnancy. Certain women develop a transient gestational diabetes, which may thus reflect a genetic inability to expand the B-cell mass in accordance with the increased insulin requirement. Indeed, women with gestational diabetes are prone to develop NIDDM with advancing age [50]. Against this background it appears worthwhile to study further the capacity and regulation of B-cell proliferation and the role of this process in the etiology and pathogenesis of both NIDDM and gestational diabetes.

Acknowledgement. The authors are grateful to Mrs AGNETA SNELLMAN for skillfully typing the manuscript.

References

1. Abu-Bakare A, Taylor R, Gill GV, Alberti KGMM (1986) Tropical or malnutrition-related diabetes: a real syndrome? Lancet 1: 1135-1138
2. Alumets J, Håkansson R, Sundler F (1983) Ontogeny of endocrine cells in porcine gut and pancreas. Gastroenterology 85: 1359-1372
3. Andersson A (1983) The influence of hyperglycaemia, hyperinsulinaemia and genetic background on the fate of intrasplenically implanted mouse islets. Diabetologia 25: 269-272
4. Andersson A, Eriksson U, Petersson B, Reibring L, Swenne I (1981) Failure of successful intrasplenic transplantation of islets from lean mice to cure obese-hyperglycemic mice, despite islet growth. Diabetologia 20: 237-241
5. Andersson I, Billig H, Fryklund L, Hansson H-A, Isaksson O, Isgaard J, Nilsson A, Rozell B, Skottner A, Stemme S (1986) Localization of IGF-I in adult rats. Immunohistochemical studies. Acta Physiol Scand 126: 311-312
6. Ashcroft SJH, Bassett JM, Randle PJ (1972) Insulin secretion mechanisms and glucose metabolism in isolated islets. Diabetes 21 [Suppl 2]: 538-545
7. Ashcroft SJH, Bunce J, Lowry M, Hansen SE, Hedeskov CJ (1978) The effects of sugars on (pro)insulin biosynthesis. Biochem J 174: 517-526
8. Ashworth MA, Kerbel MC, Haist RE (1952) Effect of chronic caloric insufficiency on the growth of the islets of Langerhans. Am J Physiol 171: 25-28
9. Asplund K (1973) Dynamics of insulin release from the foetal and neonatal rat pancreas. Eur J Clin Invest 3: 338-344
10. Asplund K (1973) Effects of intermittent glucose infusions in pregnant rats on the functional development of the foetal pancreatic B-cells. J Endocrinol 59: 285-293
11. Asplund A, Andersson A, Jarousse C, Hellerström C (1975) Function of the fetal endocrine pancreas. Israel J Med Sci 11: 581-590
12. Ballinger WF, Lacy PE (1972) Transplantation of intact pancreatic islets in rats. Surgery 72: 175-186
13. Bell GI, Pictet RL, Rutter WJ, Cordell B, Tischer E, Goodman HM (1980) Sequence of the human insulin gene. Nature 284: 26-32
14. Bell G, Santerre RF, Mullenbach GT (1983) Hamster preproglucagon contains the sequence of glucagon and two related peptides. Nature 302: 716-718
15. Bonner-Weir S, Trent DF, Honey RN, Weir GC (1981) Responses of neonatal rat islets to streptozotocin. Limited B-cell regeneration and hyperglycemia. Diabetes 30: 64-69
16. Bonner-Weir S, Trent DF, Zmachinski CJ, Clore ET, Weir GC (1981) Limited B-cell regeneration in a B-cell deficient rat model: studies with dexamethasone. Metabolism 30: 914-918
17. Bonner-Weir S, Trent DF, Weir GC (1983) Partial pancreatectomy in the rat and subsequent defect in glucose-induced insulin release. J Clin Invest 71: 1544-1553
18. Bonnevie-Nielsen V, Steffes MW, Lernmark Å (1981) A major loss in islet mass and B-cell function precedes hyperglycemia in mice given multiple low doses of streptozotocin. Diabetes 30: 424-429
19. Boquist L (1968) Alloxan administration in the Chinese hamster. II. Ultrastructural study of degeneration and subsequent regeneration of the pancreatic islet tissue. Virchows Arch (Cell Pathol) 1: 169-181
20. Brown J, Molnar I, Clark W, Mullen Y (1974) Control of experimental diabetes mellitus in rats by transplantation of fetal pancreases. Science 184: 1377-1379
21. Bucchini D, Ripoche M-A, Stinnakre MG, Desbois P, Loré D, Montehioux E, Absil J, Lepesant J-A, Pictet R, Jami J (1986) Pancreatic expression of human insulin gene in transgenic mice. Proc Natl Acad Sci USA 83: 2511-2515
22. Bunnag SC (1966) Postnatal neogenesis of islets of Langerhans in the mouse. Diabetes 15: 480-491
23. Burch PT, Berner DK, Leontire A, Vogin A, Matschinsky BM, Matschinsky FM (1984) Metabolic adaptation of pancreatic islet tissue in aging rats. J Gerontol 39: 2-6
24. Cahill GF (1977) Diabetes and nutrition: Charaka lecture. In: Bajaj JS (ed) Diabetes. Excerpta Medica, Amsterdam, pp 32-35
25. Cantenys D, Portha B, Dutrillaux MC, Hollande E, Rozé C, Picon L (1981) Histogenesis of

the endocrine pancreas in newborn rats after destruction by streptozotocin. Virchows Arch (Cell Pathol) 35: 109-122
26. Chick WL, Like AA (1971) Effects of diet on pancreatic beta cell replication in mice with hereditary diabetes. Am J Physiol 221: 202-208
27. Clark A, Grant AM (1983) Quantitative morphology of endocrine cells in human fetal pancreas. Diabetologia 25: 31-35
28. Clark A, Brown E, King R, Vanhegan RI, Turner RC (1982) Islet changes induced by hyperglycemia in rats. Effects of insulin or chlorpropamide therapy. Diabetes 31: 319-325
29. Coleman DL (1978) Obese and diabetes: two mutant genes causing diabetes-obesity syndromes in mice. Diabetologia 14: 141-148
30. Coleman DL, Leiter EH, Schwizer RW (1982) Therapeutic effects of dehydroepiandrosterone (DHEA) in diabetic mice. Diabetes 31: 830-833
31. Coleman DL, Leiter EH, Applezwig N (1984) Therapeutic effects of dehydropiandrosterone (DHEA) metabolites in diabetes mutant mice (C57BL/KsJ-db/db). Endocrinology 115: 239-243
32. Cordell B, Bell GI, Tischer E, DeNoto FM, Ullrich A, Pictet R, Rutter WJ, Goodman HM (1979) Isolation and characterization of a cloned rat insulin gene. Cell 18: 533-543
33. Crace CJ, Swenne I, Milner RDG (1986) Protein deprivation in weanling rats permanently impairs growth and insulin secretory response to glucose (abstract). Diabetologia 59: 530A
34. DeClerq L, Schmidt G, Delaere P, Remacle C (1980) Nuclear events in B-cells of young and senescent rat islets in organ culture. Cell Biol 4: 817-827
35. DeGasparo M, Faupel M (1986) Chromatographic characterization of adult and foetal rat insulin. J Chromatogr 357: 139-146
36. DeGasparo M, Milner GR, Norris PD, Milner RDG (1978) Effects of glucose and amino acids on foetal rat pancreatic growth and insulin secretion in vitro. J Endocrinol 77: 241-248
37. D'Ercole AJ, Stiles AD, Underwood LE (1984) Tissue concentrations of somatomedin C: further evidence for multiple sites of synthesis and paracrine or autocrine mechanisms of action. Proc Natl Acad Sci USA 81: 935-939
38. Diabetes mellitus. Report of a WHO study group (1985) Technical report series 727. World Health Organization, Geneva, pp 20-25
39. Dixit PK, Cheng Kaung H-L (1985) Rat pancreatic B-cells in protein deficiency: a study involving morphometric analysis and alloxan effects. J Nutr 115: 375-381
40. Drawnin B, Steinberg JP, Leitner JW, Sussman KE (1985) The nature of insulin secretory defect in aging rats. Diabetes 34: 1168-1173
41. Dutrillaux MC, Portha B, Rozé C, Hollande E (1982) Ultrastructural study of pancreatic B-cell regeneration in newborn rats after destruction by streptozotocin. Virchows Arch (Cell Pathol) 39: 173-185
42. Edlund T, Walker MD, Barr PJ, Rutter WJ (1985) Cell-specific expression of the rat insulin gene: evidence for role of two distinct 5' flanking elements. Science 230: 912-916
43. Edström C (1971) Alloxan sensitivity of rats at various intervals following ligation of the pancreatic ducts. Acta Soc Med Upsal 76: 77-86
44. Efendić S, Luft R, Wajngot A (1981) Aspects of the pathogenesis of type 2 diabetes. In: Boström H, Ljungstedt N (eds) Recent trends in diabetes research. Almqvist and Wiksell, Stockholm, pp 75-84
45. Eisenbarth GS (1984) Autoimmune B-cell insufficiency - diabetes mellitus type I. Triangle 23: 111-124
46. Eriksson U, Andersson A, Efendić S, Elde R, Hellerström C (1980) Diabetes in pregnancy: effects on the foetal and newborn rat with particular regard to body weight, serum insulin concentration and pancreatic contents of insulin, glucagon and somatostatin. Acta Endocrinol 94: 354-364
47. Eriksson U, Hellerström C, Andersson A (1981) Diabetes in pregnancy: effects on the maturation of (pro)insulin biosynthesis in fetal and neonatal rat islets. Diabète Metab 7: 243-249
48. Falkmer S (1981) Experimental diabetes research in fish. Acta Endocrinol 37 [Suppl 59]: 1-122
49. Foulis AK, Stewart JA (1984) The pancreas in recent-onset type I (insulin-dependent) diabetes mellitus: insulin content of islets, insulitis and associated changes in the exocrine acinar tissue. Diabetologia 26: 456-461

50. Freinkel N (ed) (1985) Proceedings of the second international workshop-conference on gestational diabetes mellitus. Diabetes 34 [Suppl 2]: 1-30
51. Freinkel N, Lewis NJ, Johnson R, Swenne I, Bone AJ, Hellerström C (1984) Differential effects of age versus glycemic stimulation on the maturation of insulin stimulus-secretion coupling during culture of fetal rat islets. Diabetes 33: 1028-1038
52. Fuji S (1979) Development of pancreatic endocrine cells in the rat fetus. Arch Histol Jpn 42: 467-479
53. Gapp DA, Leiter EH, Coleman DL, Schwizer RW (1983) Temporal changes in pancreatic islet composition in C57BL/6J-db/db (diabetes) mice. Diabetologia 25: 439-443
54. Gates RJ, Hunt MJ, Smith R, Lazarus NR (1972) Return to normal of blood-glucose, plasma-insulin, and weight gain in New Zealand obese mice after implantation of islets of Langerhans. Lancet 2: 250-253
55. Gepts W (1984) The cytotoxic pathology of the islets of Langerhans in juvenile diabetes. In: Brolin SE, Hellman B, Knutsson H (eds) The structure and metabolism of the pancreatic islets. Pergamon, Oxford, pp 513-520
56. Gepts W (1965) Pathologic anatomy of the pancreas in juvenile diabetes mellitus. Diabetes 14: 619-633
57. Gepts W (1972) Pathology of islet tissue in human diabetes. In: Steiner DF, Freinkel N (eds) Handbook of physiology, section 7, vol 1. American Physiological Society, Washington DC, pp 289-303
58. Gepts W, LeCompte PM (1985) The pathology of type I (juvenile) diabetes. In: Volk BW, Arquilla ER (eds) The diabetic pancreas, 2nd edn. Plenum, New York, pp 337-365
59. Gepts W, Christophe J, Mayer J (1960) Pancreatic islets in mice with the obese-hyperglycemic syndrome. Lack of effect of carbutamide. Diabetes 9: 63-69
60. Gerritsen GC (1982) The Chinese hamster as a model for the study of diabetes mellitus. Diabetes 31 [Suppl 1]: 14-21
61. Girard JR, Cuendet GS, Marliss EB, Kervran A, Rieutort M, Assan R (1973) Fuels, hormones, and liver metabolism at term and during the early postnatal period in the rat. J Clin Invest 52: 3190-3200
62. Grumbach MM, Kaplan SL, Sciarra JJ, Burr IM (1968) Chorionic growth hormone-prolactin (CGP): secretion, deposition, biological activity in man and postulated function as the "growth hormone" of the second half of pregnancy. Ann N Y Acad Sci 148: 501-531
63. Haist RE (1949) Factors affecting the volume of the islets of Langerhans. Proc Am Diabetes Assoc 9: 53-62
64. Haist RE, Pugh EJ (1948) Volume measurement of the islets of Langerhans and the effects of age and fasting. Am J Physiol 152: 36-41
65. Heard CRC, Stewart RJC (1971) Protein-calorie deficiency and disorders of the endocrine glands. Hormones 2: 40-64
66. Hedeskov CJ (1980) Mechanism of glucose-induced insulin secretion. Physiol Rev 60: 442-509
67. Hegre OD (1985) Islet cell transplantation. In: Volk BW, Arquilla ER (eds) The diabetic pancreas, 2nd edn. Plenum, New York, pp 513-542
68. Hellerström C (1977) Growth pattern of pancreatic islets in animals. In: Volk BW, Wellman KF (ed) The diabetic pancreas. Plenum, New York, pp 61-97
69. Hellerström C (1984) The life story of the pancreatic B-cell. Diabetologia 26: 393-400
70. Hellerström C, Swenne I (1985) Growth pattern of pancreatic islets in animals. In: Volk BW, Arquilla ER (eds) The diabetic pancreas, 2nd edn. Plenum, New York, pp 53-79
71. Hellerström C, Lewis NJ, Borg H, Johnson R, Freinkel N (1979) Method for large-scale isolation of pancreatic islets by tissue culture of fetal rat pancreas. Diabetes 28: 769-776
72. Hellerström C, Swenne I, Eriksson UJ (1985) Is there an animal model for gestational diabetes? Diabetes 34 [Suppl 2]: 28-31
73. Hellman B (1959) The total volume of the pancreatic islet tissue at different ages of the rat. Acta Pathol Microbiol Scand 47: 35-50
74. Hellman B (1959) The effect of protracted administration of small doses of alloxan on the islets of Langerhans in rats fed on diets rich poor in carbohydrates. Acta Soc Med Upsal 64: 393-431

75. Hellman B, Petersson B (1963) Long-term changes of the A_1- and A_2-cells in the islets of Langerhans of rats with alloxan diabetes. Endocrinology 72: 238-242
76. Hellman B, Petersson B, Hellerström C (1964) The growth pattern of the endocrine pancreas in mammals. In: Brolin SE, Hellman B, Knutsson H (eds) The structure and metabolism of the pancreatic islets. Pergamon, Oxford, pp 45-61
77. Hill DE, Holt AB, Parra A, Cheek DB (1970) The influence of protein-calorie versus calorie restriction on the body composition and cellular growth of muscle and liver in weanling rats. John Hopkins Med J 127: 146-163
78. Hultquist GT, Olding LB (1981) Endocrine pathology of infants of diabetic mothers. Acta Endocrinol 97 [Suppl 241]: 1-202
79. Jacob S (1977) Regeneration of the islets of Langerhans in the guinea pig. Cell Tissue Res 181: 277-286
80. King DL, Chick WL (1976) Pancreatic beta cell replication: effects of hexose sugars. Endocrinology 99: 1003-1009
81. King DL, Chick WL, Kitchen KC (1977) Pancreatic beta cell replication. In: Wasielewski EV, Chick WL (eds) Pancreatic beta cell culture. Excerpta Medica, Amsterdam, pp 109-114
82. King DL, Kitchen KC, Chick WL (1978) Pancreatic B-cell replication: relation to insulin secretion. Endocrinology 103: 1321-1327
83. Klöppel G, Heitz PK (1984) Persistent hyperinsulinemic hypoglycaemia in infancy. In: Klöppel G, Heitz PU (eds) Pancreatic pathology. Livingstone, Edinburgh, pp 193-205
84. Klöppel G, Drenck CR, Aberholzer M, Heitz PU (1984) Morphometric evidence for a striking B-cell reduction at the clinical onset of type I diabetes. Virchows Arch (Pathol Anat) 403: 441-452
85. Klöppel G, Löhr M, Hablich K, Oberholzer M, Heitz PU (1985) Islet pathology and pathogenesis of type 1 and type 2 diabetes mellitus revisited. Surv Synth Path Res 4: 110-125
86. Korcáková L (1971) Mitotic division and its significance for regeneration of granulated B-cells in the islets of Langerhans in alloxan-diabetic rats. Folia Morphol 14: 24-30
87. Lazarow A (1952) Spontaneous recovery from alloxan diabetes in the rat. Diabetes 1: 363-372
88. Lazarow A, Wells LJ, Carpenter AM, Hegre OD, Leonard RJ, McEvoy RC (1973) Islet differentiation, organ culture and transplantation. Diabetes 22: 877-912
89. Leiter EH (1984) Genetic control of pathogenesis of diabetes in C3H mice. Influence of the major histocompatibility complex. Diabetes 33: 1068-1071
90. Leiter EH, Coleman DL, Hummel KP (1981) The influence of genetic background on the expression of mutations at the diabetes locus in the mouse. III. Effect of H-2 haplotype and sex. Diabetes 30: 1029-1034
91. Leiter EH, Coleman DL, Eisenstein AB, Strack E (1981) Dietary control of pathogenesis in C57BL/KsJ db/db diabetes mice. Metabolism 30: 554-562
92. Leiter EH, Coleman DL, Ingram DK, Reynolds MA (1983) Influence of dietary carbohydrate on the induction of diabetes in C57BL/KsJ-db/db diabetes mice. J Nutr 113: 184-195
93. Like AA (1985) Spontaneous diabetes in animals. In: Volk BW, Arquilla ER (eds) The diabetic pancreas, 2nd edn. Plenum, New York, pp 385-413
94. Like AA, Chick WL (1969) Mitotic divisions in pancreatic beta cells. Science 163: 941-943
95. Like AA, Chick WL (1970) Studies in the diabetic mutant mouse. II. Electron microscopy of pancreatic islets. Diabetologia 6: 216-242
96. Like AA, Rossini AA (1976) Streptozotocin-induced pancreatic insulitis. New model of diabetes mellitus. Science 193: 415-417
97. Like AA, Gerritsen GC, Dulin WE, Gaudreau P (1974) Studies in the diabetic Chinese hamster: light microscopy and autoradiography of pancreatic islets. Diabetologia 10: 501-508
98. Logothetopoulos J, Brosky G, Kern HF (1970) Islet cell proliferation in experimental and genetic diabetes. In: Falkmer S, Hellman B, Täljedal IB (eds) The structure and metabolism of the pancreatic islets. Pergamon, Oxford, pp 15-23
99. Logothetopoulus J, Valiquette N, Cvet D (1983) Glucose stimulation of beta-cell DNA replication in the intact rat and in pancreatic islets in suspension culture. Effects of alpha-ketoisocaproic acid, dibutyryl cyclic AMP, and 3-isobutyl-1-methyl-xanthine in the in vitro system. Diabetes 32: 1172-1176

100. Lomedico P, Rosenthal N, Efstratiadis A, Gilbert W, Kolodner R, Tizard R (1979) The structure and evolution of the two nonallelic rat preproinsulin genes. Cell 18: 545-558
101. McEvoy RC (1981) Changes in the A-, B- and D-cell populations in the pancreatic islets during the postnatal development of the rat. Diabetes 30: 813-817
102. McEvoy RC, Hegre OD (1977) Morphometric quantitation of the pancreatic insulin-, glucagon- and somatomedin-positive cell populations in normal and alloxan-diabetic rats. Diabetes 26: 1140-1146
103. McEvoy RC, Leung PE (1982) Tissue culture of fetal rat islets: comparison of serum-supplemented and serum free, defined medium on the maintenance, growth, and differentiation of A, B, and D cells. Endocrinology 111: 1568-1575
104. McEvoy RC, Andersson J, Sandler S, Hellerström C (1984) Multiple low-dose streptozotocin-induced diabetes in the mouse. Evidence for stimulation of a cytotoxic cellular immune response against an insulin-producing beta cell line. J Clin Invest 74: 715-722
105. Mellgren A, Schnell Landström AH, Petersson B, Andersson A (1986) The renal subcapsular site offers better growth conditions for transplanted mouse pancreatic islet cells than the liver or spleen. Diabetologia 29: 670-672
106. Milner RDG, Hill DJ (1984) Fetal growth control: the role of insulin and related peptides. Clin Endocrinol 21: 415-433
107. Nielsen JH (1982) Effects of growth hormone, prolactin, and placental lactogen on insulin content and release, and deoxyribonucleic acid synthesis in cultured pancreatic islets. Endocrinology 110: 600-606
108. Nir U, Walker MD, Rutter WJ (1986) Regulation of rat insulin 1 gene expression: evidence for negative regulation in non-pancreatic cells. Proc Natl Acad Sci USA 83: 3180-3184
109. Olsson H, Edlund T (1986) Sequence-specific interactions of nuclear factors with the insulin gene enhancer. Cell 45: 35-44
110. Patel YC, Weir GC (1976) Increased somatostatin content of islets from streptozotocin-diabetic rats. Clin Endocrinol 5: 191-194
111. Petersson B, Hellerström C, Hellman B (1960) The influence of the litter size on the postnatal growth of the islets of Langerhans in the rat. Acta Endocrinol 35: 533-540
112. Petersson B, Elde R, Efendić S, Hökfelt T, Johansson O, Luft R, Cerasi E, Hellerström C (1977) Somatostatin in the pancreas, stomach and hypothalamus of the diabetic Chinese hamster. Diabetologia 13: 463-466
113. Pictet R, Rutter WJ (1972) Development of the embryonic endocrine pancreas. In: Steiner DF, Freinkel N (eds) Handbook of physiology, sect 7, vol 1. American Physiological Society, Washington DC, pp 25-66
114. Platt BS, Stewart RJC (1967) Experimental protein-calorie deficiency: histopathological changes in the endocrine glands of pigs. J Endocrinol 38: 121-143
115. Pohl MN, Swartz FJ, Carstens PHB (1981) Polyploidy in islets of normal and diabetic humans. Hum Pathol 12: 184-186
116. Portha B, Picon L (1982) Insulin treatment improves the spontaneous remission of neonatal streptozotocin diabetes in the rat. Diabetes 31: 165-169
117. Portha B, Levacher C, Picon L, Rosselin G (1974) Diabetogenic effect of steptozotocin in the rat during the perinatal period. Diabetes 23: 889-895
118. Prochazka M, Premdas FH, Leiter EH, Lipson LG (1986) Estrone treatment dissociates primary versus secondary consequences of "diabetes" (db) gene expression in mice. Diabetes 35: 725-728
119. Rabinovitch A, Quigley C, Russel T, Patel Y, Mintz DH (1982) Insulin and multiplication stimulating activity (an insulin-like growth factor) stimulate islet B-cell replication in neonatal rat pancreatic monolayer cultures. Diabetes 31: 160-164
120. Rabinovitch A, Quigley C, Rechler MM (1983) Growth hormone stimulates islet B-cell replication in neonatal rat pancreatic monolayer cultures. Diabetes 32: 307-312
121. Rahier J, Wallon J, Henquin JC (1980) Abundance of somatostatin cells in the human neonatal pancreas. Diabetologia 18: 251-254
122. Rahier J, Wallon J, Henquin JC (1981) Cell population in the endocrine pancreas of human neonates and infants. Diabetologia 20: 540-546
123. Rahier J, Goebbels RM, Henquin JC (1983) Cellular composition of the human diabetic pancreas. Diabetologia 24: 366-371

124. Rao RH (1984) The role of undernutrition in the pathogenesis of diabetes mellitus. Diabetes Care 7: 595-601
125. Reaven EP, Reaven GM (1981) Structure and function changes in the endocrine pancreas of aging rats with reference to the modulating effects of exercise and caloric restriction. J Clin Invest 68: 75-84
126. Reaven EP, Gold G, Reaven GM (1979) Effect of age on glucose-stimulated insulin release by the B-cell of the rat. J Clin Invest 64: 591-599
127. Reaven E, Curry D, Moore J, Reaven G (1983) Effect of age and environmental factors on insulin release from the perfused pancreas of the rat. J Clin Invest 71: 345-350
128. Reaven E, Wright D, Mondon CE, Solomon R, Ho H, Reaven GM (1983) Effect of age and diet on insulin action in the rat. Diabetes 32: 175-180
129. Reddy SN, Elliott RB (1985) Ontogeny of cells containing insulin glucagon, pancreatic polypeptide hormone and somatostatin in the bovine pancreas. Aust J Biol Sci 38: 237-243
130. Reddy S, Oliver JR, Elliott RB (1984) Immunofluorescence localization of pancreatic polypeptide hormone in the pancreas of fetal and adult sheep. Aust J Exp Biol Med Sci 62: 239-242
131. Remacle C, Hauser N, Jeanjean M, Gommers A (1977) Morphometric analysis of endocrine pancreas in old rats. Exp Gerontol 12: 207-214
132. Remacle C, DeClercq L, Delaère P, Many MC, Gommers A (1980) Organ culture of the islets of Langerhans from young and senescent rats. Cell Tissue Res 207: 429-448
133. Romanus JA, Rabinovitch A, Rechler MM (1985) Neonatal rat islet cell cultures synthesize insulin-like growth factor I. Diabetes 34: 696-702
134. Salans LB, Graham BJ (eds) (1982) Proceedings of a task force on animals appropriate for studying diabetes mellitus and its complications. Diabetes 31 [Suppl 1]
135. Sandler S, Swenne I (1983) Streptozotocin, but not alloxan, induces DNA repair synthesis in mouse pancreatic islets in vitro. Diabetologia 25: 444-447
136. Sandler S, Andersson A, Schnell A, Mellgren A, Tollemar J, Borg H, Petersson B, Groth CG, Hellerström C (1985) Tissue culture of human fetal pancreas. Development of function of B-cells in vitro and after transplantation of explants to nude mice. Diabetes 34: 1113-1119
137. Sartin JL, Chandhuri M, Farina S, Adelman RC (1986) Regulation of insulin secretion by glucose during aging. J Gerontol 41: 30-35
138. Seldon RF, Skóskiewicz MJ, Howie KB, Russel PS, Goodman HM (1986) Regulation of human insulin gene expression in transgenic mice. Nature 321: 525-528
139. Shafrir E, Renold AE (eds) (1984) Lessons from animal diabetes. Libbey, London
140. Shen LP, Rutter WJ (1984) Sequence of the human somatostatin I gene. Science 224: 168-171
141. Skoog L, Nordenskjöld B (1971) Effects of hydroxyurea and 1-darabinofuranosylcytosine on deoxyribonucleotide pools in mouse embryo cells. Eur J Biochem 19: 81-89
142. Stead RH, Brock JF (1972) Experimental protein-calorie malnutrition: rapid induction of protein depletion signs in early-weaned rats. J Nutr 102: 1357-1366
143. Stefan Y, Orci L, Malaisse Lagae F, Perrelet A, Patel Y, Unger RH (1982) Quantitation of endocrine cell content in the pancreas of nondiabetic and diabetic humans. Diabetes 31: 694-700
144. Stefan Y, Grasso S, Perrelet A, Orci L (1983) Quantitative immunofluorescent study of the endocrine cell population in the developing human pancreas. Diabetes 32: 293-307
145. Steiner H, Oelz O, Zahnd G, Froesch ER (1970) Studies on islet cell regeneration, hyperplasia and intrainsular cellular interrelations in long lasting streptozotocin diabetes in rats. Diabetologia 6: 558-564
146. Stewart RJC, Heard CRC (1959) Pancreatic islet cells and blood sugar regulation in pigs maintained on low protein diets. Proc Nutr Soc 18: X-Xi
147. Strautz RL (1970) Studies of hereditary-obese mice (ob/ob) after implantation of pancreatic islets in Millipore filter capsules. Diabetologia 6: 306-312
148. Sutherland DER (1981) Pancreas and islet transplantation. I. Experimental studies. Diabetologia 20: 161-185
149. Svenningsen A, Bonnevie-Nielsen V (1984) Effects of fasting on B-cell function, body fat islet volume, and total pancreatic insulin content. Metabolism 33: 612-616

150. Swenne I (1982) Role of glucose in the in vitro regulation of cell cycle kinetics and proliferation in fetal pancreatic B-cells. Diabetes 31: 754-760
151. Swenne I (1983) Effects of ageing on the regenerative capacity of the pancreatic B-cell of the rat. Diabetes 32: 14-19
152. Swenne I (1984) The cell cycle and growth regulation of pancreatic B-cells. In: Larner J, Pohl S (eds) Methods in diabetes research, vol I: laboratory methods, part B. Wiley, New York, pp 175-191
153. Swenne I (1985) Glucose-stimulated DNA replication of the islets during development of the rat fetus: Effects of nutrients, growth hormone and triiodothyronine. Diabetes 34: 803-807
154. Swenne I, Andersson A (1984) Effect of genetic background on the capacity for islet cell replication in mice. Diabetologia 27: 464-467
155. Swenne I, Bone AJ (1981) Effects, in tissue culture, of serum from obese mice on the DNA synthesis of the pancreatic B-cell. Cell Biol Int Reports 5: 647-652
156. Swenne I, Bone AJ, Howell SL, Hellerström C (1980) Effects of glucose and amino acids on the biosynthesis of DNA and insulin in fetal rat islets maintained in tissue culture. Diabetes 29: 686-692
157. Swenne I, Hill DJ, Strain AJ, Milner RDG (1987) Growth hormone regulation of somatomedin C/insulin-like growth factor I production and DNA replication in fetal rat islets in tissue culture. Diabetes 36: 288-294
158. Tejning S (1949) Dietary factors and quantitative morphology of the islets of Langerhans. Acta Med Scand 128 [Suppl 198]: 1-154
159. Tuch BE, Jones A, Turtle JR (1985) Maturation of the response of human fetal pancreatic explants to glucose. Diabetologia 28: 28-31
160. Weinkowe C, Weinkowe E, Timme A, Pimstone B (1977) Pancreatic islets of malnourished rats. Quantitative histologic and electron microscopic findings. Arch Pathol Lab Med 101: 266-269
161. Weir GC, Leaky JL, Bonner-Weir S (1986) Experimental reduction of B-cell mass: implications for the pathogenesis of diabetes. Diabetes/Metabolism Rev 2: 125-161
162. Westermark P, Wilander E (1978) The influence of amyloid deposits on the islet volume in maturity onset diabetes mellitus. Diabetologia 15: 417-421
163. Westman J, Andersson A, Hellerström C, Petersson B (1970) Ultrastructure of monolayer cultures of pancreatic islet cells. Acta Diabetol Lat 7: 557-589
164. Wirdman PK, Milner RDG (1981) Quantitation of the B and A cell fractions in human pancreas from early fetal life to puberty. Early Human Develop 5: 299-399
165. Wissler RW, Findley JW, Frazier LE (1949) Pancreatic islet hyperplasia in rats force fed high carbohydrate diets. Proc Soc Exptl Biol Med 71: 308-313
166. Woerner CA (1938) Studies of the islands of Langerhans after continuous intravenous injection of dextrose. Anat Rec 71: 33-57
167. Yoshinari M, Daikoku S (1982) Ontogenetic appearance of immunoreactive endocrine cells in rat pancreatic islets. Anat Embryol 165: 63-70
168. Yoshino G, Kazumi T, Kobayashi N, Terashi K, Morita S, Saba S (1979) Insulin and glucagon relationship during aging in rats. Endocrinol Jpn 26: 325-329

Islet Cell Tumors and Diabetes Mellitus

G. Somers and M. De Vroede

The human endocrine pancreas is composed of four major cell types, A-, B-, D-, and PP-cells, which are distinguished by routine staining procedures, immunocytochemistry and electron microscopy. The A-cells secrete glucagon and contain round and dense granules. The B-cells produce insulin. They make up the core of the islet and are characterized by the presence of rectangular insulin-containing granules. The D-cells, which are responsible for the secretion of somatostatin, contain large and pale granules. PP-cells produce pancreatic polypeptide (PP) and have dark and small granules [91, 109, 110, 111]. The PP-cells, but not the other endocrine cell types, have also been reported to be scattered within the exocrine pancreas [87].

The biochemical, physiological, and pharmacological properties of the hormones produced by each of the four islet cell types have been identified. This information allowed prediction of signs and symptoms which could possibly be associated with an excessive production of these hormones. As a result, patients with islet cell tumors were identified and a clinical and pathological profile of the different endocrine syndromes associated with these tumors has emerged.

Islet cell tumors belong to the family of endocrine tumors considered as "apudomas." In fact, islet cells display the typical cytochemical characteristics of APUD (*a*mine *p*recursor *u*ptake and *d*ecarboxylation) cells as described by Pearse [117].

The classification of islet cell tumors is often based on either clinical findings (the existence of a particular symptom or increased hormone levels) or pathological criteria (the positivity in immunocytochemistry for a particular cell type). Information yielded by the two disciplines is complementary. Specific clinical signs together with an increased plasma concentration of an islet cell hormone should alert the clinician to the existence of an islet cell tumor. Morphological assessment of the predominance of a particular cell type in the tumor allows the pathologist to further delineate the tumors and to indicate appropriate treatment. The clinician conceives the importance of this islet cell pathology in as far as it is associated with clinical syndromes, amongst which glucagonoma, insulinoma and somatostatinoma syndrome are the best known [47]. Interestingly, tumoral proliferation of PP-cells does not seem to give rise to any particular syndrome [46, 86]. Other tumors of the endocrine pancreas are considered "inappropriate" as they consist of cell types that are not encountered in normal islets of Langerhans, and are sometimes associated with a particular syndrome (gastrinoma, vipoma, ACTH-ADH-calcitonin, neurotensin-PTH-GRF containing tumors, carcinoid tumors) [47].

Clinical diagnosis of these tumors is not always easy. The symptoms and signs associated with pancreatic islet cell tumors can vary extensively. One reason is that these tumors are often composed of a mixture of different cell types [8, 85, 89, 108, 116]. This can even result in changing patterns of hormone secretion [107]. In addition, there is considerable variability in the extent of hormone synthesis and secretion by the tumor and in the bioactivity of the secreted hormone, which is often different from the expected normal activity. The detection of increased hormone levels in the context of a particular clinical syndrome may suggest a causal relationship between the elevated substances and that syndrome. However, discrepancies are possible between the bioactivity of the hormone produced by the tumor and the hormone levels measured by radioimmunoassay. This may be due to the predominant release of prohormones which display altered antibody interactions compared to the native hormone [120, 162, 163]. In contrast, elevated plasma hormone levels are not always indicative for a tumoral pathology. Indeed, increased glucagon secretion is also documented in familial hyperglucagonemia [19, 112], diabetes mellitus, acute pancreatitis, renal failure, acute trauma, cirrhosis, burn injury, Cushing's syndrome [90], and following administration of steroidal ethisterone derivatives such as danazol and oxymetholone [182]. Stimulatory or inhibitory tests are sometimes needed to disclose the tumoral origin of elevated hormone levels. They are crucial if symptoms are atypical and basal hormone levels normal. In spite of a better understanding of the pathophysiology of these tumors and of the refinement of the diagnostic aids, early detection is still hampered by the complexity of the tumor endocrinopathology and the characteristics of endocrine tumoral growth. In addition the real effectiveness of a chemotherapeutic intervention is difficult to assess, since many endocrine tumors of the apudoma family grow slowly. The early diagnosis of the tumor prior to the occurrence of metastases and the determination of its composition in order to select appropriate therapy remain the ultimate goal of the clinician. The specific therapeutic approach to an endocrine pancreatic tumor should incite the clinician to investigate thoroughly any clinical syndrome with endocrine features for its relationship with a possible pancreatic tumor.

As for the clinical data, several pitfalls can occur in the interpretation of pathological results [69]. Morphological examination can be impaired by the irregular distribution of immunoreactive tumor cells. This implies that the intensity of immunoreactivity in the part of the tumor that was examined cannot be extrapolated to the whole tumor. Likewise, a negative result obtained in one part of the tumor does not completely rule out a tumoral overproduction of peptides. Complete analysis of tumors through serial sections is therefore imperative to give definite answers. Another potential problem in the interpretation of morphological data arises from the observation that tumor cells often display a decreased hormone storage capacity compared to normal hormone-producing cells [33]. Therefore, poor granulation of the tumoral cells can preclude both immunocytochemical and ultrastructural identification of the tumor. In addition, when hormones are present in tumoral cells, they are often stored as promolecules. Since prohormones often fail to interact well with hormone antibodies, they can remain undetected in routine immunocytochemistry [173].

Diabetes as Part of an Islet Cell Tumor-Related Syndrome

Glucose intolerance and diabetes have been reported to occur in patients bearing islet cell tumors. These tumors may affect glucose homeostasis through an excessive release of pancreatic hormones. Tumor-induced hyperglucagonemia results in hyperglycemia through an increase in glycogenolysis and gluconeogenesis [29, 159]. In contrast, hyperglycemia associated with an excessive secretion of somatostatin results from a direct inhibition of insulin and glucagon release [2, 3, 53, 54, 56]. Diabetes has been described as part of the glucagonoma and somatostatinoma syndrome. In addition to neoplasms associated with these major pancreatic hormones, tumoral processes have been reported that release peptides which are barely detectable or even absent in normal islets, such as vasoactive intestinal peptide (VIP), adrenocorticotropic hormone (ACTH), corticotropin-releasing factor (CRF), and growth-hormone-releasing factor (GRF) [24, 26, 27, 47, 64, 70]. These peptides can disturb glucose metabolism through mechanisms involving insulin secretion or by interfering with the peripheral activity of the hormone.

A-Cell Tumors and Diabetes

The Glucagonoma Syndrome

A distinct clinical syndrome has been associated with glucagon-producing islet cell tumors of the pancreas [95, 96]. The clinical features include a necrolytic migratory erythematous rash, glossitis, stomatitis, diarrhea, weight loss, depression, deep vein thromboses and diabetes. Laboratory data reveal increased serum glucagon levels, normochromic-macrocytic anemia, hypercholesterolemia, hypoproteinemia, and hypoaminoacidemia. Review papers that cover almost all reported cases of glucagonoma provide possible explanations for these clinical signs [11, 17, 63, 90, 92, 94, 183]. Mild diabetes or glucose intolerance is encountered in about 80% of the reported cases. There is, however, poor correlation between the degree of hyperglucagonemia and that of hyperglycemia. The following possible explanations can be advanced for this observation:

1. The secretion by the tumor of glucagon immunoreactivity with different molecular weights.
   Four molecular weight species of glucagon have been detected in normal plasma (big glucagon M_r >90000 daltons; proglucagon >9000 daltons; glucagon 3500 daltons) and low-M_r material (3000 daltons). In patients with a tumor, both the high-M_r (>90000) and low-M_r (<3500) forms are predominantly found [36, 121, 133, 176, 179].
2. The variability in insulin secretion observed in these patients.
   Insulin output is often decreased because of the massive replacement of the normal pancreas by the tumor. In contrast, elevated insulin levels may originate in the tumor itself or result from excessive stimulation of insulin output by tumoral glucagon [90].

3. The concomitant secretion by the tumor of other polypeptides (PP, insulin, ACTH, VIP, calcitonin, gastrin, neurotensin and somatostatin), of which some interfere directly or indirectly with glucose metabolism [8, 13, 20, 44, 48, 51, 62, 71, 108 126, 180, 181, 186].
4. The presence of hepatic metastases, which may weaken the gluconeogenetic effect of high glucagon levels [90].

Ketoacidotic decompensation in general does not occur in this syndrome, probably because absolute insulin deficiency is rather infrequently encountered [52].

Removal of the tumor is usually associated with normalization of the glucose intolerance [72]. In case of failure, chemotherapy or oral hypoglycemic agents may be efficient in controlling glucose levels. The occurrence of diabetic complications has till now not been reported, presumably because as soon diabetes is manifest, the clinical course of the entity is too rapid to allow complications to develop. Finally a few cases were reported of glucagonoma associated with multiple endocrine neoplasia [34, 35, 184]. However, in these particular conditions, there was no evidence that the glucagonoma was functionally active, underlining again the need to develop specific diagnostic tests for these tumors.

Tumor Characteristics

The following classification of glucagonoma is based on pathological examination of the islet cell tumor and immunocytochemical and ultrastructural demonstration of predominantly glucagon-containing cells [140]:

1. Glucagonomas associated with the typical clinical syndrome are usually single pancreatic tumors of considerable size, 80% being larger than 5 cm (within the diagnostic scope of radiological imaging) [21]. These glucagonomas are predominantly found in the tail of the pancreas. The rate of malignancy is high [11, 21, 71, 90]: in about 60% of the cases, liver metastases are present.
2. A-cell tumors identified in the absence of the typical glucagonoma syndrome, but diagnosed on the basis of biochemical and morphological data, were described in well-defined conditions, such as:
   - solitary malignant A-cell tumors associated or not with diabetes
   - glucagonomas associated with other pancreatic tumors
   - glucagonomas occurring in multiple endocrine neoplasia
   - single microadenomas found post mortem in elderly patients

   A-cell tumors presenting with the clinical syndrome show no common cellular pattern [21, 183]. Trabecular solid or diffuse growth patterns are found. Tumoral cells appear multinucleated with granular and abundant cytoplasm. Electron microscopic examination reveals medium-sized, dense, round granules which are different from the normal A-cell granules and may resemble the human fetal A-cell granules. Evidence is however available from immunofluorescence and extraction studies that these granules do contain glucagon. A-cell tumors not presenting with the typical clinical syndrome are usually small and have typical A-type secretory granules [21, 34].

Tests

The work-up of a patient who is suspected to have an islet cell tumor requires specific laboratory tests. Testing is important for the diagnosis of an A-cell tumor when basal glucagon levels are normal or when the clinical presentation is atypical, for example diabetes mellitus alone. Table 1 lists various stimulating and inhibitory tests. These tests take advantage of the observation that factors reported to stimulate or inhibit glucagon secretion in normal men display different effects on glucagon output in patients with glucagonoma. Indeed, paradoxical increases of glucagon following oral glucose, mixed meal, or tolbutamide were observed in patients with glucagonoma. IV glucose reduced plasma glucagon, but only partially. Other stimuli, such as IV arginine [171] and epinephrine [75, 178], provoked an exaggerated secretion of glucagon in glucagonoma patients.

Table 1. Clinical tests of glucagon secretion

Stimulus/inhibitor	Effect on normal subjects (plasma level of glucagon)	Glucagonoma
Oral glucose	↓	Paradoxical increase
IV glucose	↓	Partial decrease
Mixed meal	↑, ↓ or no effect	Paradoxical increase
Tolbutamide	No effect	Paradoxical increase

Normal subjects: [2, 67, 106, 118, 168, 169, 171]
Glucagonoma patients: [20, 90]

D-Cell Tumors and Diabetes

The Somatostatinoma Syndrome

After the isolation and characterization of somatostatin from the hypothalamus [142] its presence was demonstrated in other parts of the brain [23, 113], in sensory neurons [113], in the gastrointestinal tract [5], in the endocrine pancreas [5, 40] and thyroid [38], and in plasma [84, 122]. Immunofluorescence techniques have localized this peptide in the D-cell of the islet of Langerhans [127]. This 14 amino acid cyclic peptide was reported to exert a wide spectrum of effects most of which are inhibitory [55, 114, 149]. In regard to glucose metabolism, it inhibits the release of a variety of peptides, including insulin, glucagon, and growth hormone [3, 53, 54, 56, 177]. Indirect effects on glucose metabolism result from somatostatin-induced inhibition of gastrointestinal motility and nutrient absorption [148]. Further research expanded the concept of somatostatin to a group of somatostatin-related peptides, including somatostatin-14 (S-14), somatostatin-28 (S-28) [100], and several species-specific variants and high molecular weight (presumably prohormone) forms [31, 134]. Somatostatin-28 was isolated from the porcine intestine [128] and hypothalamus [153] and was also reported in pancreatic islet cells and in the epithelial cells of the duodenum [152]. Since the C-terminal amino acid sequences of

Table 2. Published cases of Pancreatic somatostatinoma

Author(s)	Age, sex	Diabetes	Diarrhea, steatorrhea, gastrointestinal signs	Gallbladder disease	Other clinical features	Other tumoral hormones
Larsson et al. [88]	55 F	+	+	+	Flush, achlorhydria	–
Ganda et al. [51]	46 F	+	–	+	Anemia, abdominal pain	–
Kovacs et al. [89]	54 M	+	NR	NR	Hypertension, hypokalemic alkalosis	ACTH
Pipeleers et al. [124, 125]	63 F	+	+	+	Anemia, hypochlorhydria	–
Galmiche et al. [49, 50]	70 F	+	+	+	Achlorhydria	Calcitonin
Krejs et al. [83] Conlon et al. [30] Lowry et al. [93]	52 M	+	+	+	Anemia, abdominal pain, achlorhydria	Calcitonin
Gerlock et al. [57] Stacpoole et al. [158]	36 F	+	+	+	Flush, emotional lability, labile blood pressure	Calcitonin, PP, VIP, gastrin, PGE_2
Penman et al. [119] Wright et al. [185]	36 F	–	NR	–	Hyperpigmentation, anemia, hypoglycemia, hypokalemia	Insulin, thyroxine, glucagon, C-peptide, PP, 5-OH-IAA
Penman et al. [119]	32 M	+	NR	–	Cushing's syndrome, hypokalemic alkalosis	ACTH
Asa et al. [6]	68 F	+	+	NR	Anemia	Endorphin, calcitonin, ACTH, gastrin
Axelrod et al. [7]	54 F	+	+	(+)	Anemia	–
Berger et al. [10]	67 F	NR	+	NR	–	–
English et al. [42]	32 M	+	+	NR	–	–
Schuzdiarra et al. [150]	30 F	+	+	+	Achlorhydria	–
Pipeleers et al. [125]	54 M	–	–	–	Hypoglycemia	Insulin
	47 M	–	–	–	Hypoglycemia	Insulin
	84 F	IGT	–	–		Insulin/glucagon
Roberts et al. [138]	62 M	–	+	+	Abdominal pain	–
Kelly et al. [80]	48 F	+	+	+	Hypochlorhydria	–

Table 2. continued

Author(s)	Age, sex	Dia- betes	Diarrhea, steatorrhea, gastro- intestinal signs	Gall- bladder disease	Other clinical features	Other tumoral hormones
Sakazaki et al. [141] Taruya et al. [166]	66 F	IGT	NR	+	Goiter	Gastrin-releasing polypeptide (bombesin)
Nakanome et al. [102, 103]		+	+	+	–	PP
Chadenas et al. [27, 28] Pinsard et al. [123]	47 F	+	+	+	Acromegaly	GRF

+, present; –, absent; NR, not reported; IGT, impaired glucose tolerance

S-28 are identical to S-14, S-28 might be a precursor of S-14. S-28 possesses the same target organ as S-14 [157, 175]. Differences in relative potency between S-14 and S-28 have been described [98, 147]. No biological effect of $S\text{-}28_{1\text{-}12}$ fragment has been described [115].

The insight into the physiopathology and biochemistry of this group of peptides has led to the detection of D-cell tumors. Vice versa, the studies on endocrine tumoral material have further expanded the knowledge of this peptide. Since 1977 several cases of somatostatinoma of the pancreas (Table 2) or of the gastrointestinal tract [4, 25, 37, 58, 59, 61, 76, 78, 79, 97, 99, 158, 164] have been reported. The diagnosis was based on a high plasma somatostatin immunoreactivity (SIR) or on the demonstration of SIR in the tumors. The presentation of these cases was interpreted in the light of the reported pharmacological effects of somatostatin and resulted in the description of a "somatostatinoma syndrome" [83].

The main characteristics of this syndrome as proposed by Krejs and coworkers include non-ketosis-prone diabetes mellitus, steatorrhea, and cholelithiasis [83]. In 22 cases of documented pancreatic somatostatinoma, the "somatostatinoma" triad was reported in less than 50% (10/22), whereas diabetes was found in about 77% (17/22).

Impairment of glucose levels may occur through several mechanisms. Indeed, somatostatin inhibits insulin, glucagon, and growth hormone release and controls the nutrient uptake at the gastrointestinal level. Unger suggested that a physiological role of somatostatin is to regulate, through paracrine secretion, the amount of insulin and glucagon, and their relative proportion, released into the systemic circulation [170]. These physiological bases may explain the infrequent occurrence of ketosis and the limited fluctuation of plasma glucose in conditions of hypersomatostatinemia. Diabetes is thus reported to be mild, even in the absence of insulin treatment, as a result of the complete suppression of diabetogenic hormones such as glucagon and growth hormone and delayed nutrient uptake. Incomplete inhibition of these hormones can occur if the tumor releases high amounts of SIR with low bioactivity [7, 125]. In some patients with diabetes, concomitant secretion of another hyperglycemic hormone, namely ACTH, was described. In addition to ACTH, production of glucagon, calcitonin, serotonin, endorphins, and GRF has been disclosed, which may also impair glucose concentrations and result in variable clinical features. Significant ketosis was found only in one patient with somatostatinoma and attributed to a lack of inhibition by the tumoral secretory products on glucagon release [7]. AXELROD et al. found a graded relationship between the plasma somatostatin-like immunoreactivity level and the biologic effects of endogenous somatostatin produced by an islet cell tumor. They concluded that the immunoreactivity level and its biologic effect, such as inhibition of arginine-induced glucagon and growth hormone secretion, is different for various tumoral somatostatin-like peptides [7].

The inhibition by somatostatin of gastrointestinal endocrine and exocrine function [144, 174], intestinal motility and absorption [16, 18], pancreatic exocrine function [32, 66], and gallbladder contraction [12, 136] results in diarrhea and steatorrhea. Reduced gallbladder contraction in addition leads to the formation of gallstones. Other clinical signs in patients with islet tumors consisting predominantly of D-cells include achlorhydria due to the inhibition of the gastric acid output [15], abdominal pain, and anemia.

The clinically delineated association between this reported triad and somatostatin-producing tumors can, however, be questioned in the light of cases presenting with ketoacidotic diabetes, hypoglycemia, cushingoid symptoms, or flushing [125, 158]. In particular, the so-called typical somatostatinoma syndrome appeared to be present in only one of 15 somatostatin-producing tumors of extrapancreatic origin [58], and diabetes was reported in only three of 15 cases [25, 37, 58]. In one patient with the somatostatinoma syndrome no primary localization was identified [135].

Analysis of the secretory products of pancreatic somatostatinoma showed the presence of S-14 and/or S-28 and probably prohormonal forms with presumably different biological activity. Different inhibitory effects on glucagon and insulin secretion and on intestinal metabolism and motility have indeed been reported for S-14, S-28, and synthetic somatostatin analogues [81].

The SIR measured in our patients with pancreatic somatostatinoma corresponded to components of different molecular weight. Only 5 to 60% of total SIR occurred under form of S 14, while the remaining SIR was detected at higher molecular weights varying from Mr. 3000–4000 to more than 12000 (Table 3). A similar variability was described in other case reports [30, 115, 119].

However, no correlation could be found between the existence of a clinical somatostatinoma syndrome and the distribution or circulating levels of these various hormonal forms. In some patients with somatostatinoma, but without diabetes or the "classical" clinical syndrome, a predominant secretion of SIR with high M_r is reported. Absence of diabetes in these patients might be due to the secretion of a high M_r inactive somatostatin, to a reduced inhibition of insulin secretion, or to the absence of any paracrine effects of the tumor products.

Tumor Characteristics

Pancreatic somatostatinomas are usually very large tumors and are predominantly located in the head of the pancreas. At the time of diagnosis most of the patients already have liver metastases. Yet, three benign tumors have been described [51, 80, 125]. The histologic appearance of the tumor tissue of patients with or without somatostatinoma syndrome is similar. The tumor is composed of cells with an eosinophilic granular cytoplasm and round nuclei with prominent nucleoli. Cells are arranged in cords and clusters, separated by thin fibrovascular septa. Staining with the HELLERSTRÖM-HELLMAN silver method produces a characteristic granular stain in most tumor cells. On electron microscopy the tumor cells display many large secretory granules of variable size and electron density characteristic for D-cells. The ultrastructural features of typical D-cell granules were reported [88, 124], but in the majority of cases the ultrastructural aspect is not distinctive for any endocrine cell type. In some tumors, immunocytochemistry disclosed the concomitant presence of other peptide hormones (ACTH, GRF, insulin, glucagon, calcitonin, endorphins, thyroxine, bombesin, VIP, gastrin, PP) and of PGE_2 and serotonin.

In the tumor tissue of patients with the so-called typical somatostatinoma syndrome, calcitonin, PP, VIP, gastrin, PGE_2, and GRF could be detected (Table 2). In one patient with an adenoma presenting with hypoglycemia, insulin was detected and tumor cells displayed small secretory granules which were not typical for any of the previously described islet cell types [125]. Finally, one tumor appeared to be composed of mixed exocrine and endocrine cells [125]. One somatostatinoma has been described as part of multiple endocrine neoplasms (MEN) presenting with pheochromocytoma and neurofibromatosis [25]. In four of 22 cases calcitonin was found in the D-cell tumor. Interestingly, in medullary thyroid carcinoma somatostatin has been identified in calcitonin-producing cells [172].

Diagnostic Tests

In view of the heterogeneity in clinical signs, early detection of a somatostatin-producing tumor may be difficult. Moreover, basal plasma SIR levels are not consistently elevated. Obviously these findings point to the need for provocative diagnostic tests.

In normal human subjects, arginine infusion raises plasma SIR levels only moderately. In somatostatinoma patients, a two- to fourfold increase in plasma SIR was found following a 30-min infusion of 20-30 g arginine [7]. In animal studies tolbutamide induced a release of somatostatin from the pancreas [73]. IV tolbutamide was reported to increase dramatically peripheral SIR levels in somatostatinoma patients [124, 158] while no response was seen in normal or diabetic controls [124]. The SIR response to tolbutamide decreased after chemotherapeutic treatment, indicating the usefulness of this test in determining the extent of the tumoral process and in evaluating the treatment [124]. The combined intravenous injection of calcium (2 mg/kg body weight) and pentagastrin (0.5 mg/kg body weight), which both stimulate somatostatin release in vitro and in animal studies [74], also induced a significant increase in plasma SIR levels in patients with a pancreatic

Table 3. Molecular weight of SIR in plasma and tumor of 3 patients with pancreatic somatostatinoma [125]

	Case 1	Case 2	Case 3
Age	55	54	84
Sex	F	M	F
Major clinical symptom	"Somatostatinoma syndrome"	Hypoglycemia	Impaired glucose tolerance, obstructive jaundice
Somatostatin immunoreactivity			
Plasma	M_r 1600 (45%) M_r 3000–4000 (25%) M_r 6000–7000 (30%)	M_r 1600 (20%) M_r 8000–12000 (80%)	M_r 1600 (5%) M_r 6000–7000 (20%) High M_r (75%)
Tumor	M_r 1600 (32%) M_r 6000–7000 (68%)	M_r 1600 (60%) M_r 6000–7000 (35%) M_r 8000–12000 (5%)	M_r 1600 (10%) M_r 6000–7000 (80%) High M_r (10%)

somatostatinoma [125, 155] and in one patient with a duodenal somatostatinoma [156]. An exaggerated somatostatin response to secretin administration has been described in a single patient [28]. In one patient a paradoxical decrease in plasma SIR was observed following an IV bolus injection or infusion of glucagon (unpublished data).

A diazoxide infusion test was performed in certain patients with a D-cell tumor and induced a rather particular effect. Diazoxide exerts its hypotensive action only after a bolus injection. Continuous infusion of diazoxide gives rise to hardly any change in blood pressure in normal subjects. During diazoxide infusion in patients with high SIR levels, a partial decrease of these high levels is induced by the drug [124], but prolonged hypotension is also noted. This effect could be due to the pharmacokinetic interaction between diazoxide and somatostatin resulting in an increase in the period of diazoxide availability. It could also be the result of an inhibition by somatostatin of the pressure-restoring mechanism such as the release of renin [101]. Administration of diazoxide to partially suppress tumoral somatostatin release should therefore be performed with caution, since its hypotensive effect may endure for several hours.

Other Pancreatic Endocrine Tumors Associated with Diabetes

Growth-hormone-releasing factor (GRF), a 44-amino-acid peptide, that was recently characterized, was initially isolated from pancreatic tumors of patients presenting with acromegaly [22, 137, 143] and subsequently located in the brain [14]. The diabetic state observed in these patients resulted from an excessive growth hormone secretion, since, paradoxically, GRF itself has been reported to stimulate insulin secretion [60]. Some pancreatic tumors have been described to produce ACTH and/or CRF, thereby influencing glucose homeostasis [26, 47, 70]. VIP-secreting islet cell tumors result in a Verner-Morrison syndrome in which hypokalemia might impair insulin secretion [47]. Tumoral PP secretion has been reported but no diabetes has been associated with elevated plasma PP level. This is somewhat surprising, since infusion of PP in vivo does elevate postprandial glycemia [1].

Markers for Islet Cell Tumors

Early diagnosis of the islet cell tumor by specific tests or by detection of serum-markers specific for endocrine tumoral growth remains imperative. Neuron-specific enolase (NSE), a glycolytic enzyme found exclusively in neural and neuroendocrine cells [145, 146], human pancreatic polypeptide (PP) [126], human chorionic gonadotropin (hCG) [68, 77], and alpha-1-antitrypsin [132] have been proposed as markers for diagnosis and management of apudomas. Although islet cell tumors were reported to contain alpha-1-antitrypsin, serum alpha-1-antitrypsin appeared elevated in only three of 16 cases of proven endocrine pancreatic tumors [132]. Thus alpha-1-antitrypsin does not seem to be a very sensitive tumor marker for islet cell tumors. NSE immunoreactivity was detected in all the endocrine cells of the pancreas [129, 165]. Increased serum levels of NSE have been reported in a number of patients with nonfunctioning islet cell carcinoma and decreased after tumor resection [131]. In a study by PRINZ et al., elevated NSE levels were found in the only somatostatinoma, in one of three insulinomas, and in all of six gastrinoma patients, but not in three glucagonoma patients [130].

The physiologic role of human PP remains unclear and no definite clinical picture associated with PP hypersecretion has been advanced [43]. However, PP has been suggested as a possible tumor marker for pancreatic islet cell tumors and intestinal carcinoid tumors [45, 104, 126, 151]. POLAK et al. reported PP to be elevated in 18 of 28 patients with islet cell tumors [126]. These findings were confirmed by OBERG et al. in nine of 16 patients with pancreatic tumors [104]. In some series, pancreatic polypeptide levels were elevated in more than 50% of the patients with glucagonoma [126]. This increase reflects either concomitant tumoral PP secretion or is due to PP cell stimulation. In some patients with somatostatinoma high PP levels were noted [103], but in the majority of patients PP levels were low, probably due to the inhibitory effect of somatostatin on PP secretion [123, 124]. The increase in PP secretion reported by POLAK in gastrinomas was not confirmed by TAYLOR et al., who found elevated PP levels in only four of 141 patients with Zollinger-Ellison syndrome [167]. Finally, PP deserves a special interest in the monitoring of patients with MEN I syndrome [43].

Human chorionic gonadotropin, hCG, a glycoprotein hormone, and its subunits have been found to be increased in several endocrine neoplasms including pancreatic islet cell tumors and intestinal carcinoids [68, 77, 105]. Elevation of hCG or its subunits has been proposed as a marker for malignancy for all types of pancreatic endocrine tumors [105]. From the actual clinical studies it is apparent that NSE, hPP, and hCG (or its subunits) levels are not elevated in all patients with pancreatic islet cell carcinoma, and their usefulness in the screening for endocrine tumors is questioned. However, when elevated these markers proved valuable in the monitoring of therapy and in the estimation of the prognosis.

Localization of the Tumor

The modalities to localize and image endocrine pancreatic tumors include abdominal angiography, ultrasonography, computerized tomography, portal vein catheterization and blood sampling for hormone determination [39, 65], isotope studies, and recently nuclear magnetic resonance [160]. A-cell and D-cell tumors presenting with their typical clinical syndrome are large and can usually be detected on CT examination or angiography. However, CT may fail to visualize tumors less than 4 cm in diameter [41, 161]. Ultrasound examination proved effective in the evaluation of non-B-cell tumors [154] and can even be used intraoperatively [139]. Isotope scanning is primarily useful in detection of liver metastases. New techniques should thus be developed for the early detection of the tumor prior to the occurrence of metastases. High expectations are nourished for nuclear magnetic resonance scanning as a very sensitive diagnostic tool. Another potential approach for earlier imaging is the development of radioisotope-tagged specific antibodies to islet cell components.

Conclusion

The diagnosis and management of islet cell tumors have benefited enormously from the improved radioimmunological and immunocytochemical techniques, from a better understanding of hormone activities and from more precise insights in the physiological interaction within the islets. The imbalance in the secretion of the islet cell hormones can result in alteration of glucose homeostasis. The exaggerated secretion of a particular islet cell hormone may lead to a well-defined clinical syndrome. However, the multihormonicity of the tumoral output and the secretion of precursor hormones often give rise to a broad variety in symptoms. Typical clinical symptoms and/or radiological detection of pancreatic tumoral growth should lead to measurement of basal and/or post-stimulation circulating islet cell hormone levels.

In diabetes, peripheral concentrations of somatostatin, glucagon, and other hyperglycemic hormones should be evaluated not only for a better understanding of the islet cell perturbation in type 1 or type 2 diabetes, but also for the detection of the more rare but often overlooked endocrine pancreatic tumors.

In addition to the plasma hormone determinations, some tumoral serum markers might be of diagnostic and prognostic aid. In the early detection of slowly growing islet cell tumors, novel imaging techniques may prove to be sensitive noninvasive investigational tests.

References

1. Adrian TE, Greenberg GR, Barnes AJ, Christofides ND, Alberti KGMM, Bloom SR (1980) Effect of pancreatic polypeptide on motilin and circulating metabolites in man. Eur J Clin Invest 10: 235-240
2. Aguilar-Parada E, Eisentraut AM, Unger RH (1969) Pancreatic glucagon secretion in normal and diabetic subjects. Am J Med Sci 257: 415-419
3. Alberti KGMM, Christensen SE, Hansen AP, Iversen J, Lundbaeck K, Seyer-Hansen K, Orskov H (1973) Inhibition of insulin secretion by somatostatin. Lancet II: 1299-1301
4. Alumets J, Ekelund G, Håkanson R, Ljungberg O, Lundqvist V, Sundler F, Tibblin S (1978) Jejunal endocrine tumour composed of somatostatin and gastrin cells and associated with duodenal ulcer disease. Virchows Arch [A] 578: 17-22
5. Arimura A, Sato H, Dupont A, Nishi N, Schally AV (1975) Somatostatin: abundance of immunoreactive hormone in rat stomach and pancreas. Science 189: 1007-1009
6. Asa SL, Kovacs K, Killinger DW, Marcon N, Platts M (1980) Pancreatic islet cell carcinoma producing gastrin, ACTH, α-endorphin, somatostatin and calcitonin. Am J Gastroenterol 74: 30-35
7. Axelrod L, Bush MA, Hirsh HJ, Loo SWH (1981) Malignant somatostatinoma: clinical features and metabolic studies. J Clin Endocrinol Metab 52: 886-896
8. Belchetz PI, Brown CL, Marein HLJ, Traflord DJH, Mason AS, Bloom SR, Ratcliffe JG (1973) ACTH, glucagon and gastrin production by a pancreatic islet cell carcinoma and its treatment. Clin Endocrinol 2: 307-316
9. Bencosme SA, Liepa F (1955) Regional differences of the pancreatic islets. Endocrinology 57: 588-593
10. Berger G, Berger F, Guillaud MM, Frappart L, Patricol LM, Buerlet J (1979) Immunocytochémie des apudomes pancréatiques et pancréatico-duodénaux. Ann Anat Pathol 24: 215-230
11. Binnick AN, Spencer SK, Dennison WL Jr, Horton ES (1977) Glucagonoma syndrome. Report of two cases and literature review. Arch Dermatol 113: 749-754
12. Bjork S, Svanvik J (1984) The influence of somatostatin on gallbladder response to intraduodenal acid and autonomic nerve stimulation in the cat. Scand J Gastroenterol 19: 173-177
13. Blackburn AM, Bryant MG, Adrian TE, Bloom SR (1981) Pancreatic tumors produce neurotensin. J Clin Endocrinol Metab 52: 820-822
14. Block B, Brazeau P, Ling N, Bohlen P, Esch F, Wehrenberg W, Benock R, Bloom F, Guillemin R (1983) Immunocytochemical detection of growth hormone releasing factor in brain. Nature 301: 607-609
15. Bloom SR, Mortimer CH, Thorner MO, Besser GM, Hall R, Gomez-Pan A, Roy VM, Russel RCG, Coy DH, Kastin AJ, Schally AV (1974) Inhibition of gastrin and gastric acid secretion by growth hormone release inhibiting hormone. Lancet II: 1106-1109
16. Bloom SR, Ralphs DN, Besser GH, Hall R, Coy DH, Kastin AJ, Schally AV (1975) Effect of somatostatin on motilin levels and gastric emptying. Gut 16: 834
17. Bloom SR, Polak JM (1978) The glucagonoma syndrome. Adv Exp Med Biol 106: 183-194
18. Boden G, Jacob HJ, Staus A (1976) Somatostatin interacts with basal and carbachol stimulated antral and duodenal motility. Gastroenterology 70: 961
19. Boden G, Owen OE (1977) Familial hyperglucagonaemia - an autosomal dominant disorder. N Engl J Med 296: 534-538
20. Boden G, Owen OE, Rezvani I, Elfenbein BI, Quickel KE (1977) An islet cell carcinoma containing glucagon and insulin. Diabetes 26: 128-137
21. Bordi C, Ravazzola M, Baetens D, Gorden P, Unger RH, Orci L (1979) A study of glucagonomas by light and electron microscopy and immunofluorescence. Diabetes 28: 925-936
22. Bostwick DG, Quan R, Hoffman AR, Webber RJ, Chang JK, Bensch KG (1984) Growth-hormone releasing factor immunoreactivity in human endocrine tumors. Am J Pathol 117: 167-170
23. Brazeau P, Vale W, Burgus R, Lung W, Butcher M, Guillemin R (1973) Hypothalamic polypeptide that inhibits the secretion of immunoreactive pituitary growth hormone. Science 179: 77-79

24. Burkinshaw JH, O'Brien D, Pendower JEH (1967) Cushing's syndrome associated with an islet-cell tumour of the pancreas in a boy aged 2 years. Arch Dis Child 42: 525-531
25. Cantor AM, Rigby CC, Beck PR, Mangion D (1982) Neurofibromatosis, phaeochromocytoma and somatostatinoma. Br Med J 285: 1618-1619
26. Carey RM, Varma SK, Drake CR Jr, Thorner MO, Kovacs K, Rivier J, Vale W (1984) Ectopic secretion of corticotropin-releasing factor as a cause of Cushing's syndrome: a clinical, morphologic, and biochemical study. N Engl J Med 311: 13-20
27. Chadenas D, Pinsard D, Melliere D, Trouillas J, Zafrani ES, Pradayrol L, Sassolas G, Li Y, Girod C, Aumaitre J (1985) Tumeur pancréatique endocrine sécrétant de la somatostatine et de la somatocrinine. Presse Med 14: 2129-2134
28. Chadenas D, Pinsard D, Dutilleux P, Monod R, Bastenaire F, Villeneuve A (1986) The secretin test in a case of pancreatic somatostatinoma (letter). Presse Med 15: 119
29. Claus TH, Park CR, Pilhis SJ (1983) Glucagon and gluconeogenesis. In: Lefèbvre PJ (ed) Glucagon I. Springer, Berlin Heidelberg New York, pp 311-360
30. Conlon JM, McCarthy D, Krejs G, Unger RH (1981) Characterization of somatostatin-like components in the tumour and plasma of a patient with a somatostatinoma. J Clin Endocrinol Metab 52: 66-72
31. Conlon JM (1981) Molecule forms of somatostatin. In: Bloom SR, Polak JM (eds) Gut hormones. Livingstone, Edinburgh, pp 354-361
32. Creutzfeldt W, Lankisch PG, Fölsch UR (1975) Hemmung der Sekretin- und Cholezystokinin-Pankreozymin induzierten Saft- und Enzymsekretion des Pankreas und der Gallenblasenkontraktion beim Menschen durch Somatostatin. Dtsch Med Wochenschr 100: 1135-1138
33. Creutzfeldt W (1977) Endocrine tumors of the pancreas. In: Volk BW, Wellmann KF (eds) The diabetic pancreas. Baillière Tindall, London, p 551
34. Croisier JC, Lehy T, Zeitoun P (1971) A_2-cell pancreatic microadenomas in a case of multiple endocrine adenomatosis. Cancer 28: 707-713
35. Croughs RJM, Hulsmans HA, Israel DE, Hackeng WHL, Schopman W (1972) Glucagonoma as a part of the polyglandular syndrome. Am J Med 52: 690-698
36. Danforth DN, Triche T, Doppman JL, Beazley RM, Perrino PV, Recant L (1976) Elevated plasma proglucagon-like component with a glucagon-secreting tumor. N Engl J Med 295: 242-245
37. Dayal Y, Doos WG, O'Brien MJ, Nunnemacher G, DeLellis RA, Wolfe HJ (1983) Psammomatous somatostatinomas of the duodenum. Am J Surg Pathol 7: 653-665
38. Deftos LJ, Bone HG, Parthemore JG (1980) Immunohistological studies of medullary thyroid carcinoma and C-cell hyperplasia. J Clin Endocrinol Metab 51: 857-862
39. Dodds WJ, Wilson SD, Thorsen MK, Stewart ET, Lawson TL, Foley WD (1985) MEN I syndrome and islet cell lesions of the pancreas. Semin Roentgenol XX (1): 17-63
40. Dubois MP (1975) Immunoreactive somatostatin is present in cells of the endocrine pancreas. Proc Natl Acad Sci USA 72: 1340-1343
41. Dunnick NR, Doppman JL, Mib SR, McCarthy M (1980) Computed tomographic detection of nonbeta pancreatic islet cell tumors. Radiology 135: 117-120
42. English J, Stassen W, Keohane C, Kirwan WO, Whelton MJ (1983) Somatostatinoma in a young caucasian male. Scand J Gastroenterol [Suppl] 18: 197
43. Floyd JC, Fajans SS, Pek S, Chance RE (1977) A newly recognized pancreatic polypeptide: plasma levels in health and disease. Recent Prog Horm Res 33: 519-570
44. Friesen SR, Hermreck AS, Mantz FA (1973) Glucagon, gastrin and carcinoid tumors of the duodenum, pancreas and stomach, polypeptide "apudomas" of the foregut. Am J Surg 127: 90-101
45. Friesen SR, Kimmel JR, Tomita T (1980) Pancreatic polypeptide as a screening marker for pancreatic polypeptide apudomas in multiple endocrinopathies. Am J Surg 139: 61-72
46. Friesen SR, Stephens RL, Huard GS II (1981) Effective streptozocin therapy for metastatic pancreatic polypeptide apudoma. Arch Surg 116: 1090-1092
47. Friesen SR (1982) Tumors of the endocrine pancreas. N Engl J Med 306: 580-590
48. Galle K, Schweiß D (1983) Das Glukagonom-Syndrom - eine wenig bekannte kutane Paraneoplasie. Ein kasuistischer Bericht. Hautarzt 35: 204-209
49. Galmiche JP, Colin R, Dubois PM, Chayvialle JA, Descos F, Paulin C, Geffroy Y (1978) Calcitonin secretion by a pancreatic somatostatinoma. N Engl J Med 299: 1252

50. Galmiche JP, Chayvialle JA, Dubois PM, David L, Descos F, Paulin C, Ducastille T, Colin R, Geffroy Y (1980) Calcitonin producing pancreatic somatostatinoma. Gastroenterology 78: 1577-1583
51. Ganda OP, Weir GC, Soeldner JS, Legg MA, Chick WL, Patel YC, Ebeid AM, Gabbay KH, Reichlin S (1977) "Somatostatinoma": a somatostatin-containing tumor of the endocrine pancreas. N Engl J Med 296: 963-967
52. Ganda OP (1980) Glucagonoma and diabetic ketoacidosis. Arch Intern Med 140: 1397-1398
53. Gerich JE, Lorenzi M, Schneider V, Karam CW, Karam HJ, Guillemin R, Forsham P (1974) Inhibition of pancreatic glucagon response to arginine by somatostatin in normal man and in insulin-dependent diabetics. Diabetes 23: 870-880
54. Gerich JE, Patton G (1978) Somatostatin physiology and clinical implication. Med Clin North Am 62: 375-392
55. Gerich JE, Raptis S, Rosenthal J (eds) (1978) Somatostatin symposium. Metabolism 27 [Suppl 1]: 1133-1469
56. Gerich JE (1981) Somatostatin and diabetes. Am J Med 70: 619-626
57. Gerlock AM, Muhlethler CA, Halter S, Goucharenko V (1979) Pancreatic somatostatinoma: histologic, and angiographic features. AJR 133: 939-943
58. Ghose RR, Gupta SK (1981) Oatcell carcinoma of bronchus presenting with somatostatinoma syndrome. Thorax 36: 550-551
59. Goodman ZD, Albores-Saavedra J, Lundblad DM (1984) Somatostatinoma of the cystic duct. Cancer 53: 498-502
60. Green JC, Lo C, Crowther N, Bone L, Ray K, Wallis M (1986) Mechanism of action of growth hormone releasing factor on insulin secretion from islets of Langerhans and dispersed islet cells. Diabetologia 29: 542A
61. Grundmann R, Thul P, Krestin GP, Krueger GR (1985) Liver somatostatinoma. Leber Magen Darm 15: 81-84
62. Greider MH, Bencosme JA, Lechago J (1970) The human pancreatic islet cells and their tumours. I. The normal pancreatic islet. Lab Invest 22: 344-354
63. Guillausseau PJ, Guillausseau C, Villet R, Kaloustian E, Valleur P, Hautefeuille P, Lubetzki J (1982) Les glucagonomes. Aspects cliniques, biologiques, anatomopathologiques et thérapeutiques (revue générale de 130 cas). Gastroenterol Clin Biol 6: 1029-1041
64. Guillemin R, Brazeau P, Bohlen P, Esch F, Ling N, Wehrenberg W (1982) Growth hormone-releasing factor from a human pancreatic tumor that caused acromegaly. Science 218: 585-587
65. Günther R, Klose K, Ruckert K et al. (1985) Localization of small islet-cell tumors: preoperative and intraoperative ultrasound, computed tomography, arteriography, digital subtraction angiography, and pancreatic venous sampling. Gastrointestinal Radiol 10: 145-152
66. Hanssen LE, Hanssen KF, Myuren J (1977) Inhibition of secretin release and pancreatic bicarbonate secretion by somatostatin infusions in man. Scand J Gastroenterol 12: 371-394
67. Heding LG, Rasmussen SM (1972) Determination of pancreatic and gut glucagon-like immunoreactivity in normal and diabetic subjects. Diabetologia 8: 408-411
68. Heitz PU, Kasper M, Klöppel G, Vaitukaitis JL (1983) Glycoprotein-hormone alpha chain production by pancreatic endocrine tumors. A specific marker for malignancy. Cancer 51: 277-282
69. Heitz PU, Kasper M, Polak JM, Klöppel G (1982) Pancreatic endocrine tumors: immunocytochemical analysis of 125 tumors. Human Pathol 13: 263-271
70. Heitz PU, Kasper M, Polak JM, Klöppel G (1979) Pathology of the endocrine pancreas. J Histochem Cytochem 27: 1401-1402
71. Higgins GA (1979) Pancreatic islet cell tumors: insulinoma, gastrinoma and glucagonoma. Surg Clin North Am 59: 131-141
72. Higgins GA, Recant L, Rischman AB (1979) The glucagonoma syndrome: surgically curable diabetes. Am J Surg 137: 142-148
73. Ipp E, Dobbs RE, Arimura A, Vale W, Harris V, Unger RH (1977) Release of immunoreactive somatostatin from the pancreas in response to glucose, amino acids, pancreozymin-cholecystokinin, and tolbutamide. J Clin Invest 60: 760-765
74. Ipp E, Dobbs RE, Harris V, Arimura A, Vale W, Unger RM (1977) The effects of gastrin,

gastic inhibitory polypeptide, secretin, and the octapeptide of cholecystokinin upon immunoreactive somatostatin release by the perfused canine pancreas. J Clin Invest 60: 1216-1219
75. Iversen J (1973) Adrenergic receptors and the secretion of glucagon and insulin from the isolated, perfused canine pancreas. J Clin Invest 52: 2102-2116
76. Jensen SL, Christiansen LA, Oxholm AM, Holst JJ (1984) Duodenal somatostatinoma. Br J Surg 71: 159
77. Kahn CR, Rosen SW, Weintraub BD, Fajans SS, Gorden P (1977) Ectopic production of chorionic gonadotropin and its subunits by islet-cell tumors: a specific marker for malignancy. N Engl J Med 297: 565-569
78. Kaneko H, Toshima M, Kobayashi H, Kitzawa M (1983) Ultrastructural characteristics of duodenal somatostatinomas. I. Somatostatinoma cells and Schwann-like cells. Acta Pathol Jpn 33: 347-357
79. Kaneko H, Yanaihairi N, Ito S, Kusumoto J, Fujita T, Ishikawa S, Sumida T, Sekuya M (1979) Somatostatinoma of the duodenum. Cancer 44: 2273-2275
80. Kelly TR (1983) Pancreatic somatostatinoma. Am J Surg 146: 671-673
81. Konturek SJ, Tasler J, Jaworek J, Pawlik W, Walus KM, Schusdziarra V, Meyers CA, Coy DH, Schally AV (1981) Gastrointestinal secretory, motor, circulatory and metabolic effect of prosomatostatin. Proc Natl Acad Sci 78: 1967-1971
82. Kovacs K, Horvath E, Ezrin C, Sepp M, Elman I (1977) Immunoreactive somatostatin in pancreatic islet-cell carcinoma accompanied by ectopic ACTH syndrome. Lancet 1: 1365-1366
83. Krejs GJ, Orci L, Conlon JM, Ravazzola M, Davis GF, Raskin P, Collins SM, McCarthy DM, Baetens D, Rubenstein R, Alder TAM, Unger RH (1979) Somatostatinoma syndrome: biochemical, morphologic and clinical features. N Engl J Med 301: 285-292
84. Kronheim S, Berelowitz M, Pimstone BL (1978) The characterization of somatostatin-like immunoreactivity in human serum. Diabetes 27: 523-529
85. Larsson LI, Grimelius L, Håkanson R, Rehfeld JF, Stadel F, Holst J, Angervall L, Sundler F (1975) Mixed endocrine tumors producing several peptide hormones. Am J Pathol 79: 271-284
86. Larsson LI, Schwartz T, Lundquist G, Chance RE, Sundler F, Rehfeld JF, Grimelius L, Fahrenkrug J, Schaffalitzky de Muckadell OB, Moon N (1976) Occurrence of human pancreatic polypeptide in pancreatic endocrine tumors: possible implications in the watery diarrhea syndrome. Am J Pathol 85: 675-684
87. Larsson LI, Sundler F, Håkanson R (1976) Pancreatic poly-peptide - a postulated new hormone: identification of its cellular storage site by light and electron microscopic immunocytochemistry. Diabetologia 12: 211-226
88. Larsson LI, Holst JJ, Kühl C, Lundquist G, Hirsch MA, Ingemansson S, Lundhaer Jensen S, Rehfeld JF, Schwartz TW (1977) Pancreatic somatostatinoma. Clinical features and physiological implications. Lancet I: 666-668
89. Law DH, Liddale GW, Scott HW Jr, Tauber SD (1965) Ectopic production of multiple hormones by a single malignant tumor. N Engl J Med 273: 292-296
90. Leichter SB (1980) Clinical and metabolic aspects of glucagonoma. Medicine 59: 100-113
91. Lloyd RV, Mervak T, Schmidt K, Warner TF, Wilson BS (1984) Immunohistochemical detection of chromogranin and neuron-specific enolase in pancreatic endocrine neoplasms. Am J Surg Pathol 8: 607-614
92. Lokich J, Anderson N, Rossini A, Hadley W, Federman M, Legg M (1977) Pancreatic alpha cell tumors. Cancer 45: 2675-2683
93. Lowry S, Burt M, Brennan M (1981) Glucose turn-over and gluconeogenesis in a patient with somatostatinoma. Surgery 89: 309-313
94. Luyckx AS, Lefèbvre PJ (1981) Les glucagonomes. Diabète Metab 7: 289-300
95. Mallinson CN, Bloom SR, Warin AP, Salmon PR, Cox B (1974) A glucagonoma syndrome. Lancet II: 1-5
96. Mallinson CN, Bloom SR (1978) The hyperglycaemic cutaneous syndrome: pancreatic glucagonoma. In: Friesen SR (ed) Surgical endocrinology, clinical syndromes. Lippincott, Philadelphia, pp 171-202
97. Malone MJ, Silverman ML, Braasch JW, Jin GL, Dayal Y (1985) Early somatostatinoma of the papilla of the duct of Santorini. Arch Surg 120: 1381-1383

98. Mandarino L, Steiner D, Blanchard W, Nissen S, Gerich J, Ling N, Brazeau P, Bohlen P, Esch F, Guillemin F (1981) Selective effects of somatostatin-14-25 and 28 on in vitro insulin and glucagon secretion. Nature 291: 76-77
99. Marcial MA, Pinkus GS, Skarin A, Hinrichs HR, Warhol MJ (1983) Ampullary somatostatinoma: psammomatous variant of gastrointestinal carcinoid tumor. An immunohistochemical and ultrastructural study. Report of a case and review of the literature. Am J Clin Pathol 80: 755-761
100. Meyers CA, Murphy WA, Redding TW, Coy DH, Schally AV (1980) Synthesis and biological actions of prosomatostatin. Proc Natl Acad Sci USA 77: 6171-6174
101. Moulopolos SD, Stamatelopoulos SF, Vita L (1978) Somatostatin prolongation of the blood pressure lowering effect of diazoxide. Metabolism 27: 1365-1367
102. Nakanome C, Koizumi M, Fujiya H, Akai H, Toyota T, Goto J, Kameyama J, Miyagawa K, Harrew K, Yamagushi K, Kameya T (1983) A case of somatostatinoma syndrome. Nippon Shokalibyo Gakkai Zasshi 80: 1036-1041
103. Nakanome C, Koizuni M, Fujiya H (1984) Somatostatinoma syndrome accompanied by overproduction of pancreatic polypeptide. Tohoku J Exp Med 142/2: 201-210
104. Öberg K, Grimelius L, Lundquist G, Lörelius LE (1981) Update on pancreatic polypeptide as a specific marker for endocrine tumors of pancreas and gut. Acta Med Scand 210: 145-152
105. Öberg K, Wide L (1981) hCG and hCG subunits as tumor markers in patients with endocrine pancreatic tumors and carcinoids. Acta Endocrinol 98: 256-260
106. Ohneda A, Parada E, Eisentraut AM, Unger RH (1968) Characterization of response of circulating glucagon to intraduodenal and intravenous administration of amino acids. J Clin Invest 47: 2305-2322
107. Ohneda A, Otsuki M, Fujiya H, Yaginuma N, Kokubo T, Ohtani H (1979) A malignant insulinoma transformed into a glucagonoma syndrome. Diabetes 28: 962-969
108. O'Neal LW, Kipnis DM, Lux SA, Lacy PE, Jarett L (1968) Secretion of various endocrine substances by ACTH secretory tumors - gastrin, melanotropin, serotonin, parathormones, vasopressin, glucagon. Cancer 21: 1219-1232
109. Orci L, Unger RH (1971) Functional subdivision of islet of Langerhans and possible role of D-cells. Lancet 2: 1243
110. Orci L, Baetens D, Dubois MP (1975) Evidence for the D-cell of the pancreas secreting somatostatin. Horm Metab Res 7: 400-402
111. Orci L, Baetens D, Ravazolla M, Stefan J, Malaisse-Lagae F (1976) Pancreatic polypeptide and glucagon non random distribution in pancreatic islets. Life Sci 19: 1811-1816
112. Palmer JP, Werner L, Benson JW, Ensinck JW (1976) Dominant inheritance of large molecular weight immunoreactive glucagon. Diabetes [Suppl 1] 25: 326A
113. Patel YC, Reichlin S (1978) Somatostatin in hypothalamus, extrahypothalamic brain and peripheral tissues of the rat. Endocrinology 102: 523-530
114. Patel YC (1979) Peripheral distribution and actions of somatostatin. In: Tolis G et al. (eds) Clinical neuroendocrinology: a pathophysiological approach. Raven, New York, pp 139-146
115. Patel YC, Ganda OP, Benoit R (1983) Pancreatic somatostatinoma: abundance of somatostatin 28 (1-12)-like immunoreactivity in tumor and plasma. J Clin Endocrinol Metab 57: 1048-1053
116. Pearse AGE, Polak JM, Heath CM (1974) Polypeptide hormone production by "carcinoid" apudomas and their relevant cytochemistry. Virchows Arch [A] 16: 95-109
117. Pearse AGE (1968) Common cytochemical and ultrastructural characteristics of cells producing polypeptide hormones (the APUD series) and their relevance to thyroid and ultimobranchial C-cells and calcitonin. Proc R Soc Lond 170: 71-80
118. Pek S, Fajans SS, Floyd JC, Knopf RF, Conn JW (1972) Failure of sulfonylureas to suppress plasma glucagon in man. Diabetes 21: 216-223
119. Penman E, Lowry PJ, Wass JAM, Marks V, Dawson AM, Besser GM, Rees LH (1980) Molecular forms of somatostatin in normal subjects and in patients with pancreatic somatostatinoma. Clin Endocrinol 12: 611-620
120. Permutt MS, Biesbroeck J, Chyn R (1977) Characteristics of high molecular weight insulin in insulinoma patients. J Clin Endocrinol Metabol 44: 536-544
121. Perrino PP, Lavine RL, Bhathena SJ, Burns WA, Recant L (1975) Big glucagon in glucagonoma. Clin Res 37: 446A

122. Pimstone B, Berelowitz M, Kranold D, Shapiro B, Kronheim S (1978) Somatostatin-like immunoreactivity (SRIF-LI) in human and rat serum. Metabolism 27 [Suppl 1]: 1145-1149
123. Pinsard D, Odent S, Chadenas D (1986) Pancreatic polypeptide in somatostatinoma (letter). Dig Dis Sci 31: 445-446
124. Pipeleers D, Somers G, Gepts W, De Nutte N, De Vroede M (1979) Plasma pancreatic hormone levels in a case of somatostatinoma: diagnostic and therapeutic implications. J Clin Endocrinol Metab 49: 572-579
125. Pipeleers D, Couturier E, Gepts W, Reynders J, Somers G (1983) Five cases of somatostatinoma: clinical heterogeneity and diagnostic usefulness of basal and tolbutamide-induced hypersomatostatinemia. J Clin Endocrinol Metab 56: 1236-1242
126. Polak JM, Bloom SR, Adrian TE, Heitz Ph, Bryant MG, Pearse AGE (1976) Pancreatic polypeptide in insulinomas, gastrinomas, vipomas and glucagonomas. Lancet I: 328-330
127. Polak JM, Pearse AGE, Grimelius L, Bloom SR, Arimura A (1979) Growth hormone release inhibiting hormone in gastrointestinal and pancreatic D-cell. Lancet I: 1220-1222
128. Pradayrol L, Jornvall H, Mutt V, Ribet A (1980) N-terminally extended somatostatin: the primary structure of somatostatin-28. FEBS Lett 109: 55-58
129. Prinz RA, Marangos PJ (1982) Use of neuron-specific enolase as a serum marker for neuroendocrine neoplasms. Surgery 92: 887-889
130. Prinz RA, Bermes EW, Kimmel JR, Marangos PJ (1983) Serum markers for pancreatic islet cell and intestinal carcinoid tumors: a comparison of neuron-specific enolase, beta-human chorionic gonadotropin and pancreatic polypeptide. Surgery 94: 1019-1023
131. Prinz RA, Marangos PJ (1983) Serum neuron specific enolase: a serum marker for "nonfunctioning" pancreatic islet cell carcinoma. Am J Surg 145: 77-81
132. Prinz RA, Sandberg L (1984) Serum levels of alpha-1-antitrypsin in pancreatic islet cell tumors. J Med 15: 177-183
133. Recant L, Perrino PV, Bhathena SJ, Danforth DN Jr, Lavine RL (1976) Plasma immunoreactive glucagon fractions in four cases of glucagonoma: increased "large glucagon immunoreactivity". Diabetologia 12: 319-326
134. Reychlin S (1983) Somatostatin (first of two parts). N Engl J Med 309: 1495-1500
135. Reynolds C, Pratt R, Chan-Yan C, Boyko W, MacDonald W, Schmidt N, Rudland R (1985) Somatostatinoma: the most recently described pancreatic islet cell tumor. West J Med 142: 393-397
136. Ricci GL, Fevery J (1981) Cholestatic action of somatostatin in the rat: effect on the different fractions of bile secretion. Gastroenterology 81: 552-562
137. Rivier J, Spiess J, Thorner M, Vale W (1982) Characterization of a growth hormone-releasing factor from a human pancreatic islet tumor. Nature 300: 276-278
138. Roberts L Jr, Dunnick NR, Foster WL Jr, Halvorsen RA, Gibbons RG, Meyers WC, Feldman JM, Thompson WM (1984) Somatostatinoma of the endocrine pancreas: CT findings. J Comput Assist Tomogr 8: 1015-1018
139. Rückert K, Klotter H, Kümmerle F (1984) Intraoperative ultrasonic localization of endocrine tumors of the pancreas. Surgery 96: 1045-1047
140. Ruttman E, Klöppel G, Bommer G, Kiehn M, Heitz PU (1980) Pancreatic glucagonoma with and without syndrome. Immunocytochemical study of 5 tumor cases and review of the literature. Virchows Arch [A] 388: 51-67
141. Sakazaki S, Umeyama K, Nakagawa H, Hashimoto H, Kamino K, Mitsuhashi T, Yamaguchi K (1983) Pancreatic somatostatinoma. Am J Surg 146: 674-679
142. Schally AV, Dupont A, Arimura A, Redding TW (1976) Isolation and structure of growth hormone-release inhibiting hormone (somatostatin) from porcine hypothalami. Biochemistry 15: 505-514
143. Schernthaner BW, Carpenter PC, Block B, Brazeau P (1984) Ectopic secretion of a growth hormone-releasing factor. Am J Med 76: 605-616
144. Schlegel W, Raptis S, Harvey RF, Oliver JM, Pfeiffer EF (1977) Inhibitor of cholecystokinin-pancreozymin release by somatostatin. Lancet 2: 166-168
145. Schmeckel DE, Marangos PJ, Brightman MW (1979) Neuron specific enolase is a marker for peripheral and central neuroendocrine cells. Nature 276: 834-836
146. Schmeckel DE, Marangos PJ, Zis AP, Brightman M, Goodwin FK (1978) The brain enolases as specific marker for neuronal and glial cells. Science 199: 313-315

147. Schuit F, Pipeleers D (1986) Pancreatic A and B cells differ in their recognition of somatostatin. Diabetologia 29: 592A
148. Schusdziarra V, Zyznar E, Rouiller D, Boden G, Brown JC, Arimura A, Unger RH (1980) Splanchnic somatostatin: a hormonal regulator of nutrient homeostasis. Science 207: 530-532
149. Schusdziarra V (1983) Somatostatin: physiological and pathophysiological aspects. Scand J Gastroenterol [Suppl] 82: 69-84
150. Schusdziarra V, Grube D, Seifert H, Galle J, Etzrodt H, Beischer W, Haferkamp O, Pfeiffer EF (1983) Somatostatinoma syndrome. Clinical, morphological and metabolic features and therapeutic aspects. Klin Wochenschr 61: 681-689
151. Schwartz TW (1979) Pancreatic polypeptide (PP) and endocrine tumors of the pancreas. Scand J Gastroenterol 14: 93-100
152. Seiko I, Yukio Y, Toshihiko I, Hiroshi K, Akira S (1982) Somatostatin-28 like immunoreactivity in normal and tumor tissue from duodenum and pancreas. Acta Endocrinol 101: 421-427
153. Schally A, Huang W, Chang R, Arimura A, Redding T, Millar R, Hunkapiller M, Hood L (1980) Isolation and structure of pro-somatostatin: a putative somatostatin precursor from pig hypothalamus. Proc Natl Acad Sci USA 77: 4489-4493
154. Shawker TH, Doppman JL, Dunnick NR, MacCarthy DM (1982) Ultrasonic investigation of pancreatic islet cell tumors. J Ultrasound Med 1: 193-200
155. Somers G, Gepts W, Pipeleers D (1982) On the diagnosis of somatostatinoma. Acta Gastroent Belg 45: 322-326
156. Somers G, Pipeleers-Marichal M, Gepts W, Pipeleers D (1983) A case of duodenal somatostatinoma: diagnostic usefulness of calcium-pentagastrin test. Gastroenterology 85: 1192-1198
157. Srikant CB, Patel YC (1981) Receptor binding of somatostatin-28 is tissue specific. Nature 294: 259-260
158. Stacpoole PW, Kasselberg AG, Berelowitz M, Chey WY (1983) Somatostatinoma syndrome: does a clinical entity exist? Acta Endocrinologica 102: 80-87
159. Stalmans W (1983) Glucagon and liver glycogen metabolism. In: Lefèbvre PJ (ed) Glucagon I. Springer, Berlin Heidelberg New York, pp 291-314
160. Stark D, Moss A, Goldberg H, Deveney C, Way L (1983) Computed tomography and nuclear magnetic resonance imaging of pancreatic islet-cell tumors. Surgery 94: 1024-1027
161. Stark D, Moss A, Goldberg H, Deveney C (1984) CT of pancreatic islet cell tumors. Radiology 150: 491-494
162. Steiner DF, Oyer PE (1967) The biosynthesis of insulin and a probable precursor of insulin by a human islet cell adenoma. Proc Natl Acad Sci USA 57: 473-480
163. Steiner DF, Cunningham D, Spigelman L, Aten B (1967) Insulin biosynthesis: evidence of a precursor. Science 157: 697-760
164. Taccagni GL, Carlucci M, Sironi M, Cantaboni A, Di Carlo V (1986) Duodenal somatostatinoma with psammoma bodies: an immunohistochemical and ultrastructural study. Am J Gastroenterol 81: 33-37
165. Tapia FJ, Polak JM, Barbosa AJA, Bloom SR, Marangos PJ, Dermody C, Pearse AGE (1981) Neurone-specific enolase is produced by neuroendocrine tumours. Lancet I: 808-811
166. Taruya E, Hashimoto H, Sakazaki S, Umeyama K (1984) Electron microscopic study of pancreatic somatostatinoma. J Clin Electron Microsc 17: 381-388
167. Taylor IL, Rolter J, Walsh JH, Passaro D Jr (1978) Is pancreatic polypeptide a marker for Zollinger-Ellison syndrome? Lancet 1: 845-848
168. Unger RH, Aguilar-Parada E, Müller WA, Eisentraut AM (1970) Studies of pancreatic alpha cell function in normal and diabetic subjects. J Clin Invest 49: 837-848
169. Unger RH, Orci L (1976) Physiology and pathophysiology of glucagon. Physiol Rev 56: 778-826
170. Unger RH (1977) Somatostatinoma. N Engl J Med 296: 998-1000
171. Unger RH, Orci L (1981) Glucagon and the A-cell: physiology and pathophysiology. N Engl J Med 304: 1518-1524, 1575-1580
172. Van Noorden S, Polak JM, Pearse AGE (1977) Single cellular origin of somatostatin and calcitonin in the rat thyroid gland. Histochemistry 53: 243-247

173. Varndell IM, Polak JM (1985) Immunocytochemistry. In: Polak JM, Bloom SR (eds) Endocrine tumours. Livingstone, Edinburgh, pp 116-143
174. Vatn MH, Schrumpf E, Hanssen KF (1977) The effect of somatostatin on pentagastrin-stimulated gastric secretion and on plasma gastrin in man. Scand J Gastroenterol 12: 833-839
175. Vaysse N, Pradayrol L, Sucini C, Chayvialle JA, Ribet A (1981) Somatostatin 28: biological actions. In: Bloom SR, Polak JM (eds) Gut hormones. Livingstone, Edinburgh, pp 358-361
176. Villar HV, Johnson DG, Lynch PJ, Pond GD, Smith PH (1981) Pattern of immunoreactive glucagon in portal, arterial and peripheral plasma before and after removal of glucagonoma. Am J Surg 141: 148-152
177. Wahren J, Felig P (1976) Influence of somatostatin on carbohydrate disposal and absorption in diabetes mellitus. Lancet II: 1213-1216
178. Weir GC, Knowlton SD, Martin DB (1974) Glucagon secretion from the perfused rat pancreas: studies with glucose and catecholamines. J Clin Invest 54: 1403-1412
179. Weir GC, Horton ES, Aoki TT, Slovik DM (1976) Increased large glucagon immunoreactivity in the glucagonoma syndrome. Diabetes 25: 326
180. Welbourne RB, Polak JM, Bloom SR, Pearse AGE, Galland RB (1978) Apudomas of the pancreas. In: Bloom SR, Polak JM (eds) Gut hormones. Livingstone, Edinburgh, pp 561-569
181. White A, Tan K, Gray C, Roberts I, Ratcliffe JG (1985) Multiple hormone secretion by a human pancreatic glucagonoma in culture. Regul Pept 11: 335-345
182. Williams G, Ghatei M, Burnin JM, Bloom JR (1986) Severe hyperglucagonemia during treatment with oxymetholone. Br Med J 292: 1637-1638
183. Wood SM, Polak JM, Bloom SR (1983) The glucagonoma syndrome. In: Lefèbvre PJ (ed) Glucagon II. Springer, Berlin Heidelberg New York, pp 411-430
184. Woodtli W, Hedinger C (1978) Pancreatic islet-cell tumours and their syndromes. II. Zollinger-Ellison syndrome, glucagonoma syndrome, multiple endocrine adenomatosis and islet-cell tumours not obviously provable. Schweiz Med Wochenschr 108: 1997-2007
185. Wright J, Abollathi A, Penman E, Marks V (1980) Pancreatic somatostatinoma presenting with hypoglycemia. Clin Endocrinol 12: 603-608
186. Yano T, Yamamoto N, Fujimori K, Inamori S, Hayashi H, Mizumoto R (1982) Glucagon-secreting pancreatic islet cell carcinoma containing insulin and somatostatin, with hypoglycemic attack. Am J Gastroenterol 77: 387-391

Insulin Secretion in Diabetes Mellitus*

E. Cerasi

Introduction: Diabetes Mellitus – Insulin Deficiency or Insulin Resistance?

Endocrinologists, by tradition, think of disease in terms of hyper- or hypofunctioning of glands. The soundness of this "old-fashioned" thinking has been established repeatedly; type 1, insulin-dependent diabetes mellitus (IDDM) exemplifies this. Indeed, complete agreement exists that IDDM is the consequence of severe insulin deficiency caused by B-cell destruction. Doubt that the situation is as simple in type 2, non-insulin-dependent diabetes mellitus (NIDDM) was voiced as early as 1936 [1], and gained momentum after the studies of YALOW and BERSON [2], when it was shown that plasma insulin in NIDDM could be as high as in control subjects. Since then, numerous studies have confirmed these observations and shown that the plasma insulin values after an oral glucose load or following meals are often higher in NIDDM patients than in controls [3-5]. These observations led to the logical hypothesis that NIDDM is due to resistance to the action of insulin, rather than to reduction in insulin secretion [6]. Many studies over the past decade, mainly employing the euglycemic clamp technique, have indeed demonstrated that sensitivity to insulin is reduced in lean as well as obese NIDDM patients [for review see 7, 8].

It is not my intention to discuss in detail the issue of insulin resistance as the prime pathophysiologic phenomenon of NIDDM. However, for the intelligibility of the topic under discussion, some clarifications seem necessary. Judged from data from euglycemic clamp experiments, the insulin resistance of NIDDM patients, especially if obese, should be quite pronounced [6, 9, 10]. Still, recent studies show that in NIDDM almost complete normalization of the blood glucose level can be achieved within days by insulin treatment [11-13]. From the data of two North American studies [11, 12], where patients were moderately to severely obese, the mean daily insulin dose needed to maintain normoglycemia was calculated to be 1.2-1.6 U/kg.24 h. In our study [13] smaller doses were sufficient (0.6 U/kg.24 h). If one takes into consideration the presence of obesity, which is a well-established cause of insulin resistance, and the normal insulin production rate (0.6-1.1 U/kg.24 h) [13a], it seems evident that NIDDM patients can respond to insulin in a manner not strikingly different from patients with IDDM. Furthermore, several

* Studies performed during recent years in my laboratory were mainly supported by the Yad Hanadiv Foundation and the Juvenile Diabetes Foundation International.

studies have demonstrated that insulin resistance diminishes or disappears after a period of normoglycemia whatever the therapeutic means utilized [11, 12, 14–17], which suggests that insulin resistance is secondary to chronic hyperglycemia. We and others [18–20] have presented evidence indicating that glucose downregulates its own transport; it is therefore possible that the decreased peripheral glucose uptake in diabetic subjects is the consequence of adaptation of muscle and adipose tissue to chronic hyperglycemia. Thus it is unlikely that insulin resistance is the initiator of the diabetic process. This is not to deny that some reduction in insulin sensitivity may exist even in the early stages of diabetes [21–23]; however, I believe that its pathophysiologic role has been exaggerated.

Consideration of insulin resistance as the main causal factor for hyperglycemia relies on the fact that NIDDM patients are hyperinsulinemic. However, since the early 1960s at least as many studies have claimed that insulin secretion is reduced in NIDDM as have stated the contrary [for a short discussion of this controversy, see 24]. Although the patient materials studied have not always been comparable, and heterogeneity of insulin secretion certainly exists, in most instances the interpretation of hypersecretion of insulin in NIDDM has been due to experimental artefact, for the following reasons.

As has been discussed recently, the assessment of insulin secretion in man is difficult [25]. This difficulty stems mainly from two factors. First, insulin release in vivo is estimated from peripheral insulin levels, with the assumption that the hepatic extraction and peripheral clearance of insulin are constant; however, it has been shown convincingly that this is not the case [26–29]. Methods for calculating the insulin secretion rate by concomittant C-peptide measurement [30] or C-peptide infusion [31], and by a variety of mathematical manipulations of varying complexity [32–34] have been described; however, their use has been the exception rather than the rule. Despite these limitations, however, a recent study shows that peripheral insulin levels may reflect the systemic delivery rate of insulin [35].

The second difficulty relates to the correlation between stimulus and response. The basic fact that insulin response cannot be quantified unless it is related to the magnitude of the stimulus applied to the B-cell has been almost universally ignored in clinical studies. Because the sensitivity of the B-cell to i.v. glucose is modest, ignoring the magnitude of the stimulus (within reasonable limits) may not be critical in those studies where glucose was injected as a bolus or given as an infusion. However, in most studies oral glucose loads or meals were used; under these conditions the synergistic interaction between glucose and "incretins" [36] is very large, and minute differences in blood glucose may have extraordinary effects on the plasma insulin concentration. This point is illustrated in Fig. 1, where a dose-response study for oral glucose loads was performed in control subjects and mild NIDDM patients [37]. It is clearly seen that at a critical blood glucose range, increasing the level by as little as 10 mg/dl in healthy subjects may be sufficient to increase the insulin response by 50%–70%. The lowering and shift to the right of the dose-response curve in NIDDM is evident. Considered against this background, it becomes apparent that the insulin response of a hyperglycemic person, if similar to that of a normoglycemic one, in reality indicates severe impairment of the insulin secretion. To illustrate this point, it was shown in a recent study that Asian Indian control subjects showed twice as high insulin responses to oral glu-

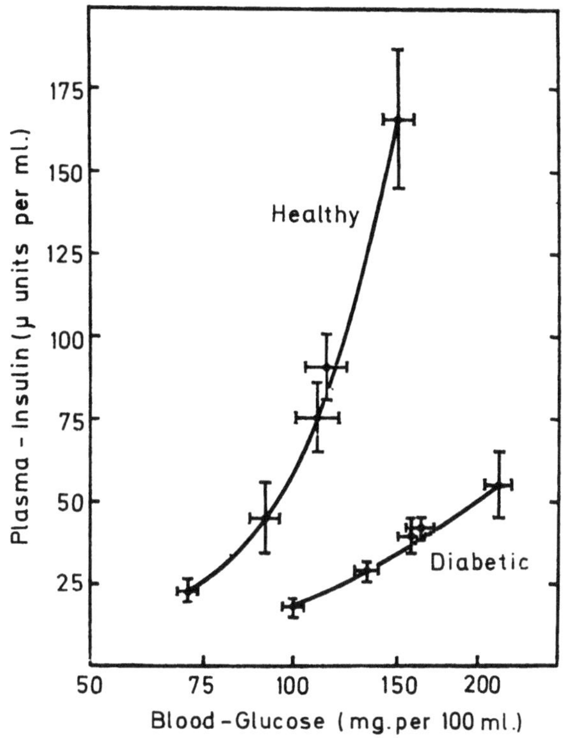

Fig. 1. The dose-response relationship for glucose-induced insulin release during oral glucose tolerance testing. Glucose was ingested at doses of 0.35, 0.7, and 1.4 g/kg, and 1.4 g/kg combined with i.v. infusion of 5 mg/kg·min from 0 to 60 min. The data refer to peak blood glucose and plasma insulin values. *Horizontal and vertical bars* stand for the SE of the mean glucose and insulin levels respectively. (From 25)

cose as Europeans, the data being interpreted to indicate racial differences in B-cell function [38]. However, peak blood glucose was one mmol/l higher in the Indians (statistically not significant), a difference which, assessed on the dose-response curve of Fig. 1 gave a two-fold difference in the insulin values, thus suggesting that B-cell responsiveness was identical in the two groups. In the majority of studies on insulin secretion in NIDDM where a claim for normal or increased insulin secretion was made, such conclusions proved unjustified when the data were evaluated in a similar manner; it is remarkable that even the Stockholm group has been inattentive to the importance of blood glucose differences during oral glucose tolerance testing and misinterpreted the insulin levels in subjects with borderline glucose intolerance as indicative of islet hyperresponsiveness [22]. If one considers that the "incretin" effect of glucose ingestion may be reduced in NIDDM patients [39, 39a], the gap between the insulin responses of control and diabetic persons at "isoglycemic" oral loads could even be greater. For these reasons, unless full dose-response studies like those shown in Fig. 1 are performed, no quantitative information on insulin secretion can be generated from oral glucose loads.

This confusion of hyperinsulinemia with hyperresponsiveness of the B-cell has dominated the thinking on the pathophysiology of NIDDM for the past decade and a half. Thus, in populations with high risk for NIDDM (and where obesity is prominent), such as Pima Indians, Mexican Americans, and Micronesians [40-42], hyperinsulinemia in response to glucose ingestion has been associated with the "prediabetic" state, and the theory of "exhaustion" of the hyperfunctioning B-cells voiced as the cause of diabetes [41, 43]. Against the above discussion, I do not think that the information available supports such a hypothesis.

The problem of synergistic interactions is greatly reduced when glucose is given intravenously, and therefore the plasma insulin levels reflect more closely the B-cell response to glucose. In all studies where i.v. glucose was utilized, the insulin response of NIDDM patients (even when the diabetes was minimal) was found to be severely impaired [21, 44-50]. Fig. 2 illustrates the quantitative aspect of the deficient insulin response in NIDDM. In these mildly diabetic patients (fasting blood glucose ~180 mg/dl) the maximal insulin response to glucose was reduced by 80%-90% compared to weight-matched controls.

Various aspects of the deficient insulin secretion in diabetes will be discussed below. This introduction has aimed at emphasizing the fundamental role that insulin deficiency plays not only in IDDM but also in NIDDM, and stressed the extreme caution that is necessary in the interpretation of insulin secretion data in vivo.

Kinetic Aspects of Glucose-Induced Insulin Release in Diabetes

The pancreatic B-cell responds to stimuli in an oscillatory manner both in vitro and in vivo. Sudden elevations of the glucose concentration induce an immediate burst of insulin release, followed by a fall in the secretion rate. If high glucose lev-

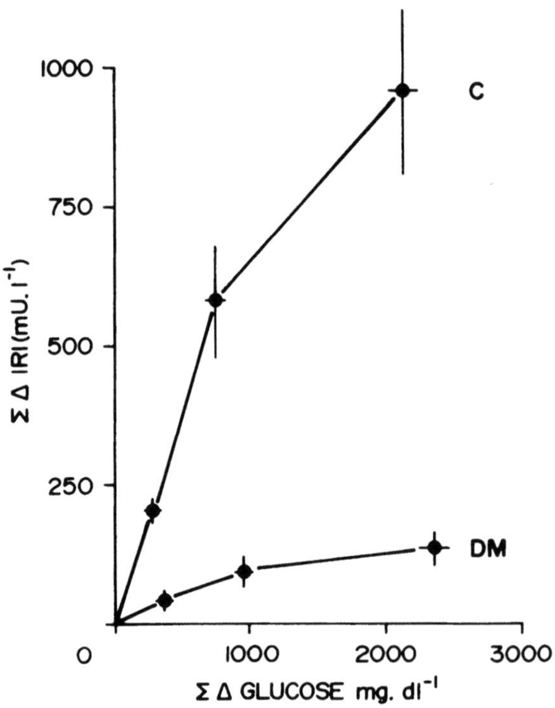

Fig. 2. The dose-response relationship for glucose-induced insulin release during intravenous glucose tolerance testing. Glucose was injected i.v. at the doses of 0.1, 0.3, and 0.9 g/kg. The data refer to the incremental plasma glucose and insulin concentrations integrated over 60 min. Symbols as for Fig. 1; *C*, control subjects; *DM*, diabetics. (From 19)

els are maintained, insulin release gradually augments to form the second-phase response. The reason for the biphasic nature of the insulin response is not clear. However, studies in man and in vitro suggest that glucose acts on insulin release at least in three distinct ways: (1) It initiates the chain of events, commonly referred to as "stimulus-secretion coupling", which are responsible for the acute secretion, and are a *conditio sine qua non* for the occurrence of release at any time. This action of glucose is very rapidly initiated, and is as rapidly reversed once the hexose falls below a threshold level. Its magnitude is best reflected by the initial, first-phase insulin response. (2) Shortly after initiation of secretion, glucose generates refractoriness in the B-cell, called "time-dependent inhibition", which reduces the secretion rate despite ongoing stimulation. This inhibitory action persists after glucose is withdrawn, with a t½ of the order of several minutes [51-53]. (3) The third event, slower in onset, amplifies the insulin response with time, and thus is responsible for the late increase in the secretion rate [54-57]. We have named this phenomenon "time-dependent potentiation"; its t½ is also quite long. Based on several lines of evidence, we have postulated that the biphasic nature of glucose-induced insulin release is due to the expression with different time courses, of both time-dependent inhibition and potentiation of the acute stimulus-secretion coupling, the sum of these positive and negative inputs resulting in the oscillation of the secretion rate [58, 58a].

This characteristic aspect of glucose-induced insulin release is important, since in NIDDM and experimental models of diabetes not all aspects of insulin secretion are equally affected, as discussed below.

Acute Insulin Response

The most pronounced defect of the insulin response to glucose in NIDDM relates to the first minutes of stimulation, first-phase release being severely reduced. Fig. 3 shows the insulin secretory pattern in a group of NIDDM patients with modest hyperglycemia; the decreased and delayed appearance of the response is striking. This pattern is observed both in overtly diabetic subjects and in persons with glucose intolerance only [for review see 22, 59]; however, the higher the fasting blood glucose of the patient, the flatter the insulin response to glucose [49]. Indeed, in several patients glucose may initially induce a fall in the plasma insulin level [60, 61]; the possible significance of this phenomenon is discussed in the contribution of Hellman in this volume.

Reduced acute insulin response to glucose is also observed in a variety of diabetes-like syndromes in animals, such as *Macaca nigra* [62], the New Zealand white rabbit [63], Chinese hamsters [64-66], C57BL/KsJ-db/db mice [67], *Acomys cahirinus* [68-71], and nonketotic Biobreeding (BB) rats [72]. It is of interest that also in diabetes induced by experimental manipulations in rats like neonatal streptozotocin injection [73-75] or partial pancreatectomy [76] the effect of glucose on acute insulin release is markedly impaired.

Only few studies exist on the dose-kinetics of glucose-induced insulin release in diabetes. In NIDDM patients, first-phase insulin response to glucose shows decreased maximal capacity (Vmax reduction) (Fig. 2) [19, 48, 77]. Second-phase re-

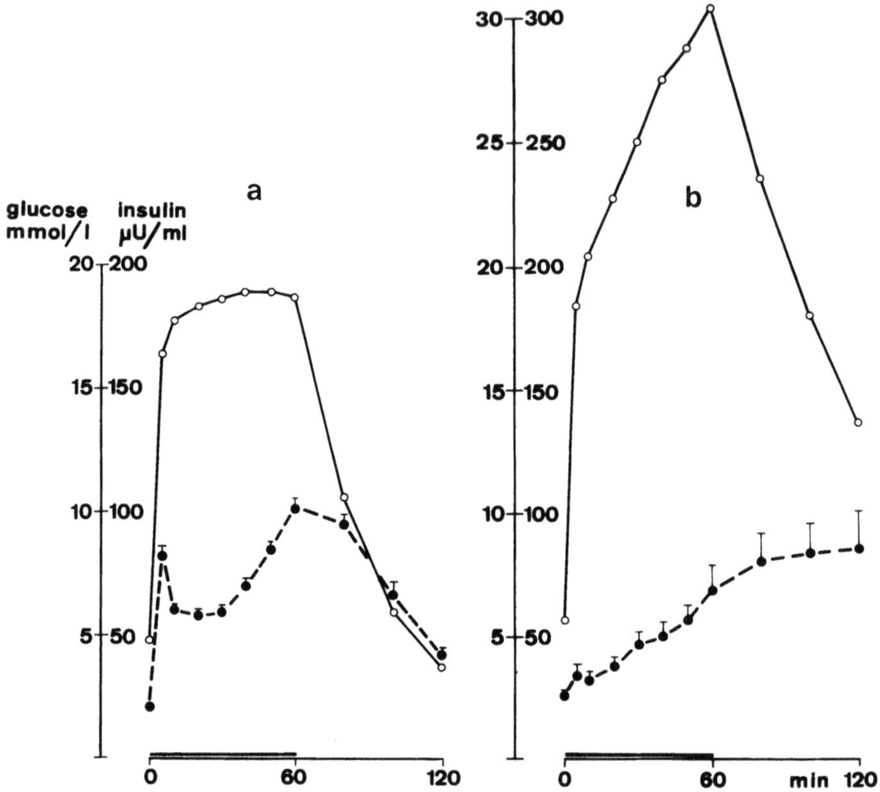

Fig. 3a, b. Plasma insulin response to glucose infusion in lean controls (**a**) and mild NIDDM (**b**). Glucose was given as an i.v. bolus (0.5 g/kg) followed by constant infusion (20 mg/kg·min, 0-60 min). *Open circles* denote the blood glucose values, *filled circles* the plasma insulin. (From 50)

sponse was found to increase with very high blood glucose levels [48], the dose-response curve thus showing a right-shift (increased apparent Km) in the glucose-insulin relationship. Since on oral glucose tolerance testing the insulin response corresponds mainly to second-phase release, a similar Km change was noted (Fig. 1) [37]. It has to be realized, however, that saturation of the insulin response to glucose is obtained only with difficulty in man, and therefore statements [48] regarding the kinetic nature of the secretory defect in diabetes (Km vs Vmax changes) should be accepted with caution. Nevertheless, findings very similar to those in NIDDM were obtained in islets isolated from *Acomys cahirinus:* full glucose dose-response studies demonstrated that, compared to rat islets, the Vmax of the first-phase response was reduced, while second-phase response showed Km changes [69].

Time-Dependent Effects of Glucose on Insulin Release

Second-phase glucose-induced insulin release is partly retained in most NIDDM patients unless their fasting blood glucose exceeds ~200 mg/dl [78]. As briefly discussed above, several lines of evidence suggest that second-phase insulin release is the expression of the ability of glucose to generate potentiation in the islet [58a, 79]. This action of glucose can be shown most efficiently by applying sequential glucose stimulations, where the insulin response to the second stimulus usually becomes two- to threefold greater. In a series of experiments, where a 1-h glucose infusion was repeated following a 40- to 60-min rest period, it could be demonstrated that the insulin response to the second stimulus was greatly amplified in subjects with NIDDM or decreased glucose tolerance [80]. Indeed, by performing complex dose-response studies, it was found that the sensitivity for the potentiating effect of glucose in NIDDM was equal to or greater than that in control subjects [80]. A more striking demonstration of the conservation of glucose-induced time-dependent potentiation in a functionally deficient islet is offered by the NIDDM model *Acomys cahirinus* [71]. As shown in Fig. 4, repeated stimulation of the *Acomys* islets by glucose not only resulted in the marked amplification of the response; the kinetics of the insulin secretion were also modified, a prominent (albeit still somewhat delayed) first-phase response becoming evident. Thus, while the acute insulin-releasing effect of glucose is greatly reduced in NIDDM, the ability of the sugar to generate time-dependent potentiation is retained and may even partly correct the secretory defect. So far only one group has attempted to exploit this effect of glucose priming in NIDDM therapeutically, with success being obtained only in some patients [81]. This issue definitely deserves further clinical trials.

The time-dependent potentiation induced by glucose was found to be reduced in the BB rat [72] and in NIDDM generated by neonatal injection of streptozotocin [75]. The latter finding may be of relevance to the observation that in this rat model of NIDDM, in contrast to findings in humans and in *Acomys*, insulin response to glucose is characteristically uniphasic, with a reduced first-phase response and almost total absence of second-phase release [73-75].

The memory of a previous stimulation in the B-cell does not always potentiate the subsequent insulin responses. Short-lasting stimulations with glucose [51] or arginine [52, 53] induce time-dependent inhibition of the release. This is illustrated in Fig. 5, where the insulin response to arginine, given 20 min after a first arginine injection, was reduced by 30%-40% in control subjects. In contrast, no time-dependent inhibition could be demonstrated in NIDDM or in glucose-intolerant obese subjects [82]. This is not due to a defect specific for diabetes; indeed, it was shown both in vitro [53] and in vivo [82] that hyperglycemia abolishes the effect of arginine on insulin inhibition through the synergistic interaction that exists between glucose and the amino acid. This is demonstrated in Fig. 5, where healthy subjects were rendered as hyperglycemic as the NIDDM patients by the glucose clamp technique. Under these conditions arginine induced much larger insulin responses; however, no inhibition of the second response could be seen. Thus, in hyperglycemic NIDDM it cannot be investigated whether the generation of a time-dependent inhibitory memory is modified. While the blood glucose level of the patient can be normalized by insulin administration, the insulin response to, for example, arginine in normoglycemic diabetics is extremely low [83], excluding the possibility to investigate inhibitory memories.

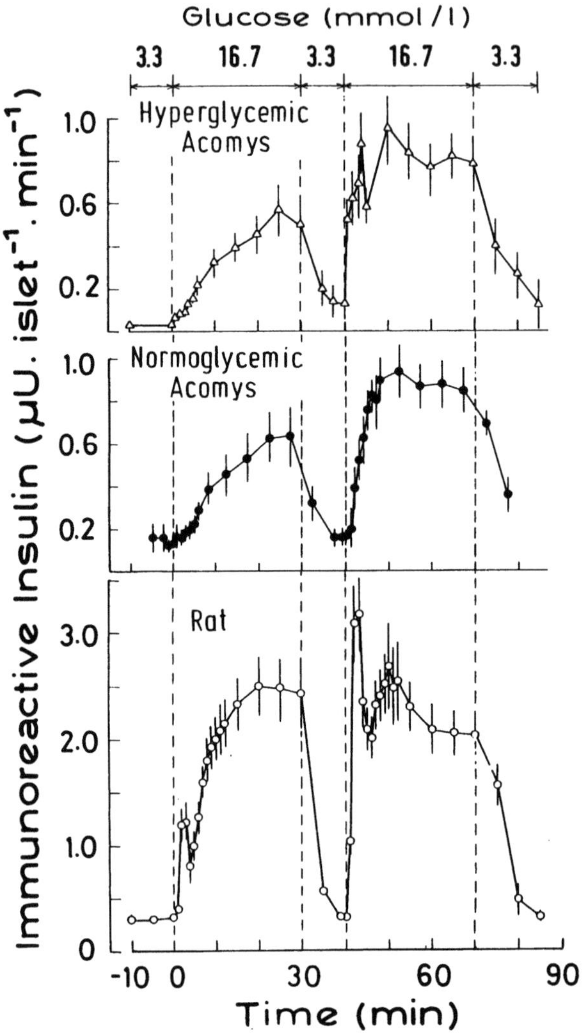

Fig. 4. Time-dependent potentiation of insulin release from rat, and normoglycemic and hyperglycemic *Acomys cahirinus*. Islets were perifused sequentially with basal (3.3 mmol/l) and stimulatory (16.7 mmol/l) glucose concentrations. (From 71)

Basal Insulin Secretion

Insulin secretion is controlled by a variety of factors, including nutrient substrates, hormones, and neurotransmitters, glucose being the dominating regulator. There is no evidence to indicate that basal insulin secretion is regulated differently from the stimulated secretion, also the basal release rate being dependent on the basal glucose concentration in this tightly coupled regulatory feedback system.

In NIDDM the basal insulin levels are variable but usually within the range of the control population [84–86]. However, since these patients are hyperglycemic,

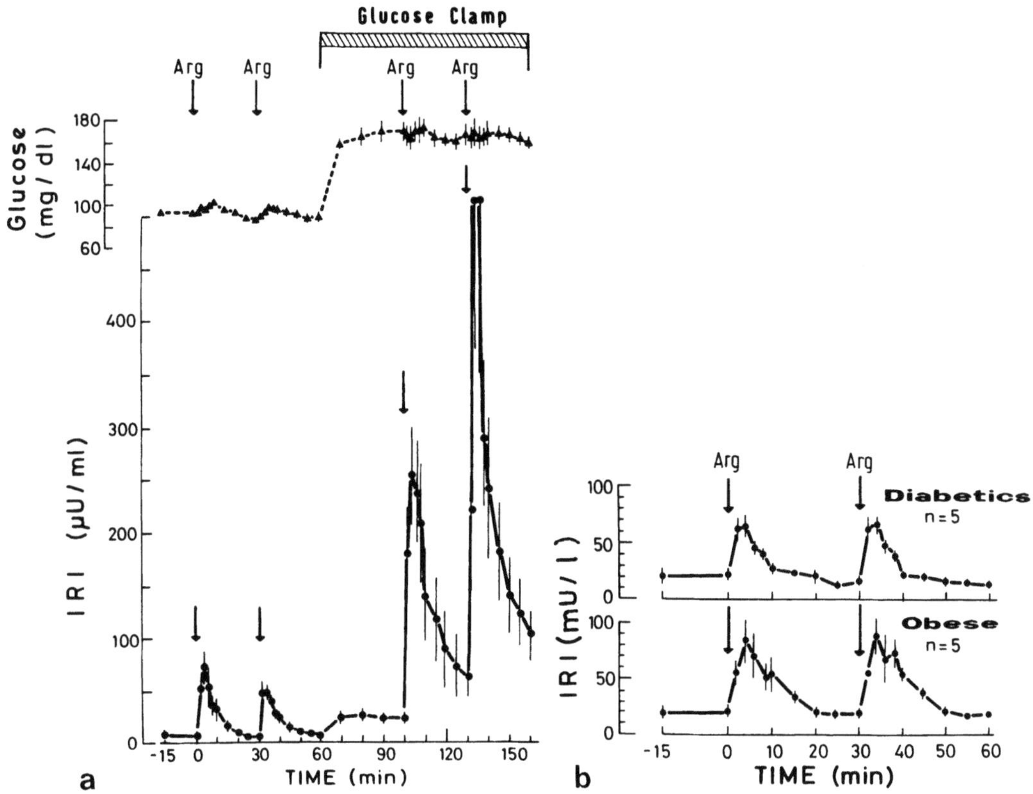

Fig. 5 a, b. Time-dependent inhibition of insulin release. Response to sequential arginine injections (75 mg/kg, *arrows*) **a** at basal state and during hyperglycemic clamp in control subjects, **b** at basal state in lean NIDDM and obese glucose intolerant subjects. (From 82)

their "basal" state in reality corresponds to a situation of glucose stimulation. That this assumption is correct has been shown by inducing normoglycemia in NIDDM patients with insulin infusion and demonstrating that the "basal" plasma insulin values then diminish markedly [87]. Furthermore, from comparison with the steady-state plasma insulin level obtained in control subjects rendered hyperglycemic by glucose infusion [83], it can be concluded that the basal insulin secretion in NIDDM is diminished to the same extent as the stimulated release. Based on these considerations an attractive hypothesis has been presented [88-90] according to which the basal insulin level in NIDDM is the result of B-cell adaptation to hyperglycemia, the degree of fasting hyperglycemia in its turn being a function of the adaptive capacity of the B-cell, the feedback regulatory system thus arriving at equilibrium.

The proportion of unconverted proinsulin that is secreted together with insulin is higher in diabetic patients [91, 92]. Therefore, RIA assays of insulin, which cross-react with proinsulin, underestimate the hypoinsulinemia of NIDDM.

Glucose Specificity of the Secretory Defect in Diabetes

Although glucose is the predominant regulator of insulin secretion, many other natural and man-made substances also act as secretagogues, and have been used as such for investigative purposes in NIDDM. The main difficulty in interpreting the results of insulin release in such studies derives from the fact that most nonglucose secretagogues show complex synergistic interactions with glucose [93-98]. These synergistic interactions can be qualitatively described as those that increase the sensitivity of the B-cell for glucose (reduction of the glucose Km), and those that amplify the action of glucose (increased Vmax). Sulfonylurea drugs are the best-known representatives of the first group [97], while arginine, a commonly used nonglucose stimulator, represents the latter group [99].

The plasma insulin response to arginine infusion [99, 100] or injection [82] in NIDDM is seemingly normal or only slightly decreased (Fig. 5). This is an artefact due to the hyperglycemia of the patients; indeed, when control subjects were hyperglycemia-matched with NIDDM patients by a glucose infusion, it became evident that the diabetic response was only 10%-15% of the matched control one (Fig. 5). Similar results were also obtained by performing arginine infusions during normo-, hypo-, and hyperglycemic clamps [101], and in two studies where the effect of arginine was superimposed on a range of glucose loads [99, 102]. The maximal insulin response to combined arginine-glucose stimulation is reduced in NIDDM, as is the glucose dose-response relationship that describes the effect of arginine at various glucose levels [99, 101, 102].

The above results may be taken to indicate that the diabetic B-cell defect includes the arginine stimulus, and therefore is not specific for glucose. Gerich's group [101] concluded that in NIDDM the response to nonglucose secretagogues is abnormal, probably due to a defective modulatory effect of glucose; Porte's group [102] stressed that the potentiating effect of glucose is diminished in NIDDM. Both groups felt that a general reduction in insulin secretory capacity best described the nature of the B-cell defect in NIDDM. The situation is, however, more complex. Because arginine almost lacks effects on the B-cell in the absence of glucose, and in kinetic terms its effect can be described as augmentation of the Vmax of glucose-induced insulin release [94, 99], my interpretation of arginine experiments in NIDDM is at variance with the above. Indeed, in all studies, arginine augmented the insulin or C-peptide level by a factor of 2-4 at all glucose concentrations, equally in controls and NIDDM patients [99, 101, 102]. Thus, instead of regarding glucose as the potentiator of arginine-induced insulin release, if one takes the physiologically correct approach of arginine as the amplifier of the glucose effect, it appears that arginine exerts a quantitatively and qualitatively normal action in the diabetic B-cell. Since glucose-induced insulin release is diminished in NIDDM (see Fig. 2), also if amplified normally by arginine the final result is low insulin response. It must be stressed, however, that no arginine dose-response study has been performed in NIDDM to evaluate whether the sensitivity to the amino acid is reduced.[1]

---

[1] We studied the effect of variable arginine doses combined with variable glucose doses in subjects with decreased insulin response but normal glucose tolerance [95]; B-cell sensitivity to arginine was not different from controls.

The therapeutically important agents of the sulfonylurea family exert their blood glucose lowering effect mainly through modulation of insulin secretion, although extrapancreatic effects have been discussed [for review, see 103]. These drugs have only a limited effect on the B-cell in the absence of glucose [104]. With increasing glucose concentrations both first-phase and second-phase insulin release are amplified, the major sulfonylurea effect being observed at medium-high levels of glucose in vitro as well as in vivo [97, 105, 106]. Both moderately hyperglycemic NIDDM patients and persons with glucose intolerance may show near-normal acute insulin responses to intravenously administered sulfonylurea [47, 97]. However, in combination with a glucose dose-response study, the ability of sulfonylureas to induce a left-shift in the dose-response curve, i.e., to increase the sensitivity of the B-cell for glucose, was found reduced in diabetic patients [97]. It is difficult to conclude from this type of acute studies whether the diabetic B-cell responds intrinsically less to sulfonylurea, or whether the lower secretory response is a reflection of deficient glucose effect on insulin release (see arginine effects). Given orally in therapeutic doses, sulfonylureas seem to retain their stimulatory effect on insulin secretion over extended periods. Thus, in two studies where patients were treated with chlorpropamide or glibenclamide and insulin secretion was measured by the hyperglycemic clamp technique at 3 days, 3 weeks, and 3 months of treatment, B-cell response was increased by 50%-100% [107, 108]. In another study [109], the plasma insulin response to a mixed meal was augmented to a variable degree after 3 and 15 months of glibenclamide treatment. Although the authors were not impressed by the insulin secretion data [109], analysis of their results (slightly augmented insulin values in the face of major reduction in the hyperglycemic response to meals) suggests that B-cell sensitivity to glucose was markedly stimulated also after 15 months of sulfonylurea treatment. Thus, under both acute and chronic exposure the diabetic islet seems to respond to sulfonylurea drugs. One difficulty in evaluating the chronic sulfonylurea effect is related to the fact that the blood glucose of the patient is reduced by the treatment, and it cannot be excluded that the improved B-cell function is the consequence of less severe hyperglycemia rather than of a direct drug effect on the B-cell (see p. 204).

The insulin responses to nonglucose stimuli in experimental or spontaneous animal models of diabetes are not always similar to the findings in man. In *Acomys cahirinus*, arginine, tolbutamide, theophylline and its derivative IBMX failed to correct the pattern of secretion, only limited synergism with glucose being observed [for review, see 110]. In nonketotic BB rats, the in vitro pancreatic response to arginine was reduced compared to controls, but less so than the insulin response to glucose [72]. In NIDDM induced by neonatal injection of streptozotocin in rats, the effect of nonglucose stimuli on insulin release seems complex; thus, the substrates glyceraldehyde and α-ketoisocaproic acid were as inefficient as glucose [75], while the insulin response to IBMX was supranormal [75, 76]. Arginine at a low perfusion glucose concentration induced supranormal insulin release; however, in contrast to findings in normal rats, at high glucose no synergistic amplification of the release occurred [76]. A point of concern for the interpretation of these results is that although the experiments in vitro were performed at identical glucose concentrations for control and streptozotocin-diabetic pancreases, the latter were removed from hyperglycemic animals, and therefore could carry over time-dependent potentiation induced in vivo, thus accounting for the high responses to IBMX and arginine [111, 112]. Whatever the explanation, some of the above defects are corrected when the high glucose background of the pancreas is reduced (see below), suggesting that these differential insulin responses to nonglucose stimuli are secondary to long-term hyperglycemia.

It should be clear from the above review of the data in human and animal NIDDM that there is no unanimity on the degree of implication of nonglucose secretagogues in the deficient insulin secretion. The complications are, first, that the absolute insulin values lack meaning due to the complex synergistic interactions with glucose; second, that few complete dose-response studies (where, for example, the effect of various arginine doses at various glucose levels were measured) exist to allow calculation of the actual degree of stimulation exerted by the nonglucose secretagogue; third, that previous exposure to a hyperglycemic milieu strongly modifies the insulin response to nonglucose stimuli [111, 112]. In my mind, however, most of the data in man and some of the in vitro results suggest that most nonglucose stimuli are normally sensed as amplifiers of the glucose action in the diabetic B-cell; the resulting insulin response is reduced because the glucose signal itself is limited.

Mechanisms of the Deficient Insulin Response

A low response of the peripheral insulin level in NIDDM in theory could be caused by one of the following mechanisms: normal B-cell response but supranormal metabolism of insulin, e.g., increased extraction at the liver; normal function of individual B-cells but reduced B-cell mass; functional defects in a normal mass of B-cells.

It was shown quite early that the prehepatic, portal vein insulin response was as reduced as the peripheral one in NIDDM and in subjects with glucose intolerance [113, 114]. Although in these studies with portal vein catheterization blood flows were not measured, and technical problems relating to the representativeness of the portal blood samples for total pancreatic venous efflux certainly existed, it seems reasonable to assume that in NIDDM the insulin secretion rate is indeed reduced.

The finding of reduced maximal insulin response to glucose (see Fig. 2) and to the synergistic interaction of, for example, arginine and glucose could suggest that the B-cell mass is reduced in NIDDM. Indeed, the "apparent Km" of the acute insulin response to glucose (Fig. 2) or that of the glucose potentiation of arginine-induced insulin release [102] is similar in NIDDM patients and healthy subjects, which could be taken to indicate that the ability of each B-cell to sense the changes in glucose concentration is normal in NIDDM. Several lines of evidence, however, do not support this hypothesis, the most important being the pathological findings in pancreases from NIDDM patients. Although in long-standing NIDDM moderate reduction in the B-cell mass does occur, this is not the case in the early stages of the disease [115] (see also Chap. 2, this volume), and under no circumstance can the morphological changes account for the observed 80%–90%

decrease in insulin response. Furthermore, second-phase insulin release in mild NIDDM shows reduced sensitivity to glucose, very high sugar levels being capable of inducing substantial responses [48]. It seems therefore more likely that the deficient insulin response of NIDDM is caused by a functional deficiency of the B-cell. The B-cell biochemical defects that may cause the functional defect in insulin secretion are reviewed in detail by several authors in this volume, and therefore here the discussion will be confined to some specific topics that have interested my group.

Due to the scarcity of human islet material in general and islets from diabetics in particular, much of the information on the nature of the diabetic insulin secretory defect in man is derived from in vivo studies. The striking feature of the defect is its restriction to the acute initiatory signal of glucose, while modulatory factors are recognized normally. Among the latter are the ability of glucose to amplify the secretion by the mechanism of time-dependent potentiation (p. 196) and the synergistic effect of arginine on glucose-induced insulin secretion (p. 200). Furthermore, when the glucose-insulin dose-response relationships in obese and lean NIDDM of similar hyperglycemia were compared, the obese patients showed a threefold increase in the Vmax of the response, which was identical to the Vmax differences between matched obese and lean controls [115a]. Thus also the modulatory effect of obesity on B-cell function is normally sensed in NIDDM.

In terms of understanding the biochemical nature of the diabetic B-cell defect, the most relevant observation, to my mind, is the normal recognition of glucose for the generation of time-dependent potentiation [80]. This observation, taken together with the in vivo [52, 111] and in vitro [56] findings that glucose induces time-dependent potentiation even when its acute insulin-releasing effect is blocked, and the demonstration that the calcium requirements of time-dependent potentiation are different from those of the acute release [116, 116a], indicates that in the B-cell, glucose utilizes different mechanisms to generate on the one hand an acute stimulus-secretion coupling signal and on the other a signal that modulates the secretory rates with time. Seen in this light, the defect in NIDDM would be restricted to the highly specialized function of glucose, namely its recognition with high sensitivity as the inducer of the rapid initiation of release; more "primitive" functions of glucose (insulin synthesis, slow amplification of release) would be conserved, at least in the early stages of the disease.

For several years we have been interested in cyclic AMP as a component of the acute secretory signal of glucose [117]; we also showed that it is not primarily involved in time-dependent potentiation [56]. It was therefore felt that changes in cyclic AMP could be a likely candidate for the defect in NIDDM. In an early study in man no effect of aminophylline on insulin response was found in NIDDM, although the first-phase response was amplified in subjects with low insulin response to glucose [118]. In contrast to these indirect and inconclusive in vivo studies, we found that in islets from nonketotic Chinese hamsters [65] and *Acomys cahirinus* [70] glucose induced only minimal cyclic AMP responses even in the presence of phosphodiesterase inhibitors. Recent studies with *Acomys* islets show that nonglucose stimulators of adenylate cyclase such as forskolin are capable of generating major cyclic AMP responses [119]. Thus in this model of NIDDM the islet cyclase does not seem to be defective; rather, the coupling of the glucose stimulus to cyclic AMP generation is deficient. However, the *Acomys* islet defect is not restricted to the generation of cyclic AMP, since phosphodiesterase inhibitors, forskolin, and exogenous cyclic AMP all failed to restore the glucose-induced first-phase insulin release despite adequate elevations in the intracellular cyclic AMP concentration [119]. From these in vitro studies it appears that at least in some animal models of diabetes, pre- and postcyclic AMP defects may be related to the deficient insulin release. The exact nature of these defects awaits further investigation. Obviously, their relation to the human diabetic islet is only conjectural.

Another islet biochemical defect that has been discussed in NIDDM relates to prostaglandin metabolism. Several studies have shown that agents which inhibit the endogenous PGE synthesis partially correct the insulin response to glucose and to other secretagogues in patients with NIDDM [120-123]. In view of the recent interest in the role that arachidonic acid metabolites play in the control of insulin secretion [124, 125] these observations are most significant; however, their exact relation to the pathogenic defect of diabetes cannot be understood unless appropriate in vitro studies are performed in islets from diabetic animals.

As already said, a factor that further obstructs the understanding of the mechanisms responsible for the B-cell defect in diabetes is chronic hyperglycemia. It is indeed known that in vitro exposure of normal islets to high glucose concentrations for prolonged periods results in the exhaustion of the insulin response [126]. That a similar situation may exist in vivo has been shown recently: insulin secretion in the isolated pancreas from rats rendered hyperglycemic by a 48-h glucose infusion was markedly diminished [127]. The extent to which the hyperglycemia in diabetic man or animals contributes to the deficient insulin secretion is not completely clear; however, several studies show that at least part of the defect is secondary to hyperglycemia. Using the experimental rat NIDDM model of neonatal streptozotocin injection, it could be demonstrated that treatment of the animals with insulin normalized the in vitro insulin responses to arginine and IBMX; the acute response to glucose remained either unchanged [75, 128] or was improved [128a]. Treatment also restored the ability of glucose to generate time-dependent potentiation [75]. Interestingly, B-cell function could be ameliorated in vitro by the simple exposure of the pancreas to a glucose-free medium for 40 min [129]. Furthermore, when islets of LANGERHANS were isolated from the diabetic rats, the defect in glucose-induced insulin release was found to be less pronounced than in vivo or in the perfused pancreas [130] (V. GRILL, personal communication), suggesting that during the islet isolation procedure part of the metabolic defect generated by the in vivo hyperglycemia was reversed.

In one study, islets were isolated from the pancreas of human diabetics and the in vitro insulin secretion compared with the in vivo insulin response; the in vitro response was found to be almost normal [131]. It is obviously impossible to conclude from this limited study that no intrinsic abnormality exists in the B-cell of NIDDM patients; however, it does stress the role that the in vivo milieu plays for insulin release. This has been shown clearly by a number of recent studies, where NIDDM patients were treated by diet [16], physical exercise [17], or insulin [11-13, 132-134]. In all studies, the insulin response of the patients was markedly improved, although not normalized. Two studies [133, 134] suggest that 20-72 h normoglycemia is sufficient to improve B-cell function in NIDDM. In addition, 2 weeks normoglycemia normalized the elevated proinsulin/C-peptide ratio, indicating that the treatment indeed reduced the stress on B-cell function (B. GLASER et al., manuscript in preparation). From this discussion it becomes evident that to investigate the various aspects of B-cell function in patients with NIDDM, at least a short period of normoglycemia is necessary in order to obtain a true picture of the intrinsic B-cell defect. Probably many of the investigations reviewed here, unless performed in very mild diabetics, should be repeated following short-term normalization of the glycemia.

Evolution of the Insulin Deficiency in Diabetes

The demonstration that hyperglycemia per se induces B-cell dysfunction poses the dilemma of the chicken and the egg: does the negative relationship that exists between degree of hyperglycemia and degree of insulin response [78] indicate that the poorer the islet function the more severe becomes the diabetic state, or is it the severe diabetic state that precipitates further impairments of islet function?

In all studies to date where blood glucose was brought to near-normal in NIDDM, insulin secretion, while improved, remained markedly abnormal suggesting that only part of the secretory deficiency is caused by the chronic hyperglycemic stress. Furthermore, even in patients with minimal fasting hyperglycemia (see Fig. 3) or with glucose intolerance only, insulin response to glucose is markedly diminished [22, 135]. Obviously, however, both in insulin-treated NIDDM and in subjects with glucose intolerance blood glucose is not entirely normal over the day, and therefore it cannot be excluded that this minimal chronic hyperglycemia suffices to induce some impairment in B-cell function.

The transition from impaired glucose tolerance to manifest NIDDM seems to develop on the basis of an impaired insulin response. The most convincing evidence for this statement was offered by KADOWAKI et al. [136] who followed a large group of subjects with glucose intolerance for a mean period of 8 years. The majority of the subjects who developed clinical diabetes had initially decreased insulin responses to glucose; indeed, the insulin response was a predictive factor for the development of diabetes independently of other risk factors like body weight. Subjects who had glucose intolerance and high insulin responses did not progress to diabetes. Similar results were obtained also in other studies, albeit on smaller numbers of subjects [22, 137, 138]. These results definitely contradict the idea that NIDDM develops as a consequence of the exhaustion of hyperfunctioning B-cells [139, 140]. The question remains, however, whether the transition from glucose intolerance to overt diabetes is caused by progressive reduction of the already low insulin response, or whether a developing insulin resistance tips the balance toward diabetes. Our experience is that the insulin response is lower in patients with hyperglycemia than in subjects with impaired glucose tolerance only; however, no detailed follow-up study exists on the insulin secretion of individuals during transition to diabetes, neither has the secondary effect of hyperglycemia on islet function been taken into consideration.

There is indirect though convincing evidence to suggest that also glucose intolerance develops on the basis of decreased B-cell function. This was studied by assessing islet function in groups of subjects in whom the risk of developing diabetes is very high. Thus, in nondiabetic identical twins of diabetic patients, the insulin response of the healthy twin was found to be as decreased as in the diabetic twin [141, 142]. Similarly, in the offspring of conjugal diabetic parents, where the prevalence of glucose intolerance can be as high as 62% [143], the insulin response was found markedly diminished in many subjects [144] (C. NORYNBERG et al., manuscript in preparation). Of even greater interest is the demonstration that women who had a history of gestational diabetes but were normoglycemic at the time of study had decreased insulin response to glucose administration [145, 146] (S. EFENDIC et al., manuscript in preparation). Since these women were previously diabetic during the stress of pregnancy, and it is known that a high proportion of such women later develop NIDDM [147], the finding of impaired B-cell function at a time of normal glucose tolerance strongly suggests that decreased insulin secretion precedes the appearance of glucose intolerance and hyperglycemia.

We described the presence of subjects with low insulin response to glucose also in the normal population [21, 44, 50, 148]. Since the insulin response was distributed without evidence of population admixture [21, 50], it is difficult to define the limit between low and high responses; nevertheless, there was complete overlap between the responses of 90% of patients with mild NIDDM and 20% of control subjects with normal glucose tolerance [50]. Examples of the insulin responses in such subjects are given in Fig. 6. It has to be stressed, however, that although the insulin response to glucose infusion in these subjects seems as low as in the diabetics shown in Fig. 3, B-cell function in reality is less deficient; thus, intravenous and oral glucose dose-response studies showed that "low insulin responders" had insulin response curves intermediary between those of the control "high responders" and the diabetics [37, 48]. Indeed, first-phase response to intravenous glucose in this group showed a right-shift (increased Km) [48] rather than the decreased Vmax observed in NIDDM (Fig. 2). Low insulin responders were observed at roughly similar frequencies in all age groups studied [50], including children [149].

The low insulin response in subjects with normal glucose tolerance is not the consequence of B-cell adaptation to increased insulin sensitivity, since measured both directly and indirectly, peripheral sensitivity to insulin was not different from control, and the mean Kg on intravenous glucose tolerance testing was lower in these subjects than in high insulin responders [22, 50]. In one study [150], the plasma glycerol and nonesterified fatty acid responses to muscular exercise were higher in low insulin responders than in control subjects, suggesting that despite normal glucose tolerance there may be metabolic consequences to the reduction of insulin secretion. However, the most marked consequence of a low insulin response seems to be predisposition to later development of glucose intolerance and diabetes. Two 10-year follow-up studies in Stockholm showed that clinical diabetes occurred only in low insulin responders, and that the frequency of glucose intolerance was fivefold greater in these subjects [22, 151]. Thus, low insulin response to glucose in a normal subject seems to be a risk factor for later development of glucose intolerance, as the low insulin response of glucose-intolerant subjects is for transition to diabetes [136]. Because of the segmentary nature of

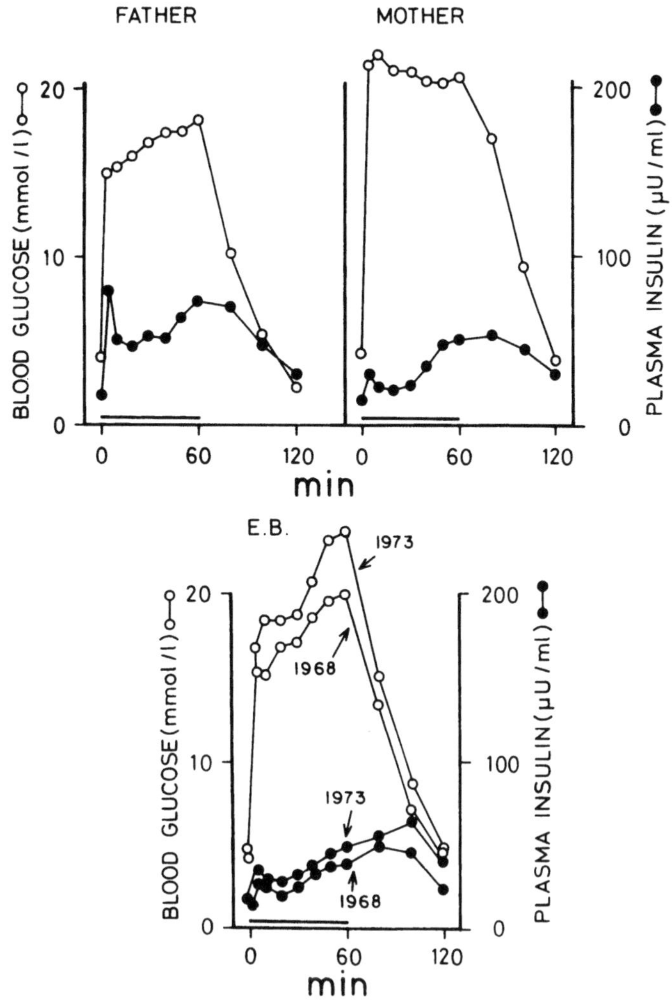

Fig. 6. Insulin response to glucose infusion in "low responders". For symbols see Fig. 3. Note the similarity of the insulin response in the mother and son (E. B.), and its reproducibility in the son over a 5-year period. E. B. is now a diabetic on insulin treatment (ICA-negative at the time of study)

the above studies [22, 151] it is not possible to give exact risk factor ratios for diabetes in low insulin responders; a study has been initiated for recalling all nondiabetics studied in Stockholm since 1963 (well over 1000 subjects) to assess more conclusively the role played by the low insulin response in the development of glucose intolerance and clinical diabetes.

Sporadic observations suggest that insulin secretion is further decreased in low insulin responders when glucose intolerance develops; however, the scarcity of data does not allow us to clarify whether the reduction in islet function is primary, or the consequence of the increasing glucose stress. The animal models that resemble NIDDM also offer only partial information. The model that mimics best the above description of the sequence of events from low insulin response to glucose intolerance and diabetes is *Acomys cahirinus*. Indeed, the majority of these animals show a low insulin response to glucose both in vivo and in vitro [152], even when young and lean and living at liberty [153]. It was shown that when obesity (and severe insulin resistance) develops in these animals, the insulin response shows only minimal adaptation, and hyperglycemia ensues [153]. However, due to technical difficulties, only end-points were studied and therefore it cannot be excluded that the apparent lack of adaptation of B-cell function to insulin resistance was in fact hyperglycemia-induced downregulation of an adequately adapted insulin release. As seen in Fig. 4, the in vitro insulin release patterns were quite similar in hyperglycemic and normoglycemic *Acomys*, perhaps supporting the view that extrapancreatic factors are of importance for the transition to glucose intolerance. A minority of the animals show normal insulin responses (with conserved first-phase release); these have not been studied longitudinally to assess the frequency of glucose intolerance. In another attractive model of NIDDM, *Macaca nigra*, the acute insulin response to glucose definitely shows a gradual decrease during the development of diabetes [62]. In this model, however, there seems to be a continuous loss of B-cells due to amyloid deposition; it is therefore difficult to evaluate its relevance for the transition from low insulin response to glucose intolerance in man.

Genetic Control of Insulin Release

A genetic connection in diabetes has long been acknowledged [154]. Because B-cell function plays such a prominent role in the development of glucose intolerance, it is logical to assume that the genetic factors responsible for NIDDM express themselves at the level of insulin release. The pattern of insulin response in man is quite stable over several years [151] (Fig. 6), suggesting that despite the recognized effect of environmental factors, and despite the sampling of insulin at a site remote from the B-cell, the response, as measured under everyday conditions, could be a genetically regulated function. The finding of low insulin response in the nondiabetic identical twins of diabetics [141] and the demonstration that in two families with NIDDM in many generations, the high frequency of low insulin responses in the F_1 generation was diluted in the following generations [155] certainly support the assumption that at least low insulin response may be a genetic trait. The heritability of the normal and deficient insulin responses has been studied in detail by Lindsten and coworkers [156-158]. In 111 control families, 96 families where the propositus was diabetic, and 24 pairs of monozygotic and 29 pairs of dizygotic healthy twins (a total of 880 subjects) the insulin response to glucose infusion was measured and the results subjected to sophisticated genetic analyses. From these studies it could be concluded unequivocally that several aspects of the insulin response to glucose are under considerable genetic influence, whereas environmental factors are of lesser importance. However, the heritability of insulin secretion was more marked in the children's generation than in the generation of the parents, suggesting that additional (genetic or nongenetic) factors modify the insulin response later in life [157, 158]. In families where one parent had diabetes, the insulin response of the children was not different from that of the appropriate controls [158]. Thus, both the normal insulin response and the low insulin response are genetically controlled, albeit in a complex manner. In some families no sophisticated methods were necessary to visualize the inheritance of the insulin release pattern; this is shown for a low insulin responder in Fig. 6.

From the above discussion I feel justified in concluding that a low insulin response is an inherited trait, and could be the factor that expresses the heritability of NIDDM. Low insulin responses have been observed in children [149], and therefore it is clear that this trait occurs relatively early in life. However, the insulin response of infants has not been studied to ascertain a similar frequency of low responders very early in life, and both the intergenerational differences in the heritability of the insulin response [157, 158], and the fact that insulin release is further impaired in glucose-intolerant subjects (see above) indicate that the response may change with time. Therefore it cannot be excluded that a low insulin response is the result of an extremely slow but continuous impairment of B-cell function, caused by as yet unknown factors (in analogy with the "prediabetic period" of IDDM).

Conclusions

It should be clear from this review that, if assessed correctly with due reference to the physiology of B-cell function, insulin secretion is found universally decreased in diabetic patients. The reduction in B-cell function is of such a magnitude (over 80%) that it should be sufficient to explain the deranged carbohydrate metabolism. Of special interest is the marked reduction in first-phase release that occurs early in the evolution of the disease. The first-phase response has a definite physiologic role; it has indeed been shown that early "priming" of the peripheral receptor sites with insulin is important for eliciting optimal metabolic response to the hormone [159, 159a]. This could explain why, despite considerable second-phase release, the postprandial glucose elevation is abnormal in subjects with glucose intolerance [for discussion, see 160].

Proper analysis of the hundreds of studies that have been performed since the 1960s on diabetics of all degrees of clinical severity indicates unequivocally that no evidence supports the hypothesis of B-cell exhaustion secondary to chronic hyperresponsiveness. On the one hand, insulin release is already reduced markedly at a stage when glucose tolerance and insulin sensitivity are only marginally modified; on the other hand, in pathologic conditions accompanied by severe insulin resistance and hyperinsulinism like morbid obesity, acromegaly and iatrogenic Cushing's syndrome, the majority of subjects remain nondiabetic. Therefore I feel compelled to repeat statements made two decades ago [161] to the effect that glucose intolerance and diabetes develop in subjects with limited B-cell function, either when insulin release deteriorates further, or when "additional factors" like insulin resistance aggravate the insulin deficiency of the subject.

No conclusive evidence exists yet to indicate that a low insulin response in normal subjects is the sole determinant of future diabetes. In the study of Efendic et al. [22], "low insulin responders" that later developed diabetes had either normal or moderately decreased sensitivity to physiologic levels of insulin. The role that such mild insulin resistance may play for eliciting glucose intolerance in the face of decreased B-cell function is not known. Neither has it been investigated whether B-cell function deteriorates in a continuous manner from the stage of low insulin responder to clinical diabetes over impaired glucose tolerance. The analogy with the "prediabetic" stage of IDDM, where a gradual reduction of the early-phase insulin response in subjects with anti-islet antibodies (and in animal models of IDDM) has been shown to precede the appearance of glucose intolerance and diabetes [162-165], is certainly tempting. Although in IDDM the B-cell mass is progressively destroyed, islet-cell antibodies can also block the insulin secretion [166, 167]; the presence of similar humoral factors in NIDDM, albeit not likely, cannot be excluded a priori. The role of hyperglycemia as a "B-cell toxin" has been discussed.

Unless and until future studies determine that low insulin responders segregate as a distinct population, the responsiveness of the B-cell seems to be distributed as a continuous variable. I propose, therefore, that the risk of developing diabetes is in inverse correlation (with, in all probability, a nonlinear relationship) with the genetically determined functional capacity of the B-cell. The lower the insulin secretory capacity, the greater the probability that either further impairment of the B-cell function, or insulin resistance, or both, generate a deficit in global insulin effect and therefore precipitate glucose intolerance. One could visualize a situation where in a low insulin responder any sustained stress, or age, could reduce the insulin secretion or otherwise cause minimal elevation of blood glucose, which gradually impairs the insulin response, thus leading to further elevation of the postprandial glycemia. At this stage glucose-induced reduction of glucose uptake in peripheral tissues [18, 20] would generate insulin resistance, further compromising the glucose tolerance. A normal B-cell copes with this situation by massive augmentation of the insulin secretion rate; the low insulin responder would find himself in an increasing insulin deficit, this vicious circle generating progressive B-cell deficiency and insulin resistance until full-blown diabetes ensues.

Until genetic manipulation of the defective B-cell becomes a reality, for practical purposes future research should concentrate on clarifying the mechanisms that govern the acute secretory effect of glucose, in distinction from those that regulate time-dependent amplification of release in the normal B-cell. The effect of oral hypoglycemic agents of the sulfonylurea type is limited, and therapeutic success unimpressive, probably because the defect of the acute stimulus-secretion coupling mechanism in the diabetic B-cell is too advanced to be amenable to pharmacological modulation. Since in diabetes islet potentiatory mechanisms are better conserved, agents that amplify these events could have more significant effects on insulin secretion. A goal-oriented search for such pharmacological agents should have very high priority, since success could lead to amelioration of the metabolic state in an estimated world population of one hundred million non-insulin-dependent diabetics.

Acknowledgments. My sincere thanks to Dr. RAFAEL NESHER for his help, and to Ms. LIZA GRANOT for the preparation of the manuscript.

References

1. Himsworth HP (1936) Diabetes mellitus: its differentiation into insulin-sensitive and insulin-insensitive types. Lancet 1: 127
2. Yalow RS, Berson SA (1960) Immunoassay of endogenous plasma insulin in man. J Clin Invest 39: 1157
3. Reaven GM, Shen SW, Silvers A, Farquhar JW (1971) Is there a delay in the plasma insulin response of patients with chemical diabetes mellitus? Diabetes 20: 416
4. Reaven GM, Bernstein R, Davis B, Olefsky JM (1976) Nonketotic diabetes mellitus: insulin deficiency or insulin resistance. Am J Med 60: 80
5. Liu G, Coulston A, Chen YDI, Reaven GM (1983) Does day-long absolute hypoinsulinemia characterize the patient with non-insulin-dependent diabetes mellitus? Metabolism 32: 754
6. Olefsky JM (1981) Insulin resistance and insulin action. An in vitro and in vivo perspective. Diabetes 30: 148
7. Olefsky JM, Kolterman OG (1981) Mechanism of insulin resistance in obesity and noninsulin-dependent (type II) diabetes. Am J Med 70: 151
8. Kahn CR (1985) The molecular mechanism of insulin action. Annu Rev Med 36: 429
9. DeFronzo RA, Simonson D, Ferrannini E (1982) Hepatic and peripheral insulin resistance: a common feature of type II (non-insulin-dependent) and type I (insulin-dependent) diabetes mellitus. Diabetologia 23: 313
10. Rizza RA, Mandarino LJ, Gerich JE (1981) Mechanism and significance of insulin resistance in non-insulin-dependent diabetes mellitus. Diabetes 30: 990
11. Andrews WJ, Vasquez B, Nagulesparan M, Klimes I, Foley J, Unger R, Reaven GM (1984) Insulin therapy in obese, non-insulin-dependent diabetes induces improvements in insulin action and secretion that are maintained for two weeks after insulin withdrawal. Diabetes 33: 634
12. Garvey WT, Olefsky JM, Griffin J, Hamman RF, Kolterman OG (1985) The effect of insulin treatment on insulin action in type II diabetes mellitus. Diabetes 34: 222
13. Glaser B, Leibovich G, Nesher R, Cerasi E (1986) Intensive insulin treatment in type 2 diabetes mellitus - effect on beta cell function and implications for long term management. Medicographia [Suppl 1] 9: 91

13a. Kruszynska YT, Home PD, Hanning I, Alberti KGMM (1987) Basal and 24-h C-peptide and insulin secretion rate in normal man. Diabetologia 30: 16

14. Foley JE, Kashiwagi A, Verso MA, Reaven GM, Andres J (1983) Improvement in in vitro insulin action after one month of insulin therapy in obese noninsulin-dependent diabetics: measurements of glucose transport and metabolism, insulin binding and lipolysis in isolated adipocytes. J Clin Invest 72: 1901
15. Scarlett JA, Kolterman OG, Ciaraldi TP, Kao M, Olefsky JM (1983) Insulin treatment reverses the postreceptor defect in adipocyte 3-0-methylglucose transport in type II diabetes mellitus. J Clin Endocrinol Metab 56: 1195
16. Henry RR, Scheaffer L, Olefsky JM (1985) Glycemic effects of intensive caloric restriction and isocaloric refeeding in non-insulin-dependent diabetes mellitus. J Clin Endocrinol Metab 61: 917
17. Krotkiewski M, Lönnroth P, Mandroukas K, Wroblewski Z, Rebuffé-Scrive M, Holm G, Smith U, Björntorp P (1985) The effect of physical training on insulin secretion and effectiveness and on glucose metabolism in obesity and Type 2 (non-insulin-dependent) diabetes mellitus. Diabetologia 28: 881
18. Sasson S, Cerasi E (1986) Substrate regulation of the glucose transport system in rat skeletal muscle: characterization and kinetic analysis in isolated soleus muscle and skeletal muscle cells in culture. J Biol Chem 261: 16827
19. Sasson S, Edelson D, Cerasi E (1987) In vitro autoregulation of glucose utilization in rat soleus muscle. Diabetes 36: 1041

20. Van Putten JMP, Krans MJ (1985) Glucose as a regulator of insulin-sensitive hexose uptake in 3T3 adipocytes. J Biol Chem 260: 7996
21. Cerasi E, Luft R (1967) Plasma insulin response to glucose infusion in healthy subjects and in diabetes mellitus. Acta Endocrinol 55: 278
22. Efendic S, Luft R, Wajngot A (1984) Aspects of the pathogenesis of type 2 diabetes. Endocrinol Rev 5: 395
23. Shen SW, Reaven GM, Farquhar JW (1970) Comparison of impedance to insulin-mediated glucose uptake in normal subjects and in subjects with latent diabetes. J Clin Invest 49: 2151
24. Ferner RE, Alberti KGMM (1986) Why is there still disagreement over insulin secretion in non-insulin-dependent diabetes? Diabetic Med 3: 13
25. Cerasi E, Nesher R (1986) Assessment of insulin secretion dynamics. In: Clarke WL, Larner J, Pohl SL (eds) Methods in diabetes research, vol II. Wiley, New York, p 77
26. Polonsky K, Jaspan J, Emmanouel D, Holmes K, Moossa AR (1983) Differences in the hepatic and renal extraction of insulin and glucagon in the dog: evidence for saturability of insulin metabolism. Acta Endocrinol 102: 420
27. Ferrannini E, Wahren J, Faber OK, Felig P, Binder C, DeFronzo RA (1983) Splanchnic and renal metabolism of insulin in human subjects - a dose response study. Am J Physiol 244: E517
28. Meistas MT, Margolis S, Kowarski AA (1983) Hyperinsulinemia of obesity is due to decreased clearance of insulin. Am J Physiol 245: E155
29. Eaton RP, Allen RC, Schade DS (1983) Hepatic removal of insulin in normal man: dose response to endogenous insulin secretion. J Clin Endocrinol Metab 56: 1294
30. Polonsky KS, Rubenstein AH (1984) C-peptide as a measure of the secretion and hepatic extraction of insulin: pitfalls and limitations. Diabetes 33: 486
31. Polonsky KS, Licinio-Paxao J, Given BP, Pugh W, Rue P, Galloway J, Kanorsen T, Frank B (1986) Use of biosynthetic human C-peptide in the measurement of insulin secretion rates in normal volunteers and Type I diabetic patients. J Clin Invest 77: 98
32. Cerasi E, Fick G, Rudemo M (1974) A mathematical model for the glucose induced insulin release in man. Eur J Clin Invest 4: 267
33. Bergman RN, Finegood DT, Ader M (1985) Assessment of insulin sensitivity in vivo. Endocrinol Rev 6: 45
34. Hosker JP, Matthews DR, Rudenski AS, Burnett MA, Darling P, Pown EG, Turner RC (1985) Continuous infusion of glucose with model assessment: measurement of insulin resistance and β-cell function in man. Diabetologia 28: 401
35. Polonsky KS, Given BD, Pugh W, Licinio-Paixao J, Thompson JE, Karrison T, Rubenstein AH (1986) Calculation of the systemic delivery rate of insulin in normal man. J Clin Endocrinol Metab 63: 113
36. Creutzfeldt W, Ebert RE (1985) New developments in the incretin concept. Diabetologia 28: 565
37. Cerasi E, Efendic S, Luft R (1973) Dose-response relationship of plasma insulin and blood glucose levels during oral glucose loads in prediabetic and diabetic subjects. Lancet 1: 794
38. Mohan V, Sharp PS, Cloke HR, Burrin JM, Schumer B, Kohner EM (1986) Serum immunoreactive insulin responses to a glucose load in Asian Indian and European Type 2 (non-insulin-dependent) diabetic patients and control subjects. Diabetologia 29: 235
39. Nauck M, Stockmann F, Ebert R, Creutzfeldt W (1986) Reduced incretin effect in Type 2 (non-insulin-dependent) diabetes. Diabetologia 29: 46
39a. Krarup T, Saurbrey N, Moody AA, Kühl C, Madsbad S (1987) Effect of porcine gastric inhibitory polypeptide on B-cell function in type I and type II diabetes mellitus. Metabolism 36: 677
40. Aronoff SL, Bennett PH, Gorden P, Rushforth N, Miller M (1977) Unexplained hyperinsulinemia in normal and "prediabetic" Pima Indians compared with normal Caucasians: an example of racial differences in insulin secretion. Diabetes 26: 827
41. Haffner SM, Stern MP, Hazuda HP, Pugh JA, Patterson JK (1986) Hyperinsulinemia in a population at high risk for non-insulin-dependent diabetes mellitus. N Engl J Med 315: 220
42. Balkau B, King H, Zimmet P, Raper LR (1985) Factors associated with the development of diabetes in the Micronesian population of Nauru. Am J Epidemiol 122: 594

43. Modan M, Karasik A, Halkin H, Fuchs Z, Lusky A, Shitrit A, Modan B (1986) Effect of past and concurrent body mass index on prevalence of glucose intolerance and Type 2 (non-insulin-dependent) diabetes and on insulin response. Diabetologia 29: 82
44. Cerasi E, Luft R (1963) Plasma insulin response to sustained hyperglycaemia induced by glucose infusion in human subjects. Lancet 2: 1359
45. Perley JM, Kipnis DM (1967) Plasma insulin response to oral and intravenous glucose: studies in normal and diabetic subjects. J Clin Invest 46: 1954
46. Seltzer HS, Allen EW, Herron A, Brennan MT (1967) Insulin secretion in response to glycemic stimulus: relation of delayed initial release to carbohydrate tolerance in mild diabetes. J Clin Invest 46: 323
47. Varsano-Aharon N, Echemendia E, Yalow RS, Berson SA (1970) Early insulin response to glucose and to tolbutamide in maturity onset diabetes. Metabolism 19: 409
48. Cerasi E, Luft R, Efendic S (1972) Decreased sensitivity of the pancreatic beta cells to glucose in prediabetic and diabetic subjects. A glucose dose-response study. Diabetes 21: 224
49. Brunzell JD, Robertson RP, Lerner RL, Hazzard WR, Ensinck JW, Bierman EL, Porte D (1976) Relationships between fasting plasma glucose levels and insulin secretion during intravenous glucose tolerance tests. J Clin Endocrinol Metab 42: 222
50. Efendic S, Cerasi E, Elander I, Thornqvist C, Fick G, Berglund B, Luft R (1979) Studies on low insulin responders. Glucose tolerance and insulin response to intravenous and oral glucose challenges in 226 normal subjects and 25 subjects with mild or chemical diabetes. Acta Endocrinol [Suppl 224] 90: 5
51. Cerasi E (1975) Feed-back inhibition of insulin secretion in subjects with high and low insulin response to glucose. Diabete Metab 1: 73
52. Efendic S, Lins PE, Cerasi E (1979) Potentiation and inhibition of insulin release in man following priming with glucose and with arginine - effect of somatostatin. Acta Endocrinol 90: 259
53. Nesher R, Waldman L, Cerasi E (1984) Time-dependent inhibition of insulin release: glucose-arginine interactions in the perfused rat pancreas. Diabetologia 26: 146
54. Grodsky GM, Curry D, Landahl H, Bennett LL (1969) Further studies on the dynamic aspects of insulin release in vitro with evidence for a two-compartmental storage system. Acta Diabetol Lat [Suppl 1] 6: 554
55. Cerasi E (1975) Potentiation of insulin release by glucose in man. I. Quantitative analysis of the enhancement of glucose induced insulin secretion by pretreatment with glucose in normal subjects. Acta Endocrinol 79: 483
56. Grill V, Adamson U, Cerasi E (1978) Immediate and time-dependent effects of glucose on insulin release from rat pancreatic tissue. Evidence for different mechanisms of action. J Clin Invest 61: 1034
57. Grill V, Adamson U, Rundfeldt M, Andersson S, Cerasi E (1979) Glucose memory of pancreatic B and A_2 cells. J Clin Invest 64: 700
58. Cerasi E (1981) Differential actions of glucose on insulin release: reevaluation of a mathematical model. In: Cobelli C, Bergman RN (eds) Carbohydrate metabolism. Wiley, London, p 3
58a. Nesher R, Cerasi E (1987) Biphasic insulin release as the expression of combined inhibitory and potentiating effects of glucose. Endocrinology 121: 1017
59. Ward WK, Beard JC, Halter JB, Pfeifer MA, Porte D (1984) Pathophysiology of insulin secretion in non-insulin-dependent diabetes mellitus. Diabetes Care 7: 491
60. Metz SA, Halter JB, Robertson RP (1979) Paradoxical inhibition of insulin secretion by glucose in human diabetes mellitus. J Clin Endocrinol Metab 48: 827
61. Hellman B, Hallgren R, Abrahamsson H, Bergsten P, Berne C, Gylfe E, Rorsman P, Wide L (1985) The dual action of glucose on the cytosolic Ca^{2+} activity in pancreatic β cells. Demonstration of an inhibitory effect of glucose on insulin release in the mouse and man. Biomed Biochim Acta 44: 63
62. Howard CF (1986) Longitudinal studies on the development of diabetes in individual *Macaca nigra*. Diabetologia 29: 301
63. Conaway HH, Faas FH, Smith SD, Sanders LL (1981) Spontaneous diabetes mellitus in the New Zealand white rabbit: physiological characteristics. Metabolism 30: 50

64. Frankel BJ, Gerich JE, Hagura R, Gerritsen GC, Fanska RE, Grodsky GM (1974) Abnormal secretion of insulin and glucagon by the in vitro perfused pancreas of the genetically diabetic Chinese hamster. J Clin Invest 53: 1637
65. Rabinovitch A, Renold AE, Cerasi E (1976) Decreased cyclic AMP and insulin responses to glucose in pancreatic islets of diabetic Chinese hamsters. Diabetologia 12: 581
66. Gerritsen GC (1982) The Chinese hamster as a model for the study of diabetes mellitus. Diabetes [Suppl 1] 31: 14
67. Berglund O, Frankel BJ, Hellman B (1978) Development of the insulin secretory defect in genetically diabetic (db/db) mouse. Acta Endocrinol 87: 543
68. Gutzeit A, Rabinovitch A, Studer PP, Trueheart PA, Cerasi E, Renold AE (1974) Decreased intravenous glucose tolerance and low plasma insulin response in spiny mice *(Acomys cahirinus)*. Diabetologia 10: 667
69. Gutzeit A, Rabinovitch A, Karakash C, Stauffacher W, Renold AE, Cerasi E (1974) Evidence for decreased sensitivity to glucose of isolated islets from spiny mice *(Acomys cahirinus)*. Diabetologia 10: 661
70. Grill V, Cerasi E (1979) The metabolism of cyclic AMP and glucose in isolated islets from *Acomys cahirinus*. Diabetologia 16: 47
71. Nesher R, Abramovitch E, Cerasi E (1985) Correction of diabetic pattern of insulin release from islets of the spiny mouse *(Acomys cahirinus)* by glucose priming in vitro. Diabetologia 28: 233
72. Grill V, Herberg L (1983) Glucose- and arginine-induced insulin and glucagon responses from the isolated perfused pancreas of the BB-Wistar diabetic rat. Evidence for selective impairment of glucose regulation. Acta Endocrinol 102: 561
73. Weir GC, Clore ET, Zmachinski CJ, Bonner-Weir S (1981) Islet secretion in a new experimental model for non-insulin-dependent diabetes. Diabetes 30: 590
74. Giroix MH, Portha B, Kergoat M, Bailbe D, Picon L (1983) Glucose insensitivity and amino-acid hypersensitivity of insulin release in rats with non-insulin-dependent diabetes. A study with the perfused pancreas. Diabetes 32: 445
75. Grill V, Rundfeldt M (1986) Abnormalities of insulin responses after ambient and previous exposure to glucose in streptozotocin-diabetic and dexamethasone-treated rats. Role of hyperglycemia and increased B-cell demands. Diabetes 35: 44
76. Leahy JL, Bonner-Weir S, Weir GC (1984) Abnormal glucose regulation of insulin secretion in models of reduced B-cell mass. Diabetes 33: 667
77. Hosker JP, Burnett MA, Davies EG, Matthews DR, Rudenski AS, Turner RC (1984) Loss of normal sigmoidal beta cell response curve to glucose in non-insulin-dependent diabetes. Diabetologia 27: 289A (abstract)
78. Pfeifer MA, Halter JB, Porte D (1981) Insulin secretion in diabetes mellitus. Am J Med 70: 579
79. Cerasi E (1975) Insulin secretion: mechanism of the stimulation by glucose. Quart Rev Biophys 8: 1
80. Cerasi E (1975) Potentiation of insulin release by glucose in man. III. Normal recognition of glucose as a potentiator in subjects with low insulin response and in mild diabetes. Acta Endocrinol 79: 511
81. Grill V, Adamson U, Viklund M (1985) Effects of previous intake of glucose on postprandial hyperglycemia in type 2 diabetics. Acta Med Scand 217: 41
82. Nesher R, Tuch B, Hage C, Levy J, Cerasi E (1984) Time-dependent inhibition of insulin release: suppression of the arginine effect by hyperglycaemia. Diabetologia 26: 142
83. Halter JB, Graf RJ, Porte D (1979) Potentiation of insulin secretory responses by plasma glucose levels in man: evidence that hyperglycemia in diabetes compensates for impaired glucose potentiation. J Clin Endocrinol Metab 48: 946
84. Goodner CJ, Conway MJ, Werrbach JH (1969) Control of insulin secretion during fasting hyperglycemia in adult diabetics and in nondiabetic subjects during infusion of glucose. J Clin Invest 48: 1878
85. Lerner RL, Porte D (1972) Acute and steady-state insulin responses to glucose in nonobese diabetic subjects. J Clin Invest 51: 624
86. Holman RR, Turner RC (1979) Maintenance of basal plasma glucose and insulin concentration in maturity-onset diabetes. Diabetes 28: 277

87. McCarthy ST, Harris F, Turner RC (1977) Glucose control of basal insulin secretion in diabetes. Diabetologia 13: 93
88. Turner RC, Holman RR (1976) Insulin rather than glucose homeostasis in the pathophysiology of diabetes. Lancet 1: 1272
89. Matthews DR, Hosker JP, Rudenski AS, Naybor BA, Treacher DF, Turner RC (1985) Homeostasis model assessment: insulin resistance and β-cell function from fasting plasma glucose and insulin concentrations in man. Diabetologia 28: 412
90. Kingston ME, Skoog WC (1986) Maintenance of basal insulin secretion in severe non-insulin-dependent diabetes. Diabetes Care 9: 232
91. Gorden P, Hendricks CM, Roth J (1974) Circulating proinsulin-like component in man. Diabetologia 10: 469
92. Rainbow SJ, Woodhead JS, Yue DK, Luzio SD, Hales CN (1979) Measurement of human proinsulin by an indirect two-site immunoradiometric assay. Diabetologia 17: 229
93. Floyd JC, Fajans SS, Pek S, Thiffault CA, Knopf RF, Conn JW (1970) Synergistic effect of essential amino acids and glucose upon insulin secretion in man. Diabetes 19: 109
94. Efendic S, Cerasi E, Luft R (1971) Role of glucose in arginine-induced insulin release in man. Metabolism 20: 568
95. Assan R, Efendic S, Luft R, Cerasi E (1981) Dose-kinetics of pancreatic glucagon responses to arginine and glucose in subjects with normal and impaired pancreatic B cell function. Diabetologia 21: 452
96. Cerasi E, Chowers I, Luft R, Widström A (1969) The significance of the blood glucose level for plasma insulin response to intravenously administered tolbutamide in healthy subjects. Diabetologia 5: 343
97. Cerasi E, Efendic S, Thornqvist C, Luft R (1979) Effect of two sulphonylureas on the dose kinetics of glucose-induced insulin release in normal and diabetic subjects. Acta Endocrinol 91: 282
98. Goldfine ID, Cerasi E, Luft R (1972) Glucagon stimulation of insulin release in man: inhibition during hypoglycemia. J Clin Endocrinol Metab 35: 312
99. Efendic S, Cerasi E, Luft R (1974) Quantitative study on the potentiating effect of arginine on glucose-induced insulin response in healthy, prediabetic, and diabetic subjects. Diabetes 23: 161
100. Floyd JC, Fajans SS, Conn JW, Triffault C, Knopf RF, Guntsche E (1968) Secretion of insulin induced by amino acids and glucose in diabetes mellitus. J Clin Endocrinol Metab 28: 266
101. Dimitriadis GD, Pehling GB, Gerich JE (1985) Abnormal glucose modulation of islet A- and B-cell responses to arginine in non-insulin-dependent diabetes mellitus. Diabetes 34: 541
102. Ward WK, Bolgiano DC, McKnight B, Halter JB, Porte D (1984) Diminished B cell secretory capacity in patients with noninsulin-dependent diabetes mellitus. J Clin Invest 74: 1318
103. Pfeiffer EF (ed) (1983) Rationale for sulfonylurea therapy. Excerpta Medica, Amsterdam
104. Grill V, Cerasi E (1978) Interacting effects of sulfonylurea and glucose on cyclic AMP metabolism and insulin release in pancreatic islets of the rat. J Clin Invest 61: 1346
105. Loubatières A (1968) Stimulators and inhibitors of insulin secretion. Physiological and pharmacological interferences, synergism and antagonism. Acta Diabetol Lat [Suppl 1]: 220
106. Widström A, Cerasi E (1973) On the action of tolbutamide in man. II. Modulation of glucose-induced insulin release by tolbutamide. Acta Endocrinol 72: 519
107. Simonson DC, Ferrannini E, Bevilacqua S, Smith D, Barrett E, Carlson R, DeFronzo RA (1984) Mechanism of improvement in glucose metabolism after chronic glyburide treatment. Diabetes 33: 838
108. Hosker JP, Burnett MA, Davies EG, Harris EA, Turner RC (1985) Sulphonylurea therapy doubles B-cell response to glucose in Type 2 diabetic patients. Diabetologia 28: 809
109. Kolterman OG, Gray RS, Shapiro G, Scarlett JA, Griffin J, Olefsky JM (1984) The acute and chronic effects of sulfonylurea therapy in type II diabetic subjects. Diabetes 33: 346
110. Cerasi E, Nesher R (1984) *Acomys cahirinus:* a useful model for the study of islet function in non-insulin-dependent diabetes. In: Shafrir E, Renold AE (eds) Lessons from animal diabetes. Libbey, London, p 15
111. Cerasi E (1975) Potentiation of insulin release by glucose in man. II. Role of the insulin response, and enhancement of stimuli other than glucose. Acta Endocrinol 79: 502

112. Grill V, Rundfeldt M (1979) Effects of priming with D-glucose on insulin secretion from rat pancreatic islets: increased responsiveness to other secretagogues. Endocrinology 105: 980
113. Blackard WG, Nelson NC (1970) Portal and peripheral vein immunoreactive insulin concentrations before and after glucose infusion. Diabetes 19: 302
114. Cerasi E, Hallberg D, Luft R (1970) Simultaneous determination of insulin in brachial and portal veins during glucose infusion in normal and prediabetic subjects. Horm Metab Res 2: 303
115. Rahier J, Goebbels RM, Henquin JC (1983) Cellular composition of the human diabetic pancreas. Diabetologia 24: 366
115a. Nesher R, Della Casa L, Litvin Y, Sinai J, Del Rio G, Pevsner B, Wax Y, Cerasi E (1987) Insulin deficiency and insulin resistance in type 2 (non-insulin-dependent) diabetes: quantitative contributions of pancreatic and peripheral responses to glucose homeostasis. Eur J Clin Invest 17: 266
116. Praiss M (1986) The Ca^{2+} dependency of biphasic insulin release and its time-dependent potentiation in the isolated perfused rat pancreas. M. Sc. Thesis, Hebrew University, Jerusalem
116a. Nesher R, Praiss M, Cerasi E (1988) Immediate and time-dependent effects of glucose on insulin release: differential calcium requirements. Acta Endocrinol 117: (in press)
117. Grill V, Cerasi E (1976) Effect of hexoses and mannoheptulose on cyclic AMP accumulation and insulin secretion in rat pancreatic islets. Biochim Biophys Acta 437: 36
118. Cerasi E, Luft R (1969) The effect of an adenosine-4′,5′-monophosphate diesterase inhibitor (aminophylline) on the insulin response to glucose infusion in prediabetic and diabetic subjects. Horm Metab Res 1: 162
119. Nesher R, Abramovitch E, Eylon L, Cerasi E (1986) Reduced first-phase insulin release in islets of *Acomys cahirinus:* pre- and post-cyclic AMP defects. Diabetologia 29: 575 A (abstract)
120. Robertson RP, Chen M (1977) A role for prostaglandin E in defective insulin secretion and carbohydrate intolerance in diabetes mellitus. J Clin Invest 60: 747
121. Giugliano D (1981) Acetylsalicylic acid in diabetes. Lancet 1: 560
122. Robertson RP (1983) Hypothesis: PGE, carbohydrate homeostasis and insulin secretion. A suggested resolution of controversy. Diabetes 32: 231
123. Giugliano D, Ceriello A, Saccomanno F, Quatraro A, Paolisso G, D'Onofrio F (1985) Effects of salicylate, tolbutamide, and prostaglandin E_2 on insulin responses to glucose in noninsulin-dependent diabetes mellitus. J Clin Endocrinol Metab 61: 160
124. Metz SA, Van Rollins M, Strife R, Fujimoto W, Robertson RP (1983) Lipoxygenase pathway in islet endocrine cells. Oxidative metabolism promotes insulin release. J Clin Invest 71: 1191
125. Pek SB, Walsh MF (1984) Leukotrienes stimulate insulin release from the rat pancreas. Proc Natl Acad Sci USA 81: 2199
126. Hoenig M, Macgregor LC, Matschinsky FM (1986) In-vitro exhaustion of pancreatic beta cells. Am J Physiol 250: E502
127. Leahy JL, Cooper HE, Deal DA, Weir GC (1986) Chronic hyperglycemia is associated with impaired glucose influence on insulin secretion. A study in normal rats using chronic in-vivo glucose infusions. J Clin Invest 77: 908
128. Leahy JL, Bonner-Weir S, Weir GC (1985) Abnormal insulin secretion in a streptozotocin model of diabetes. Effects of insulin treatment. Diabetes 34: 660
128a. Kergoat M, Bailbe D, Portha B (1987) Insulin treatment improves glucose-induced insulin release in rats with NIDDM induced by streptozotocin. Diabetes 36: 971
129. Grill V, Westberg M (1986) B-cell insensitivity in neonatally streptozotocin-injected diabetic rats (STZ). Effects of glucopenia, alloxan, and metabolic inhibitors. Diabetes [Suppl 1] 35: 7 A (abstract)
130. Portha B (1985) Decreased glucose-induced insulin release and biosynthesis by islets of rats with non-insulin-dependent diabetes: effect of tissue culture. Endocrinology 117: 1735
131. Lohmann D, Jahr H, Verlohen HJ, Schmidt S, Heilmann W, Zühlke H, Hartig W, Mattig H (1980) Insulin secretion in maturity-onset-diabetes. Function of isolated islets. Horm Metab Res 12: 349
132. Kosaka K, Kuzuya T, Akanuma Y, Hagura R (1980) Increase in insulin response after treatment of overt maturity-onset diabetes is independent of the mode of treatment. Diabetologia 18: 23

133. Vague P, Moulin JP (1982) The defective glucose sensitivity of the B-cell in noninsulin dependent diabetes. Improvement after twenty hours of normoglycemia. Metabolism 31: 139
134. Giugliano D, Di Pinto P, Ceriello A, Paolisso G, Saccomanno F, Torella R, D'Onofrio F (1985) Glycemic control with an artificial pancreas improves insulin responses to both oral and intravenous glucose in nonobese noninsulin-dependent diabetic subjects. Acta Diabetol Lat 22: 203
135. Efendic S, Wajngot A, Cerasi E, Luft R (1980) Insulin release, insulin sensitivity, and glucose intolerance. Proc Natl Acad Sci USA 77: 7425
136. Kadowaki T, Jiyake Y, Hagura R, Akanuma Y, Kajinuma H, Kuzuya N, Takaku F, Kosaka K (1984) Risk factors for worsening to diabetes in subjects with impaired glucose tolerance. Diabetologia 26: 44
137. Fajans SS (1980) Heterogeneity of plasma immunoreactive insulin responses in patients with impaired glucose tolerance and diabetes. Diabetologia 19: 250 (letter)
138. Wajngot A (1983) Aspects on the pathogenesis of Type 2 diabetes. Thesis, Karolinska Institute, Stockholm
139. Stern MP, Haffner SM (1986) Body fat distribution and hyperinsulinemia as risk factors for diabetes and carciovascular disease. Arteriosclerosis 6: 123
140. De Fronzo RA, Ferrannini E, Koivisto V (1983) New concepts in the pathogenesis and treatment of noninsulin-dependent diabetes mellitus. Am J Med [Suppl 1] 74: 52
141. Cerasi E, Luft R (1967) Insulin response to glucose infusion in diabetic and non-diabetic monozygotic twin pairs. Genetic control of insulin response? Acta Endocrinol 5: 330
142. Pyke DA, Cassar J, Todd J, Taylor KW (1970) Glucose tolerance and serum insulin in identical twins of diabetes. Br Med J 4: 649
143. Viswanathan M, Mohan M, Snehalatha C, Ramachadran A (1985) High prevalence of Type 2 (non-insulin-dependent) diabetes among the offspring of conjugal Type 2 diabetic parents in India. Diabetologia 28: 907
144. Boden G, Soeldner JS, Gleason RE, Marble A (1968) Elevated growth hormone and decreased serum insulin in pre-diabetic males after intravenous tolbutamide and glucose. J Clin Invest 47: 929
145. Ward WK, Johnston CLW, Beard JC, Benedetti TJ, Halter JB, Porte D (1985) Insulin resistance and impaired insulin secretion in subjects with histories of gestational diabetes mellitus. Diabetes 34: 861
146. Ward WK, Johnston CLW, Beard JC, Benedetti TJ, Porte D (1985) Abnormalities of islet B-cell function, insulin action, and fat distribution in women with histories of gestational diabetes: relationship to obesity. J Clin Endocrinol Metab 61: 1039
147. O'Sullivan JB (1982) Body weight and subsequent diabetes mellitus. JAMA 248: 949
148. Cerasi E Luft R (1967) Further studies on healthy subjects with low and high insulin response to glucose infusion. Acta Endocrinol 55: 305
149. Cerasi E, Luft R (1970) The occurrence of low insulin response to glucose infusion in children. Diabetologia 6: 85
150. Nordlander S, Östman J, Cerasi E, Luft R, Ekelund LG (1973) Occurrence of diabetic type of plasma FFA and glycerol responses to physical exercise in prediabetic subjects. Acta Med Scand 193: 9
151. Cerasi E, Luft R (1974) Follow-up of non-diabetic subjects with normal and decreased insulin response to glucose infusion - first report. Horm Metab Res [Suppl 5]: 113
152. Rabinovitch A, Gutzeit A, Renold AE, Cerasi E (1975) Insulin secretion in the spiny mouse *(Acomys cahirinus)*. Dose and time kinetic studies with glucose in vivo and in vitro. Diabetes 24: 1094
153. Gutzeit A, Renold AE, Cerasi E, Shafrir E (1979) Effect of diet-induced obesity on glucose and insulin tolerance of a rodent with a low insulin response *(Acomys cahirinus)*. Diabetes 28: 777
154. Rondolet G (1574) Methodus curandum omnium morborum corpus humani. Montpellier
155. Ohlsén P, Cerasi E, Luft R (1971) Glucose tolerance and insulin response to glucose in two large families with diabetic mothers in the first generation. Horm Metab Res 3: 1
156. Lindsten J, Cerasi E, Luft R, Morton N, Ryman N (1976) Significance of genetic factors for the plasma insulin response to glucose in healthy subjects. Clin Genet 10: 125
157. Iselius L, Lindsten J, Morton NE, Efendic S, Cerasi E, Haegermark A, Luft R (1982) Evi-

dence for an autosomal recessive gene regulating the persistence of the insulin response to glucose in man. Clin Genet 22: 180
158. Iselius L, Lindsten J, Morton NE, Efendic S, Cerasi E, Haegermark A, Luft R (1985) Genetic regulation of the kinetics of glucose-induced insulin release in man - studies in families with diabetic and non-diabetic probands. Clin Genet 28: 8
159. Matthews DR, Naylor BA, Jones RG, Ward GM, Turner RC (1983) Pulsatile insulin has greater hypoglycemic effect than continuous delivery. Diabetes 32: 617
159a. Weigle DS (1987) Pulsatile secretion of fuel-regulatory hormones. Diabetes 36: 764
160. Kipnis DM (1970) Does diabetes begin with insulin resistance? In: Cerasi E, Luft R (eds) Pathogenesis of diabetes mellitus. Nobel symposium 13. Almqvist and Wiksell, Stockholm, p 45
161. Cerasi E, Luft R (1967) "What is inherited - what is added" hypothesis for the pathogenesis of diabetes mellitus. Diabetes 16: 615
162. Srikanta S, Ganda OP, Gleason RE, Jackson RA, Soeldner JS, Eisenbarth GS (1984) Pre-Type I diabetes. Linear loss of beta cell response to intravenous glucose. Diabetes 33: 717
163. Soeldner JS, Tuttleman M, Srikanta S, Ganda OP, Eisenbarth GS (1985) Insulin-dependent diabetes mellitus and autoimmunity. Islet cell autoantibodies, insulin autoantibodies and beta-cell failure. N Engl J Med 313: 893
164. Svenningsen A, Dyrberg T, Markholst H, Binder C, Lernmark Å (1986) Insulin release and pancreatic insulin is reduced in young prediabetic BB rats. Acta Endocrinol 112: 367
165. Kano Y, Kanatsuna T, Nakamura N, Kitagawa Y Mori H, Kajiyama S, Nakano K, Kondo M (1986) Defect of the first-phase insulin secretion to glucose stimulation in the perfused pancreas of the nonobese diabetic (NOD) mouse. Diabetes 35: 486
166. Kanatsuna T, Baekkeskov S, Lernmark Å, Ludvigsson J (1983) Immunoglobulin from insulin-dependent diabetic children inhibits glucose-induced insulin release. Diabetes 32: 520
167. Kitagawa Y (1986) Preferential inhibition of glucose-induced insulin release by immunoglobulin from islet-cell-surface antibodies-positive insulin-dependent diabetics. J Kyoto Prefect Univ Med 95: 375

Possible Sites for Deficient Glucose Recognition in Islet Cells*

W. J. Malaisse

Introduction

In certain non-insulin-dependent diabetic patients, the secretory capacity of the pancreatic B-cell appears to be more severely affected in response to stimulation by D-glucose than other secretagogues [1]. Since D-glucose represents a major, albeit not the sole, regulator of insulin release under physiological conditions [2], the mechanisms possibly responsible for impaired recognition of this hexose by islet cells are directly relevant to our understanding of the pathology of the endocrine pancreas in diabetes mellitus.

In the present report, which is based exclusively on experimental work carried out in vitro with either normal or tumoral insulin-producing cells of murine origin, I wish to consider possible sites for deficient glucose recognition in islet cells. Such a consideration will be preceded by some remarks on the normal process of glucose identification by the B-cells.

The Normal Process of Glucose Identification

The release of insulin evoked by D-glucose and other nutrient or non-nutrient secretagogues can be schematically viewed as the outcome of a sequence of three major cytophysiological events [3]. These events include the recognition of the secretagogue by the B-cell, the participation of a coupling process transferring information from the site of recognition to more distal sites in the secretory sequence, and the eventual activation of the effector system controlling the exocytosis of secretory granules.

The process of glucose identification as an insulinotropic agent appears to coincide with the metabolism of this hexose in the pancreatic B-cell [4]. In other words, the activation of distal events in the secretory sequence is thought to be causally linked to the metabolic changes evoked by a rise in the extracellular concentration of D-glucose. More precisely, the glucose-induced increase in oxidative fluxes and respiration may generate suitable factors coupling metabolic to further (e.g. ionic) events in the islet cells. This fuel concept, which probably also applies to nonglucidic nutrient secretagogues [5], is obviously at variance with the view that the

* This work was supported, in part, by grants from the Belgian Foundation for Scientific Medical Research and the NATO Scientific Affairs Division.

molecule of D-glucose itself acts as a signal for insulin release through interaction with a stereospecific glucoreceptor [6].

Within the framework of this fuel concept, two essential aspects of B-cell physiology consist in the regulation of D-glucose metabolism [7] and the nature of the factors acting as second messengers between metabolic and distal events in the secretory sequence [8]. The present account is restricted to the first of these two issues.

The pancreatic B-cell displays, in terms of the regulation of D-glucose metabolism, specific features which are well suited for it to act as a glucose-sensor unit. Two examples will be cited. First, the efficiency of the hexose carrier located in the B-cell plasma membrane is such that the concentration of D-glucose inside the cell is virtually, and immediately, in equilibrium with its extracellular concentration. Second, the presence in the B-cell of a glucose-phosphorylating enzyme with a high Km for the hexose, i.e. glucokinase, allows the rate of D-glucose phosphorylation to increase, as a function of the hexose concentration, within the physiological range of variations in glycemia.

The latter attribute led some investigators to propose that glucokinase acts in the B-cell as a glucoreceptor [9]. I have two objections to such a view. First, the word "glucoreceptor" has been and is still used in different or ambiguous acceptations. Second, when considering the regulation of D-glucose metabolism in islet cells, it would be unwise to overlook regulatory steps located at sites distal to, or distinct from, the phosphorylation of the hexose [10].

Deficiency in Hexose Transport

As just mentioned, the transport of D-glucose into the normal B-cell is not looked upon as a regulatory process in the catabolism of this hexose. A different situation was recently characterized in tumoral insulin-producing cells of the RINm5F line.

The first indication for a deficiency of hexose transport in the RINm5F cells was obtained in a study of 3-*O*-methyl-D-[U-^{14}C] glucose uptake. Results obtained at different temperatures, at variable concentrations of the hexose, and over distinct times of incubation indicated that the uptake of 3-*O*-methyl-D-[U-^{14}C]-glucose represents a temperature-sensitive and saturable process, so that no rapid equilibration of hexose concentrations across the plasma membrane was reached, especially at low temperatures and/or high concentrations of 3-*O*-methyl-D-glucose. The uptake of 3-*O*-methyl-D-[U-^{14}C]-glucose was not affected by a prior loading of the cells with the unlabeled hexose, and its release from prelabeled cells was observed in the absence of any concentration gradient across the plasma membrane [11].

Based on these observations, a simple model for hexose transport across the plasma membrane was designed (Fig. 1). In this model, the relative magnitude of changes in the distribution space of the hexose, due to a difference in either temperature or hexose concentration, is critically dependent on the incubation time (Fig. 1, lower panel). When the experimental values mentioned above were compared to those derived from the model, a close correlation ($r = 0.936$; $p < 0.001$)

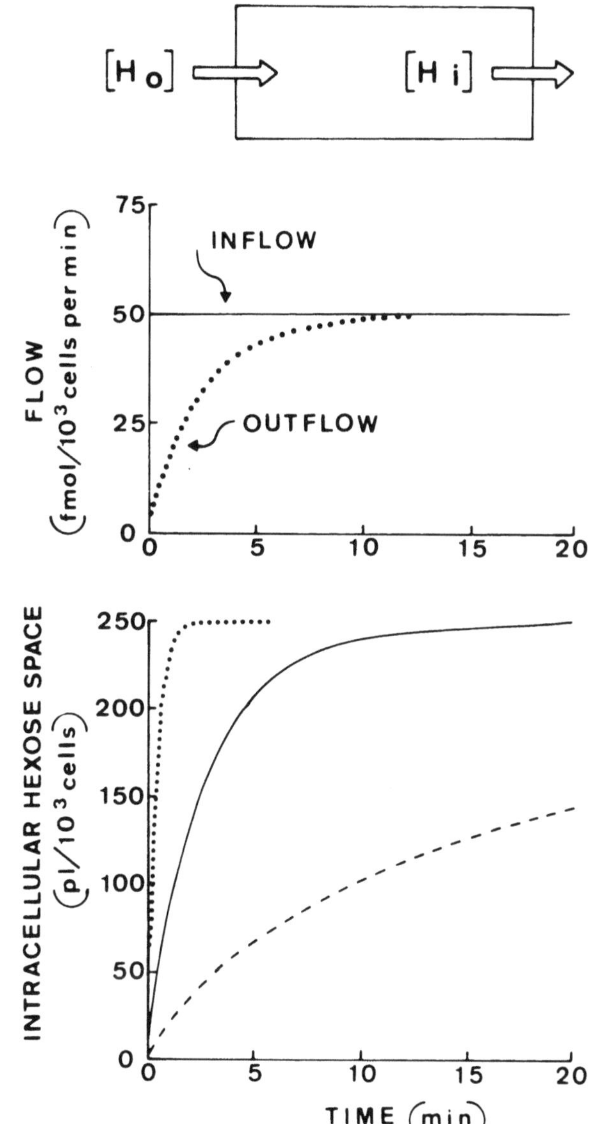

Fig. 1. Model for 3-*O*-methyl-D-glucose transport in RINm5F cells. It is assumed that the inflow and outflow of the hexose depends on its extracellular (H_o) and intracellular (H_i) concentrations, respectively, with a Km of 2.0 m*M*, a Vmax of 2.0 pmol/10^3 cells per min at 37 °C, and a coefficient of temperature (Q_{10}) of 2.0. The intracellular accessible space is taken as 250 pl/10^3 cells. The *middle panel* illustrates the time course for hexose inflow and outflow in cells exposed at 7 °C to the hexose at a concentration of 0.5 m*M*. The *solid line* in the *lower panel* indicates the corresponding values for the intracellular space. For the sake of comparison, the *dotted line* in the lower panel refers to the situation found at the same hexose concentration (0.5 m*M*) but at 37 °C instead of 7 °C, whereas the *dashed line* documents the situation found at low temperature (7 °C) in the presence of 8.0 m*M* instead of 0.5 m*M* of the hexose. The *bottom panel* illustrates the fact that the relative magnitude of changes in the intracellular hexose space, caused by a change in either temperature or hexose concentration, is closely dependent on the length of incubation

was observed between the two series of data (Fig. 2). The intercept of the regression line with the *y* axis (experimental values) yielded a distribution space which represented 18.9% of the reference value recorded over 5 min incubation at 7 °C in the presence of 1.4 m*M* 3-*O*-methyl-D-[U-^{14}C]glucose and, thus, amounted to 37 pl/10^3 cells. The latter value was virtually identical to the mean extracellular space, as judged from the distribution space of L-[1-^{14}C]glucose (41 ± 7 pl/10^3 cells). Incidentally, the decrease in the intracellular pool of 3-*O*-methyl-D-[U-^{14}C]-glucose in cells preincubated for 30 min at 7 °C in the presence of 1.4 m*M* of the labeled hexose and then incubated at 7 °C in the presence of the unlabeled hexose at the same concentration (1.4 m*M*) was compatible with a fractional outflow rate close to 0.22 min^{-1} [11], which is not vastly different from the value of 0.29 min^{-1} derived from our mathematical model. The experimental data were thus compatible with the view that the concentration of 3-*O*-methyl-D-glucose on a given side of the plasma membrane represents the major determinant of its rate of transport

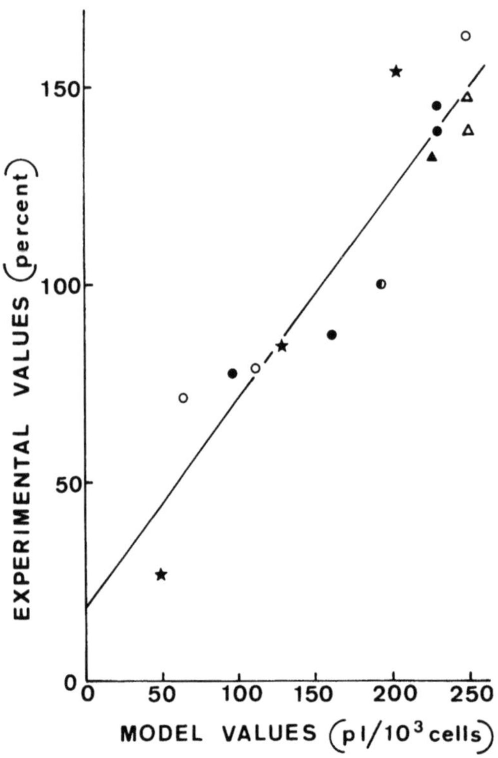

Fig. 2. Comparison between experimental values (expressed in percent of the reference value found after 5 min incubation at 7 °C in the presence of 1.4 m*M* 3-*O*-methyl-D-[U-^{14}C]glucose) and theoretical values (derived from the model depicted in Fig. 1) for the distribution space of 3-*O*-methyl-D-[U-^{14}C]glucose. The data were collected over 5 min incubation at 7 °C in the presence of increasing concentrations of the hexose *(closed symbols)*, at various times during incubation at 7 °C in the presence of 1.4 m*M* of the hexose *(open circles)*, over 1 min incubation at different temperatures in the presence of 2.8 m*M* of the hexose *(stars)* and over 5–30 min incubation at 7–37 °C in the presence of 0.14 m*M* of the hexose *(triangles)*. Note the intersection of the regression line with the ordinate

from that site to the other one, rather than each monodirectional flux being tightly dependent on the concentration gradient across the plasma membrane.

If the situation characterized with 3-*O*-methyl-D-glucose extends to D-glucose, the transport of the hexose could represent a rate-determining step in the utilization of D-glucose. The uptake of D-[U-^{14}C]glucose and the utilization of D-[5-^{3}H]glucose were indeed inhibited by 3-*O*-methyl-D-glucose, which failed, however, to affect D-[U-^{14}C]glucose oxidation [11]. At variance with the situation found in normal insulin-producing cells, the transport of D-glucose into the tumoral cells may thus play a regulatory role in its metabolism in the RINm5F cells.

The latter view was further investigated by measuring the uptake of D-[U-^{14}C]-glucose by the RINm5F cells [12]. Data collected over 5 min incubation at either 7 °C or 37 °C in the presence of increasing concentrations of D-glucose (0.14–16.7 m*M*) again suggested that the uptake of the hexose by RINm5F cells represents a saturable phenomenon which does not result in the rapid equilibration of the extracellular and intracellular concentrations of D-glucose.

The latter radioisotopic data could not be used, however, to assess the steady-state intracellular concentration of D-glucose, since both D-glucose and its intracellular labeled metabolites are simultaneously measured. In order to overcome such a limitation, the true D-glucose content was measured by an enzymatic procedure in RINm5F cells separated from the incubation medium by centrifugation through a layer of oil into a solution of HCl (50 m*M*) and CsCl (0.64 *M*). Even after 30 min incubation at 37 °C, the apparent distribution space of D-glucose (2.8–50.0 m*M*), although higher than that of L-[1-^{14}C]glucose, remained much lower than that of $^{3}H_2O$ [13]. As a matter of fact, the intracellular D-glucose space represented no more than 38% of the intracellular $^{3}H_2O$ space. This implies that the intracellular concentration of D-glucose may never be sufficiently high to allow for an optimal participation of glucokinase in the phosphorylation of this hexose.

The findings so far outlined led us to investigate whether the transport of molecules structurally related to D-glucose may also be altered in the RINm5F cells. For this purpose, rat pancreatic islets and RINm5F cells were incubated for 5 min at 7 °C or 23 °C in media containing $^{3}H_2O$ and either L-[1-^{14}C]glucose or [2-^{14}C]alloxan. In the islets, the intracellular distribution space of [2-^{14}C]alloxan represented, at 7 °C and 23 °C respectively, 11.4% ± 1.0% and 25.5% ± 2.3% of the intracellular $^{3}H_2O$ space. In the RINm5F cells, the distribution space of [2-^{14}C]alloxan failed to be affected significantly by the ambient temperature and represented, after correction for extracellular contamination, no more than 5.2% ± 0.5% of the intracellular $^{3}H_2O$ space. Preincubation for 30 min at 7 °C in the presence of alloxan (10 m*M*) failed to affect subsequent D-[U-^{14}C]glucose oxidation in the tumoral cells, whilst causing a 70% inhibition of glucose oxidation in the islets. These results were interpreted to indicate that RINm5F cells are resistant to the cytotoxic action of alloxan, this being attributable, at least in part, to poor uptake of the diabetogenic agent [14].

Comparable findings were collected in RINm5F cells exposed to streptozotocin [15]. Thus, when pancreatic islets were exposed for 60 or 120 min to streptozotocin (3.8 m*M*), both the utilization of D-[5-^{3}H]glucose and oxidation of D-[U-^{14}C]glucose were impaired (Fig. 3). However, under identical conditions, the RINm5F cells appeared resistant to the cytotoxic action of streptozotocin. At this point, it

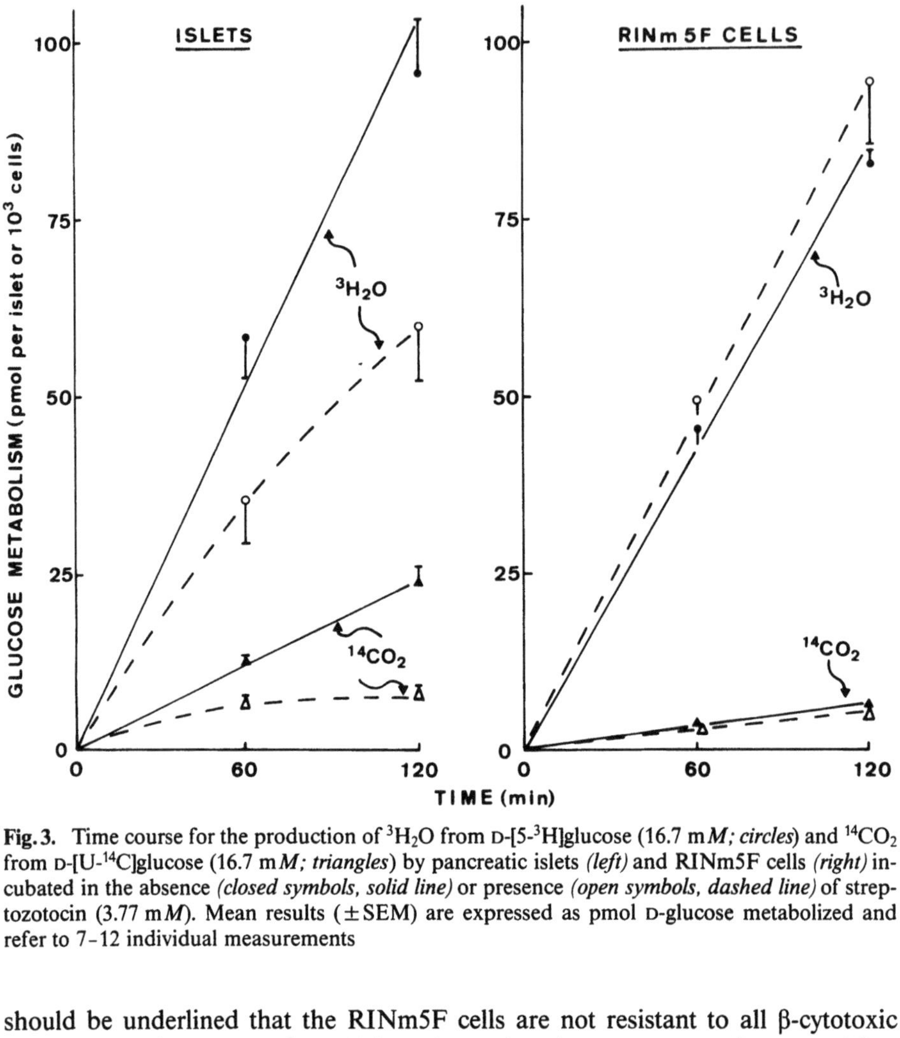

Fig. 3. Time course for the production of ^3H_2O from D-[5-^{3}H]glucose (16.7 m*M; circles*) and $^{14}CO_2$ from D-[U-^{14}C]glucose (16.7 m*M; triangles*) by pancreatic islets *(left)* and RINm5F cells *(right)* incubated in the absence *(closed symbols, solid line)* or presence *(open symbols, dashed line)* of streptozotocin (3.77 m*M*). Mean results (±SEM) are expressed as pmol D-glucose metabolized and refer to 7-12 individual measurements

should be underlined that the RINm5F cells are not resistant to all β-cytotoxic agents. For instance, after 20 h culture in the presence of pentamidine (5-500 μ*M*), a dose-related decrease in both insulin output and D-[5-^{3}H]glucose utilization was observed in pancreatic islets (Table 1). Under identical conditions, pentamidine also caused a dose-related destruction of RINm5F cells and, in the remaining cells, impaired D-[5-^{3}H]glucose utilization. As judged by the latter metabolic criterion, RINm5F cells appeared even somewhat more sensitive to pentamidine than normal pancreatic islet cells [15].

In the last set of experiments in this series, we have investigated whether a known inhibitor of hexose transport, namely cytochalasin B, would affect D-glucose transport in normal rat islets and RINm5F cells to different extents [16]. Cytochalasin B (17 μ*M*) virtually abolished 3-*O*-methyl-D-[U-^{14}C]glucose uptake and D-[5-^{3}H]glucose utilization in the RINm5F cells. This coincided with a marked decrease in D-[U-^{14}C]glucose oxidation and suppression of the stimulant action of D-glucose upon insulin release. Cytochalasin B, however, augmented basal insulin

Table 1. Effect of pentamidine upon islet cell function

Pentamidine (μM)	Pancreatic islets		RINm5F cells	
	Insulin output[a] (μU/90 min per islet)	^3H_2O production[b] (pmol/90 min per islet)	Cell number[c] (10^6 per dish)	^3H_2O production[b] (pmol/90 min per 10^3 cells)
Nil	225.1 ± 6.0 (49)	75.1 ± 8.0 (15)	5.09 ± 0.51 (3)	74.1 ± 1.2 (30)
5	170.6 ± 17.6 (10)	80.5 ± 10.3 (16)	6.47 ± 0.66 (3)	56.5 ± 1.9 (29)
50	11.3 ± 2.8 (20)	33.5 ± 10.3 (16)	2.83 ± 0.54 (3)	25.3 ± 2.2 (30)
500	17.2 ± 3.9 (24)	9.3 ± 6.0 (16)	None (3)	Not determined

The islets or RINm5F cells were first cultured for 20 h at the stated concentration of pentamidine
[a] The release of insulin was measured over 90 min incubation in the absence of pentamidine, but presence of D-glucose (16.7 mM) and theophylline (1.4 mM)
[b] The production of ^3H_2O was measured over 90 min incubation in the absence of pentamidine, but presence of D-[5-^{3}H]glucose (16.7 mM)
[c] The RINm5F cells were harvested and counted after culture for 20 h in the presence of pentamidine

release by the tumoral cells. The RINm5F cells appeared much more sensitive than normal islet cells to cytochalasin B, as judged from the relative magnitude of inhibition in either hexose uptake or utilization (Fig. 4). In both cell types, the inhibitory action of cytochalasin B upon glucose metabolism seemed to be competitive, being more marked at low than at high glucose concentration [16].

These converging observations indicate that the carrier system for the transport of hexoses and structurally related molecules is indeed poorly efficient in RINm5F cells.

Deficiency in Hexose Phosphorylation

There are at least two situations in which an endogenous deficiency in glucose phosphorylation was proposed to participate in the altered functional response of the pancreatic B-cell.

The first situation refers to the influence of fasting upon islet function. In rat islet homogenates, fasting decreases the activity of the high-Km glucokinase-like enzymic activity [17, 18]. This coincides with a decreased secretory response to D-glucose. The insulinotropic action of other secretagogues appears less severely affected [19].

The second situation was proposed to be found in insulin-producing tumoral cells of the RINm5F line [20]. However, a number of recent reports have documented the presence of glucokinase (or a high-Km glucose-phosphorylating enzymic activity) in homogenates of RINm5F cells [21, 22, 23].

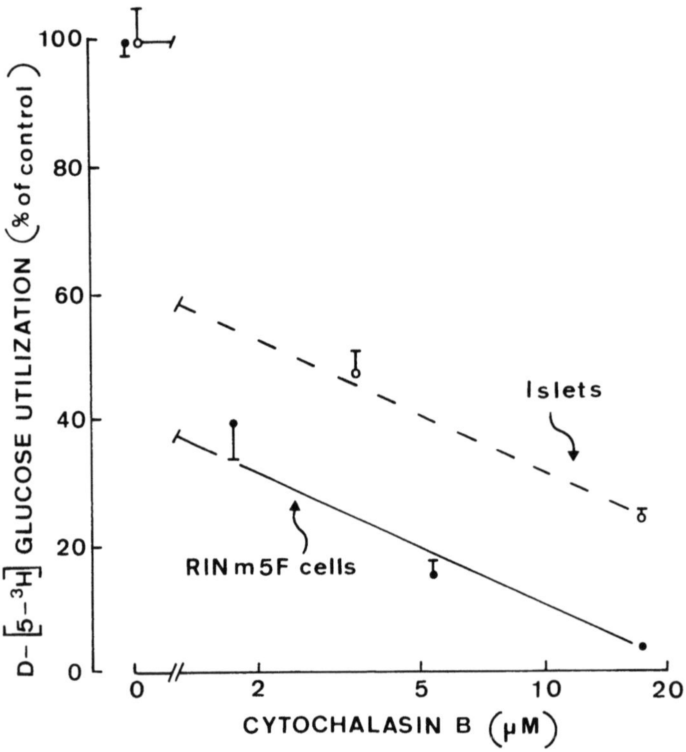

Fig. 4. Effect of increasing concentrations of cytochalasin B (logarithmic scale) upon the utilization of D-[5-^{3}H]glucose by RINm5F cells *(closed circles)* and pancreatic islets *(open circles)* incubated for 120 min in the presence of 2.8 m*M* D-glucose. Mean values (±SEM) refer to 10-16 individual determinations and are expressed in percent of the mean control measurements made in the absence of cytochalasin B

Deficiency in Phosphofructokinase Activation

Over recent years, we have defended the view that activation of phosphofructokinase in islet cells may be required for the rate of fructose 6-phosphate conversion to fructose 1,6-bisphosphate to keep pace with the rate of fructose 6-phosphate generation from glucose 6-phosphate [24, 25]. Thus, the apparent role of hexose bisphosphates, especially glucose 1,6-bisphosphate and fructose 2,6-bisphosphate, as activators of phosphofructokinase was duly emphasized [26, 27, 28]. For instance, it was proposed that the anomeric specificity of both D-glucose and D-mannose metabolism was attributable, in part, to the anomeric difference in the islet content in aldohexose bisphosphates [29, 30].

The investigation of D-glucose catabolism in islets removed from either fed or fasted rats illustrates, in our opinion, an instance in which impairment of D-glucose utilization is attributable, in part, to a deficiency in phosphofructokinase activation. The key findings in support of such a contention are summarized in Table 2.

Table 2. Effect of fasting upon islet metabolism

	Fed rats	Fasted rats	p
Glucokinase activity in islet homogenates (pmol/60 min per μg protein)			
	67.1 ± 18.2	22.3 ± 7.2	< 0.05
Glucose-1,6-P_2 islet content (fmol/islet at 30th min of incubation)			
D-Glucose (2.8 m*M*)	16.3 ± 4.5	13.2 ± 2.6	N.S.
D-Glucose (16.7 m*M*)	49.1 ± 5.1	18.0 ± 4.7	< 0.001
Lactic acid release (pmol/30 min per islet)			
D-Glucose (2.8 m*M*)	34.3 ± 2.1	49.8 ± 10.1	N.S.
D-Glucose (16.7 m*M*)	109.9 ± 7.2	44.3 ± 6.8	< 0.001
Pyruvic acid release (pmol/30 min per islet)			
D-Glucose (2.8 m*M*)	6.1 ± 0.8	6.5 ± 0.9	N.S.
D-Glucose (16.7 m*M*)	14.2 ± 2.0	5.9 ± 0.7	< 0.001

Mean values (± SEM) refer to nine or more individual observations

The activity of glucokinase is decreased in homogenates from fasted rats [17]. The values given in Table 2 were derived from measurements of glucose phosphorylation at low (0.05 m*M*) and high (20 m*M*) hexose concentration, in either the absence or presence of exogenous glucose 6-phosphate (0.33 m*M*). They suggest a 67% regression of glucokinase, this being the most severe estimation of the fasting-induced adaptative decrease in glucokinase activity among all published data [17]. Yet, in the islets from fasted rats, a rise in D-glucose concentration totally failed to enhance lactic acid and pyruvic acid output over 30 min incubation, at variance with the situation found in islets from fed animals. This coincided with a marked alteration in the capacity of D-glucose to increase the islet content in glucose 1,6-bisphosphate.

Glucose 1,6-bisphosphate can be formed in the islets from glucose 6-phosphate and a suitable phosphate donor (e.g. fructose 1,6-bisphosphate or 1,3-diphosphoglycerate) in a reaction catalyzed by phosphoglucomutase. In the islets, the activity of the latter enzyme is unaffected by fasting [31]. The fasting-induced decrease in glucose 1,6-bisphosphate synthesis is likely to be due, therefore, both to the repression of glucokinase and phosphofructokinase and to a poor activation of the latter enzyme. This interpretation is supported by the finding that in mouse islets exposed to 16.7 m*M* D-glucose, fasting decreases the tissue content in fructose 1,6-bisphosphate and triose phosphates even when the glucose 6-phosphate content appears unaffected [32, 33]. These results thus illustrate a situation in which phosphofructokinase is apparently not sufficiently activated to keep pace with the rate of glucose 6-phosphate formation.

Deficiency in Mitochondrial Oxidative Processes

We have recently taken advantage of the parallel use of D-[3,4-^{14}C]glucose and D-[6-^{14}C]glucose to measure the flow rate through the glycerol phosphate shuttle, the decarboxylation of pyruvate derived from exogenous D-glucose and the oxidation of acetyl-CoA, also derived from exogenous D-glucose, in either rat pancreatic is-

Table 3. D-glucose catabolism in rat pancreatic islets and RINm5F cells

Tissue	Pancreatic islets		RINm5F cells	
D-Glucose (m*M*)	2.8	16.7	2.8	16.7
D-[3,4-^{14}C]Glucose utilization (pmol/120 min per islet or 10^3 cells)				
	72.5 ± 5.8	228.2 ± 7.5	142.8 ± 18.1	189.2 ± 5.8
Flow through glycerol phosphate shuttle/D-[3,4-^{14}C]glucose utilization (%)				
	27.7 ± 2.9	39.9 ± 2.3	22.6 ± 3.1	19.3 ± 1.0
[^{14}C]Pyruvate decarboxylation/D-[3,4-^{14}C]glucose utilization (%)				
	19.2 ± 2.0	33.0 ± 2.1	8.3 ± 1.3	6.2 ± 0.6
Production of $^{14}CO_2$ from D-[6-^{14}C]glucose/D-[3,4-^{14}C]glucose utilization (%)				
	8.8 ± 0.9	17.1 ± 1.1	3.3 ± 0.5	1.9 ± 0.2

Mean values (± SEM) are derived from 12 or more individual observations

lets or RINm5F cells incubated at low (2.8 m*M*) and high (16.7 m*M*) concentrations of D-glucose. The results relevant to these mitochondrial oxidative processes are summarized in Table 3.

The rate of D-[3,4-^{14}C]glucose utilization was taken as the sum of the production of [^{14}C]lactate, [^{14}C]pyruvate, [^{14}C]alanine, and $^{14}CO_2$ (all expressed as glucose residues). The production of [^{14}C]lactate was measured in a neutralized perchloric acid extract through the production of $^{14}CO_2$ upon exposure to lactate oxidase from *Mycobacterium smegmatis* (EC 1.13.12.4). The production of [^{14}C]pyruvate and [^{14}C]alanine from D-[3,4-^{14}C]glucose was judged, after acidification to measure $^{14}CO_2$ production and further neutralization, by separation of amino acids through an ion-exchange resin after treatment with pig heart glutamate: pyruvate transaminase (EC 2.6.1.2) in the presence of either L-glutamate or 2-ketoglutarate. Virtually identical results were obtained for the production of [^{14}C]pyruvate, whether in the presence of D-[3,4-^{14}C]glucose or D-[6-^{14}C]glucose. The flow rate through the glycerol phosphate shuttle was assumed to correspond to the utilization of D-[3,4-^{14}C]glucose unaccounted for by the production of [^{14}C]lactate.

As shown in Table 3, the rate of D-[3,4-^{14}C]glucose utilization rose as a function of the glucose concentration in both islets ($p < 0.001$) and RINm5F cells ($p < 0.025$). The 16.7 m*M*/2.8 m*M* ratio in D-[3,4-^{14}C]glucose utilization averaged 3.14 ± 0.27 in islets as distinct from only 1.32 ± 0.17 in tumoral cells ($p < 0.001$).

In Table 3, all other metabolic variables are expressed relative to the corresponding rate of D-[3,4-^{14}C]glucose utilization. This mode of expression reveals three essential features.

First, in pancreatic islets, the flow through the glycerol phosphate shuttle, the rate of [^{14}C]pyruvate decarboxylation (as judged by the production of $^{14}CO_2$ from D-[3,4-^{14}C]glucose) and the mitochondrial oxidation of [^{14}C]acetyl-CoA residues (as judged by the production of $^{14}CO_2$ from D-[6-^{14}C]glucose) were all significantly increased ($p < 0.005$ or less) in response to the rise in D-glucose concentration, despite the fact that all results are expressed relative to the rate of D-[3,4-^{14}C]glucose utilization. It thus appears that normal islet cells are organized to favor those mitochondrial oxidative reactions yielding the major fraction of the energy generated by the catabolism of exogenous D-glucose.

Secondly, relative to D-[3,4-^{14}C]glucose utilization, the flux through the glycerol phosphate shuttle, the oxidative decarboxylation of pyruvate and the oxidation of acetyl-CoA in the Krebs cycle were all lower in RINm5F cells than in islets.

Lastly, in the tumoral cells, a rise in D-glucose concentration failed to increase the rate of mitochondrial oxidative processes, relative to the overall rate of D-glucose utilization. Actually the absolute value for D-[6-^{14}C]glucose oxidation was decreased, in the RINm5F cells, in response to the increase in D-glucose concentration ($p < 0.02$).

Two major conclusions can be drawn from these findings. First, the results obtained in normal pancreatic islets again indicate that the metabolism of D-glucose is not regulated solely at the level of hexose phosphorylation. If phosphorylation were to be the sole regulatory step, one would expect mitochondrial oxidations to proceed at a rate proportional to that of D-glucose 6-phosphate generation. Such was obviously not the case. Secondly, the results obtained in the RINm5F cells clearly document both a low efficiency of mitochondrial oxidative processes, relative to the situation found in normal islet cells, and an impaired response of such processes to an increase in extracellular D-glucose concentration.

Deleterious Effect of Sustained Hyperglycemia: The Glucotoxic Concept

All mechanisms for deficient glucose recognition by the B-cell so far presented in this report refer to situations in which a site-specific abnormality in D-glucose handling or metabolism could conceivably lead to an altered secretory response to the hexose.

Although somewhat beyond the scope of this review, it should be underlined that an abnormal functional response of the B-cell to D-glucose could also occur as a consequence of sustained hyperglycemia. Thus, it is currently believed that chronic hyperglycemia may lead to impaired insulin secretion, possibly by altering the function of the B-cell glucosensor device. A concept of glucotoxicity was even proposed [34].

It was recently suggested that prolonged exposure of the B-cell to glucose *in vitro* might cause desensitization to the hexose [35]. For reasons given elsewhere [36, 37], I feel it premature to consider this procedure as a suitable model for the alteration of B-cell function thought to result *in vivo* from sustained hyperglycemia.

To my knowledge, very little information is available as to the biochemical mechanisms possibly involved in the long-term unfavorable effect of hyperglycemia upon B-cell function. In certain models of spontaneous diabetes in animals, the B-cell may be loaded with glycogen deposit [38]. It is conceivable that such a situation plays a role in the altered function of the B-cell. By analogy with current concepts on the biochemistry of the degenerative complications of diabetes in extrapancreatic tissues, attention should also be paid to the role that sorbitol accumulation and nonenzymatic protein glycosylation in the B-cell might play in the apparent functional exhaustion of this cell.

Concluding Remarks

The present review emphasizes that a primary perturbation of D-glucose metabolism at specific locations or the metabolic consequences of sustained hyperglycemia may conceivably account for deficient glucose recognition in islet cells. It remains to investigate whether anomalies similar to those characterized in the experimental models presented in this report are indeed encountered in diabetic patients.

It should be emphasized that the present account is strictly restricted to possible mechanisms for impaired identification of D-glucose by the B-cell. This does not imply that an impaired secretory response to this hexose is necessarily attributable to its altered recognition. Indeed, it is quite conceivable that an abnormal functional response of islet cells to D-glucose and/or other secretagogues occurs as a consequence of site-specific defects located at distal sites in the secretory sequence. To cite only one among a great number of examples, an inherited or acquired lesion of the effector system for insulin release, such as the abnormality of the B-cell microtubular system in *Acomys cahirinus* [39], could obviously also result in an abnormal pattern of insulin release in response to stimulation by D-glucose.

Acknowledgements. I am indebted to M.-H. GIROIX, F. MALAISSE-LAGAE, and A. SENER for their collaboration in the experimental work presented here. I wish to thank C. DEMESMAEKER for secretarial help.

References

1. Robertson RP, Porte Jr D (1973) The glucose receptor. A defective mechanism in diabetes mellitus distinct from the beta adrenergic receptor. J Clin Invest 52: 870-876
2. Malaisse WJ (1972) Hormonal and environmental modification of islet activity. In: Steiner DF, Freinkel N (eds) Endocrine pancreas. American Physiological Society, Washington, pp 237-260 (Handbook of physiology, section 7, vol 1)
3. Malaisse WJ, Sener A, Herchuelz A, Hutton JC, Devis G, Somers G, Blondel B, Malaisse-Lagae F, Orci L (1977) Sequential events in the process of glucose-induced insulin release. In: Bajaj JS (ed) Diabetes. Excerpta Medica, Amsterdam, pp 95-102
4. Malaisse WJ, Sener A, Herchuelz A, Hutton JC (1979) Insulin release: the fuel hypothesis. Metabolism 28: 373-386
5. Malaisse WJ (1984) Insulin release: the fuel concept. Diabète Métab 9: 313-320
6. Matschinsky FM, Ellerman J, Stillings S, Raybaud F, Pace C, Zawalich W (1975) Hexoses and insulin release. In: Hasselblatt A, Bruchhausen Fv (eds) Insulin, part 2. Springer, Berlin Heidelberg New York, pp 79-114
7. Sener A, Malaisse WJ (1984) Nutrient metabolism in islet cells. Experientia 40: 1026-1035
8. Malaisse WJ, Malaisse-Lagae F, Sener A (1984) Coupling factors in nutrient-induced insulin release. Experientia 40: 1035-1043
9. Meglasson MD, Matschinsky FM (1984) New perspectives on pancreatic islet glucokinase. Am J Physiol 246: E1-E13
10. Malaisse WJ, Sener A (1985) Glucokinase is not the pancreatic B-cell glucoreceptor. Diabetologia 28: 520-527
11. Malaisse WJ, Giroix M-H, Malaisse-Lagae F, Sener A (1986) 3-O-methyl-D-glucose transport in tumoral insulin-producing cells. Am J Physiol 251: C841-C846

12. Giroix M-H, Sener A, Malaisse WJ (1986) D-Glucose transport and concentration in tumoral insulin-producing cells. Am J Physiol 251: C847-C851
13. Sener A, Giroix M-H, Malaisse WJ (1986) Impaired uptake of D-glucose by tumoral insulin-producing cells. Biochem Int 12: 913-919
14. Sener A, Malaisse WJ (1985) Resistance to alloxan of tumoral insulin-producing cells. FEBS Lett 193: 150-152
15. Sener A, Malaisse-Lagae F, Giroix M-H, Malaisse WJ (1986) Sensitivity to pentamidine but resistance to streptozotocin of tumoral insulin-producing cells (RINm5F line). Pancreas 1: 550-555
16. Malaisse WJ, Giroix M-H, Sener A (1986) Effect of cytochalasin B upon glucose uptake, utilization, oxidation and insulinotropic action in tumoral insulin-producing cells. Cell Biochem Funct 5: 183-187
17. Malaisse WJ, Sener A, Levy J (1976) The stimulus-secretion coupling of glucose-induced insulin release. XXI. Fasting-induced adaptation of key glycolytic enzymes in isolated islets. J Biol Chem 251: 1731-1737
18. Matschinsky FM, Meglasson MD, Burch PT, Berner DK, Najafi H, Vogin AP, Garfinkel D, Garfinkel L (1983) Glucokinase (ATP: D-glucose 6-phosphotransferase E.C. 2.7.1.2), the glucose sensor of pancreatic islet B-cells. In: Mngola EN (ed) Diabetes 1982. Excerpta Medica, Amsterdam, pp337-344 (International congress series 600)
19. Levy J, Herchuelz A, Sener A, Malaisse WJ (1976) The stimulus-secretion coupling of glucose-induced insulin release. XX. Fasting: a model for altered glucose recognition by the B-cell. Metabolism 25: 583-591
20. Halban PA, Praz GA, Wollheim CB (1983) Abnormal glucose metabolism accompanies failure of glucose to stimulate insulin release from a rat pancreatic cell line (RINm5F). Biochem J 212: 439-443
21. Giroix M-H, Sener A, Dufrane SP, Malaisse-Lagae F, Malaisse WJ (1985) Glucose metabolism in insulin-producing tumoral cells. Arch Biochem Biophys 241: 561-570
22. Meglasson MD, Burch PT, Hoenig M, Chick WL, Matschinsky FM (1983) Identification and significance of glucokinase in transplantable insulinomas. J Biol Chem 258: 2094-2097
23. Meglasson MD, Matschinsky FM (1984) Purification of the putative islet cell glucose sensor glucokinase from isolated pancreatic islets and insulinoma tissue. In: Larner J, Pohl SL (eds) Methods in diabetes research. Wiley, New York, pp213-226 (vol I: laboratory methods, part B)
24. Malaisse WJ, Malaisse-Lagae F, Sener A, Van Schaftingen E, Hers H-G (1981) Is the glucose-induced stimulation of glycolysis in pancreatic islets attributable to activation of phosphofructokinase by fructose 2,6-bisphosphate? FEBS Lett 125: 217-219
25. Malaisse WJ, Malaisse-Lagae F, Sener A (1982) The glycolytic cascade in pancreatic islets. Diabetologia 23: 1-5
26. Malaisse WJ, Malaisse-Lagae F, Sener A (1982) Glucose-induced accumulation of fructose-2,6-bisphosphate in pancreatic islets. Diabetes 31: 90-93
27. Sener A, Malaisse-Lagae F, Malaisse WJ (1982) Glucose-induced accumulation of glucose-1,6-bisphosphate in pancreatic islets: its possible role in the regulation of glycolysis. Biochem Biophys Res Commun 104: 1033-1040
28. Sener A, Van Schaftingen E, Van De Winkel M, Pipeleers DG, Malaisse-Lagae F, Malaisse WJ, Hers H-G (1984) Effects of glucose and glucagon on the fructose 2,6-bisphosphate content of pancreatic islets and purified pancreatic B-cells. Biochem J 221: 759-764
29. Malaisse-Lagae F, Sener A, Malaisse WJ (1982) Phosphoglucomutase: its role in the response of pancreatic islets to glucose epimers and anomers. Biochimie 64: 1059-1063
30. Malaisse WJ, Malaisse-Lagae F, Sener A (1983) Anomeric specificity of hexose metabolism in pancreatic islets. Physiol Rev 63: 321-327
31. Giroix M-H, Dufrane SP, Malaisse-Lagae F, Sener A, Malaisse WJ (1984) Fasting-induced impairment of glucose-1,6-bisphosphate synthesis in pancreatic islets. Biochem Biophys Res Commun 119: 543-548
32. Idahl L-Å (1973) Dynamics of pancreatic B-cell responses to glucose. Diabetologia 9: 403-412
33. Hedeskov CJ, Capito K (1974) The effect of starvation on insulin secretion and glucose metabolism in mouse pancreatic islets. Biochem J 140: 423-433
34. Garvey WT, Olefsky JM, Griffin J, Hamman RF, Kolterman OG (1985) The effect of insulin

treatment on insulin secretion and insulin action in type II diabetes mellitus. Diabetes 34: 222-234
35. Bolaffi JL, Heldt A, Lewis LD, Grodsky GM (1986) The third phase of in vitro insulin secretion. Evidence for glucose insensitivity. Diabetes 35: 370-373
36. Malaisse WJ, Sener A (1987) Interaction between D-glucose and Ca^{2+} in the priming of the pancreatic B-cell. Diabetes Res 4: 5-8
37. Malaisse-Lagae F, Sener A, Malaisse WJ (1987) Can desensitization of the B-cell to D-glucose be simulated in cultured pancreatic islets? Acta Diab Lat 24: 17-25
38. Malaisse WJ, Like AA, Malaisse-Lagae F, Gleason RE, Soeldner JS (1968) Insulin secretion in vitro by the pancreas of the sand rat *(Psammomys obesus)*. Diabetes 17: 752-759
39. Malaisse-Lagae F, Ravazzola M, Amherdt M, Gutzeit A, Stauffacher W, Malaisse WJ, Orci L (1975) An apparent abnormality of the B-cell microtubular system in Spiny mice *(Acomys cahirinus)*. Diabetologia 11: 71-76

Insulin Release and Islet Cell Junctions*

P. A. In't Veld

Introduction

The communication between islet cells has become an exciting research subject since the description of cell junctions in the endocrine pancreas [61]. In analogy to other tissues, the presence of these membrane specializations was considered as a likely anatomical basis for the generation of rapid and appropriate islet cell responses to nutrients and hormones.

Tight junctions (Figs. 1, 2) have been regarded as barriers in the intercellular space, which compartmentalize the islet tissue so that the released hormones diffuse along ordered channels. The existence of an interstitial organization appeared to be an attractive basis for the regulation of interactions between the various islet cell types, in particular since it could in itself be subject to modulation: tight junctions are indeed not rigid membrane specializations like desmosomes, but correspond, on the contrary, to flexible and dynamic structures which are able to rapidly adjust their density to variations in the extracellular milieu [58, 62].

Another type of cell junction, the gap junction, was also recognized between most types of islet cells. This structure was described at the same time as the islet tight junctions, with which it can form junctional complexes (Fig. 2). As in other tissues, islet gap junctions were thought to play a role in the synchronization of islet cell functions [61]. The presence of communicating junctions between the various islet cell types was, for example, associated with the phenomena of electrical coupling and dye exchange between these cells [6, 37, 49, 53]. Gap junctions could thus be considered as the structures which not only coordinate the insulin release process in an individual islet, but also adjust the functional responses of neighboring cell types.

The present chapter will review the data relating islet cell junctions to islet cell communication and function.

Islet Microanatomy

In many species the islet of Langerhans is characterized by a precise topography of its constituent endocrine cell types. In mouse, rat, or rabbit a core of insulin-containing B-cells is surrounded by a mantle of non-B-cells, while in the monkey

* This study was supported by the Belgian Fonds Geneeskundig Wetenschappelijk Onderzoek (3.0059.86).

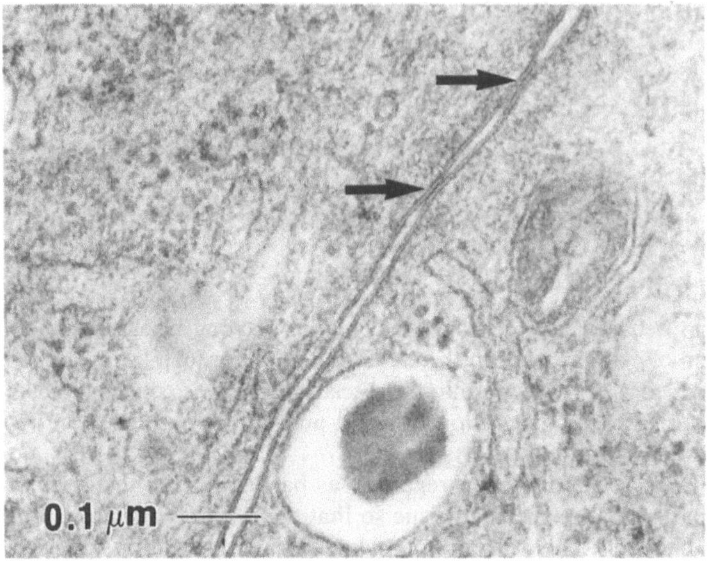

Fig. 1. Focal points of cell contact *(arrows)* between two pancreatic B-cells. Because of the small size of islet gap junctions it is difficult to distinguish between islet tight and gap junctions in conventional thin sections

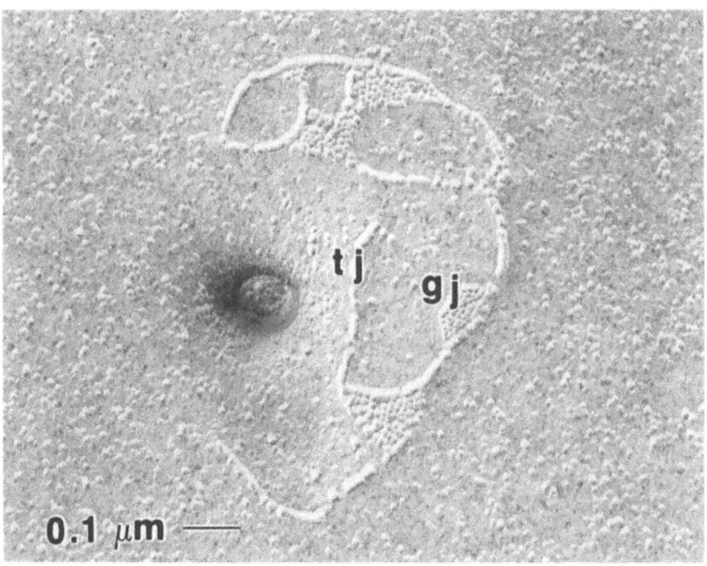

Fig. 2. Freeze fracture replica of a collagenase-isolated rat islet showing tight junctional fibrils *(tj)* associated with several small gap junctions *(gj)*. Junctional complexes incorporating both tight and gap junctions are seen only after exposure to proteolytic enzymes

and the horse a central mass of non-B-cells is covered by a layer of B-cells [13]. Similar patterns are difficult to distinguish in the human islet. Using a three-dimensional reconstruction, GRUBE et al. [20, 21] were able to demonstrate that the relative position of the human islet cells was also not random. The human islet A-, B- and D-cells were indeed found to be arranged in contiguous groups of homologous cells. All B-cells appeared in direct contact to each other, while A- and D-cells were found to be adjacent to a small proportion of B-cells. The cellular organization in man thus also exhibits the feature that some of the B-cells are in direct contact with islet non-B-cells. This particular topography of the islet cells has been considered as evidence for the modulation of insulin release by intra-islet factors [59].

Tight Junctions

Structure and Function

Islet tight junctions were first described in collagenase-isolated rat islets of LANGERHANS [61]. As in other tissues, they can be discerned in freeze fracture replicas, where they appear as continuous or discontinuous fibrils which, at high magnification, are often composed of irregular subunits. In conventional transmission electron microscopy these fibrils correspond to punctate regions of fusion between two adjacent plasma membranes. In contrast to the tight junctions in tissues such as liver and intestines, islet tight junctions do not form a continuous belt of fibrils around the apical border of the cell. No real zonula occludens capable of separating two compartments of different chemical composition is therefore present, nor can these junctions completely separate the apical membrane compartment from the basolateral one [9].

Although tight junctions have been morphologically described since 1963 [12] their chemical composition is still unclear. Traditionally, tight junctions have been considered to be composed of protein molecules which are linearly arranged so that they contact identical molecules in the apposed plasma membrane [83].

Recent data support the protein nature of the tight junction [22], but considerable evidence also favors lipid or combined protein/lipid composition [33, 90].

Modulation of Density

When isolated rat islets were exposed for 90 min to a mixture of proteolytic enzymes, the number of tight junctional fibrils increased five- to sixfold, indicating that these fibrils are dynamic structures which have the ability to rapidly increase their density [62]. Exposure to glucose also resulted in a two- to threefold increase in the amount of tight junctions [58].

It should, however, be noted that the method of collagenase isolation can in itself induce the formation of tight junction fibrils [29]. In fact, tight junctions could not be demonstrated in the in situ fixed rat or human pancreas. Only when the intact organ was perfused with trypsin did tight junction fibrils appear in the islet

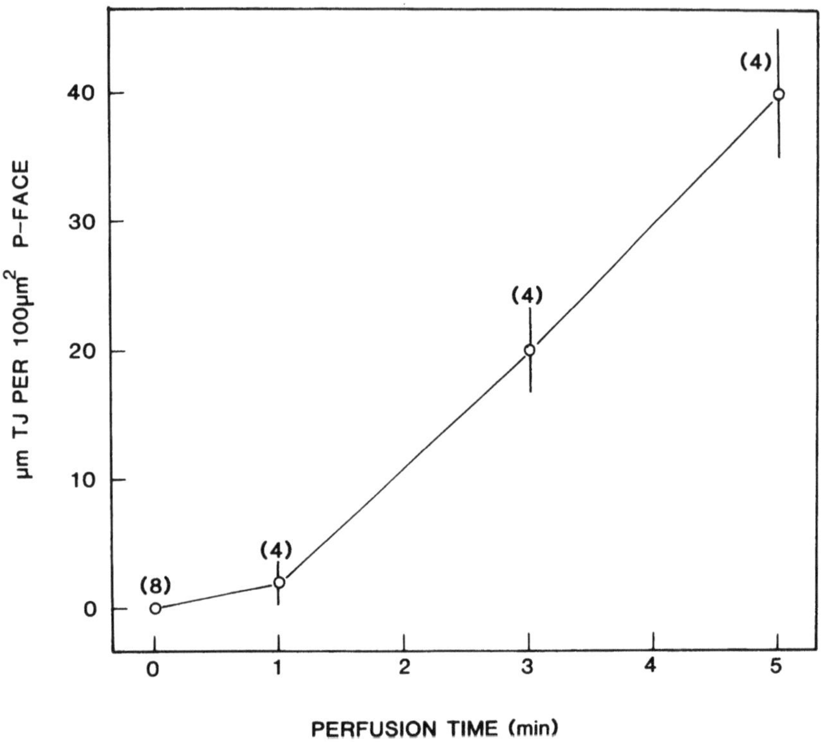

Fig. 3. Trypsin-induced tight junction *(TJ)* formation in the perfused rat pancreas. Values represent mean ± SEM of *(n)* islet replicas and were obtained after analysis of 1000-2500 μm^2 of membrane P-face

tissue. The structures were already detected after 1 min exposure; after 2 min, the tight junction density was comparable to that in collagenase-isolated rat islets (Fig. 3). Culture resulted in a gradual decrease in the number of tight junctional fibrils in isolated islets. Disassembly of these artificially induced fibrils proceeded slowly, reaching 70% of the initial amount after 2 h and 8% after 20 h culture at 5.6 m*M* glucose [29]. The reported effects of glucose on tight junction quantity in vitro [58] should therefore not necessarily be interpreted as glucose-mediated induction of tight junctional fibrils; they may also represent glucose modulation of the inductive effect of collagenase or alternatively a glucose-mediated differential breakdown rate of such fibrils.

While absent in rat and human pancreatic islets in situ [29, 93], tight junctional fibrils have been described in bovine, gerbil, guinea pig, and mouse pancreas [2, 34, 93]. In species where they are absent under basal circumstances, tight junctions can be rapidly and massively assembled, suggesting the existence of a large pool of tight junction precursors in the plasma membrane. These observations may indicate that tight junctions play a role in particular physio(patho)logic conditions, but are much less in favor of a universal role in the process of insulin release.

In view of the inducing effects of proteolytic enzymes, we have postulated that tight junctions provide protection of the islet tissue in conditions in which islet cells are exposed to activated pancreatic enzymes [29].

Role in Compartmentalization

Tight junctions, when present in islets, may seal off one part of the interstitial tissue from the other and thus establish compartmentalization of the islet intercellular space. This phenomenon may explain why islets in which tight junctions were induced by pronase and which were subsequently exposed to high glucose presented large accumulations of insulin-like material between the cells, probably because the tight junctions limited diffusion into the capillary space [62]. From the localization of these insulin deposits, it appears that B-cells in isolated islets secrete a substantial amount of insulin at their lateral borders and not (only) at their capillary pole. This is consistent with the presence of canaliculi containing many microvilli at areas of cell-to-cell contact near the capillaries [17]. It is also near these sites that most of the gap junctions, desmosomes, and tight junctions are found.

In the perfused dog pancreas KAWAI et al. (35) were able to inhibit insulin secretion by somatostatin-14 (S-14) concentrations which were significantly lower than those measured in the venous effluent. These observations led them to postulate the existence of secretory and receptor poles that are separated by a tight junction barrier. In this view, endogenously secreted somatostatin would not reach the neighboring A- or B-cells.

Although this hypothesis has several interesting aspects, it is evident that, according to this model, species that do not normally possess islet tight junctions (like rat and man) would not be able to effectively compartmentalize the islet intercellular space. The model also implicates that retrograde perfusion with somatostatin would give different results than anterograde perfusion. Recent work by the same authors seems to indicate that this is not the case [36].

Among the alternative explanations for the observed high sensitivity of the islet B-cells to S-14 is the observation that purified A-cells are 1000 times more sensitive to S-14 than are purified B-cells [74]. Since insulin secretion is stimulated by glucagon, the inhibition of insulin release by endogenous somatostatin may well be mediated through inhibition of glucagon release. The exquisite sensitivity of the B-cell to pancreatic glucagon [69], as well as the presence of high-affinity glucagon receptors on the B-cell [88], is compatible with this alternative hypothesis. This model would necessitate that sufficiently high levels of glucagon reaching the B-cell zone, either via the circulation (using the portal circulation of FUJITA [16] or the circulation pattern suggested by BONNER-WEIR [3]) or via a paracrine route. Diffusion in the intercellular space seems possible, as continuous seals of tight junctions are not present in any of the investigated species, and as injected tracers like horseradish peroxidase diffuse freely between the cells [42].

Gap Junctions

Structure and Function

Gap junctions are morphologically defined membrane specializations which can be recognized in many tissues [for review see 43]. The structures represent aggregates of particles each 9 nm in diameter and visible on freeze-fracture replicas. Form and size of the aggregates can vary considerably between the various cell types [40], but their subunits or connexons [18] always appear identical and exhibit a central channel of approximately 2 nm in diameter [76]. Two apposing connexons are sufficient to establish an intercellular channel through which ions and small molecules with an M_r up to 1200 daltons can be exchanged between the neighboring cells [79]. Using negative staining, frozen hydrated sections, and X-ray diffraction the connexons were found to be composed of six identical subunits [45, 86, 87]. These subunits have been isolated from the rat liver and shown to be composed of a protein with M_r 27000 [25].

Antibodies raised against the liver subunits permitted evaluation of their functional significance. It was shown that the addition of connexon antibodies blocks electrical coupling and dye transfer between adjacent hepatocytes [28, 92]. The antibodies cross-reacted with gap junctions in pancreas, brain, adrenals, kidney, and stomach, which is suggestive of substantial structure homology [8, 27]. However, a lack of cross-reactivity was noted for myocardium and for islets of LANGERHANS. Sequencing of the myocardial gap junction protein demonstrated considerable differences in amino acid sequences as compared to liver gap junctions. These variations appeared more pronounced between tissues than between species, indicating tissue-specific gap junctions [19, 26, 39, 57, 66]. The lack of reactivity of connexon antibodies to islet gap junctions [8, 27, 65] may similarly indicate the existence of islet-specific gap junctions.

Modulation of Permeability

The central connexon channel, characterized by a conductance of 120–165 pS, is able to open or close in milliseconds [56, 89]. Its permeability can be modulated by variations in intracellular calcium concentration, in cytoplasmic pH, and in cellular cyclic adenosine monophosphate (cAMP) levels [23, 71, 85]. However, the intracellular levels of ionized calcium which are required to induce closure of gap junction channels are usually higher than $10^{-3} M$, which is 10000 fold higher than the normal cytoplasmic calcium concentration. It seems therefore likely that the calcium-induced closure is only observed in conditions of cell damage. The sensitivity to calcium can thus be regarded as a safety mechanism, sealing off a damaged cell and separating it from its healthy neighbors [43]. On the other hand the gap junction channel is more sensitive to changes in pH. A decline of the intercellular pH from 7.6 to 7.3 has been shown to result in a 50% decrease in gap junction permeability in teleost blastomeres [81] indicating that the channels are approximately 10^4 times more sensitive to H^+ than to Ca^{2+} [82]. It should be realized, though, that the characteristics described here pertain mainly to nonexcitable cells. The electrically excitable pancreatic B-cells may well display different gap junction characteristics.

The third mechanism through which gap junction permeability can be altered seems to be mediated via cAMP-dependent phosphorylation of the connexon subunits. Such phosphorylation is associated with increased connexon permeability [72].

The mechanism of connexon permeability control has not been fully elucidated. It has been suggested that rotation of the six connexon subunits in the plane of the membrane results in the opening or closing of the connexon channel [86]. Such a change on the molecular level may result in altered connexon diameter and spacing as visualized on freeze fracture replicas [67].

Occurrence in Islets

Electrical excitability of islet cells was established some 20 years ago when it was noted that insulinotropic agents like glucose, L-leucine, and tolbutamide rapidly induced action potentials in islet B-cells [6]. Using dual impalement techniques, it was observed that 11.1 mM glucose induced synchronous electrical activity in mouse islet cells which were separated by several B-cell diameters [52]. On the basis of this finding it was proposed that, in analogy to other cell systems, islet B-cells are electrically coupled. This concept is compatible with the observation of small gap junctions in rat and human islets [61, 63].

More recently it was demonstrated, with the aid of current injections, that synchronous electrical activity existed in islet cells that were separated by approximately two B-cell diameters [10]. The degree of electrical coupling was dependent on the glucose concentration in the medium, the removal of the sugar resulting in complete disappearance of detectable electrical coupling within 60 s, while its reintroduction increased the degree of coupling. These findings in microdissected mouse islets correlate well with the rapid glucose-induced changes in gap junction morphology (Fig. 4) which occur in perfused rat pancreata [31] (Fig. 5). An increased connexon aggregation may well represent the structural counterpart of the observed changes in electrical coupling between islet B-cells.

Freeze fracture studies have indicated that gap junctions not only exist in the islet B-cell zone but are also present between B-cells and cells tentatively identified as A-cells [64]. Heterologous contacts were also observed between B- and D-cells in conventional transmission electron microscopy [15].

Dye-coupling studies using fluorescent dyes provided additional proof for the existence of heterologous coupling. Experiments on monolayer cultures of newborn rat pancreases [49] and on collagenase-isolated islets [53] showed that dye coupling occurred between most types of endocrine cells. PP-cells were not investigated in these studies.

Coupling between endocrine and nonendocrine cells was reported by ORCI et al. [60], who described focal points of cell contact between a cholinergic nerve terminal and a B-cell in lanthanum-contrasted thin sections of collagenase-isolated

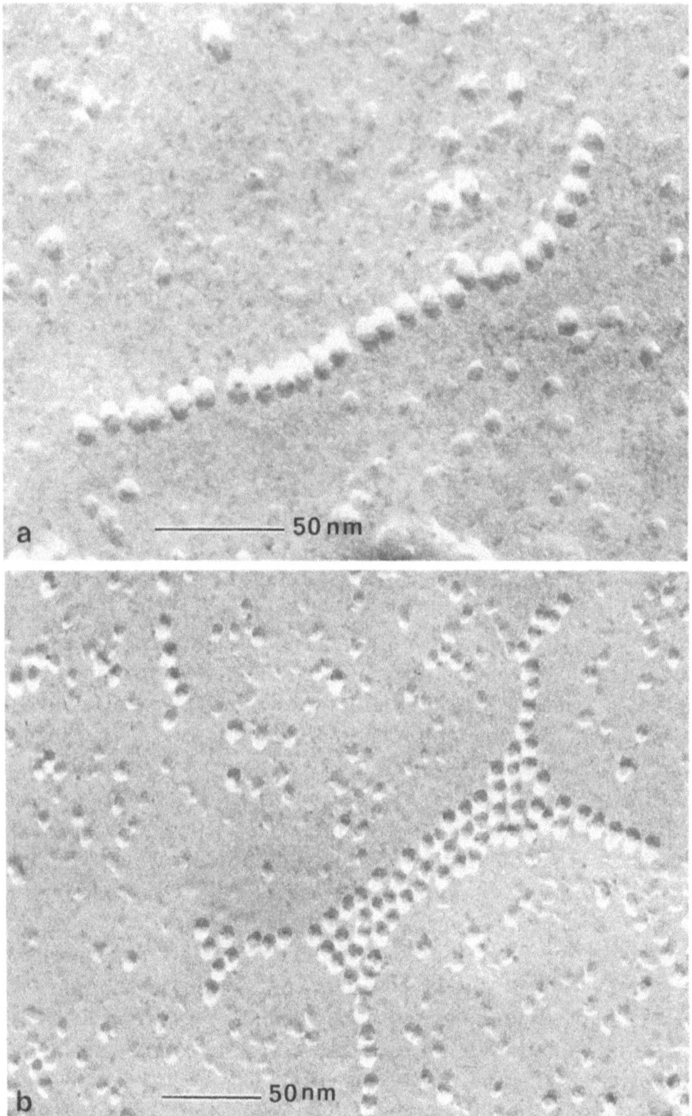

Fig. 4 a, b. Freeze fracture replicas of islet B-cells showing two types of gap junction configuration. Linear particle arrays are the most frequent type of gap junctions found in situ (**a**) although gap junctions consisting of polygonally arranged particles or composed of both linear and polygonal arrays (**b**) do also occur

rat islets and tentatively identified them as gap junctions. However, in plastic thin sections, islet gap junctions are difficult to distinguish from collagenase-induced tight junctions due to their small size. We have not observed any gap junctions between endocrine cells and nerve terminals in freeze fracture replicas, so that their existence is still controversial.

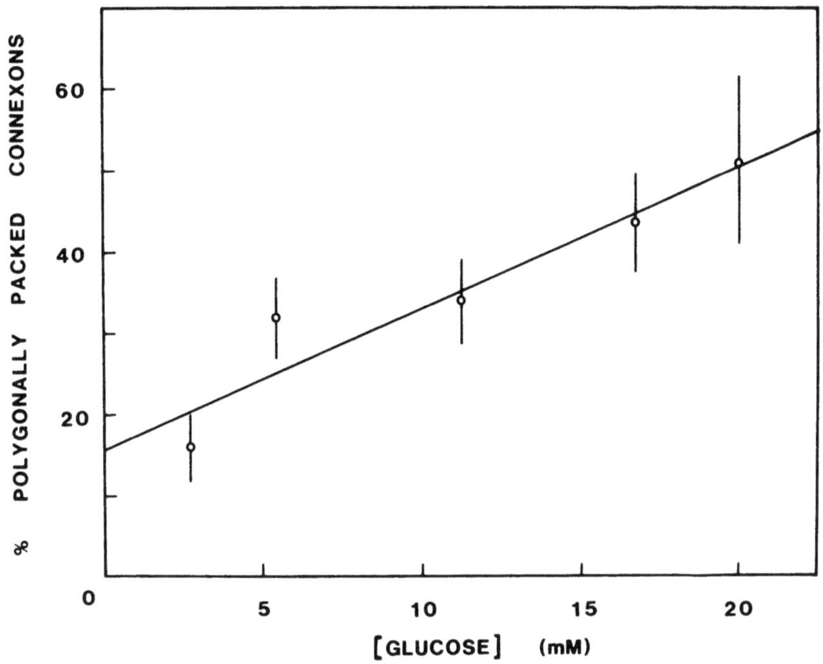

Fig. 5. Effect of glucose on gap junction morphology in the isolated perfused rat pancreas: a dose-dependent increase in the percent polygonally packed connexons was observed after 10 min of glucose stimulation. The total amount of connexons remained unchanged, indicating a glucose-induced connexon rearrangement. Reprinted from [31]

Role in Intercellular Communication

Injection of the fluorescent dye 6-carboxy-fluorescein (M_r 376) into endocrine cells from newborn rat pancreases grown in monolayer culture [37] showed that these cells were capable of exchanging dye molecules within 0.4 s, an exceptionally short time compared to other cell systems [91]. It was noted that the spreading of the dye was restricted to small regions, on average consisting of four cells. Comparable results were obtained in collagenase-isolated rat islets, where an average of five cells were dye-coupled in the center [50, 53] and only two in the periphery [53]. The lower number in the islet periphery is somewhat puzzling, as this region exhibited a higher density of gap junctions than the B-cell-enriched central area [47].

The extent of dye coupling can be modulated by a number of physiologic and pharmacologic agents, some of which were also found to alter the degree of electrical coupling or the quantity of gap junctions (Table 1). The common denominator behind these alterations is, however, not yet evident, which is not so surprising in view of the simultaneous involvement of such diverse events as connexon permeability, localization, synthesis and breakdown.

Several agents which stimulate insulin release were found to increase the amount of islet gap junctions. Using freeze fracture techniques, it was shown that rats treated for 2 days with the sulfonylurea glibenclamide exhibited significantly

Table 1. Modulation of islet cell coupling

	Gap junctional area	Dye coupling	Electrical coupling	Reference(s)
Short term (<90 min)				
Glucose	0		↑	10, 31, 46
Tetraethylammonium	↑			77
Somatostatin		↓		38
A23187		↑		38
Prolactin		↑		80
Long term				
Glucose		↑		51
Glibenclamide	↑	↑		46,50
Diazoxide	↑	↑		50
Theophylline	↑			30
IBMX		↑		38
Dibutyryl cAMP	↑			30

higher numbers of gap junctional subunits in their collagenase-isolated islets [46, 50]. This effect has been correlated with a decrease in islet insulin content [48]. According to a recent report, glibenclamide may interact with the adenosine triphosphate (ATP)-sensitive K^+ channels in B-cells [84]. It is also known that blocking the K^+ efflux with tetraethylammonium (TEA) increases gap junctional area [77]. It may therefore be interesting to examine the possible link between membrane potassium fluxes and the rate of gap junction formation or breakdown. The plasma membrane of islet B-cells is reported to contain at least two types of potassium channels: an ATP-sensitive channel [5] that may be similar to the glucose-sensitive K^+ channel [1], and a Ca^{2+}-sensitive channel [24]. A block of these channels leads to membrane depolarization, which in turn may alter membrane calcium fluxes. Whether such altered fluxes lead to changes in connexon synthesis and turnover rate is not known but might represent a pathway through which events leading to insulin secretion are linked to variations in gap junction characteristics.

Long-term in vivo exposure to glibenclamide not only increased B-cell gap junctional area but also increased the extent of dye coupling [46, 50]. Similar results were obtained with the thiazide derivative diazoxide [50]. As diazoxide is known to inhibit insulin release, a causative link between hormone secretion and islet gap junction quantity seems unlikely. The agent causes, however, an elevation in blood glucose level which may be responsible for the observed increase in islet gap junctions. Short-term in vitro exposure to high glucose levels resulted in more but smaller gap junctions in collagenase-isolated islets [46] and in a marked rearrangement of connexons in the perfused pancreas [31]. Moreover, glucose was found to increase electrical and dye coupling levels [10, 37]. In long-term exposure experiments in which blood sugar levels were artificially elevated through continuous infusion of glucose, dye coupling domains were significantly enlarged [51].

A third group of experiments that has provided insight into the underlying mechanisms of changes in cell coupling employed hormones, phosphodiesterase inhibitors, and cAMP analogs. Somatostatin, a well-known inhibitor of insulin secretion, significantly decreased dye coupling in monolayer cultures of newborn rat pancreas within 60 min [38]. The phosphodiesterase inhibitors IBMX and theophylline and the cAMP analog dibutyryl-cAMP prevented the decrease in cellular cAMP levels, in dye coupling and in gap junctional area which occurs during culture at low glucose concentrations [30, 38]. All treatments have in common the fact that they alter islet cAMP content, which, as in other cell systems, appears an important modulator of both cell coupling and gap junction quantity [14, 23].

Understanding the variations in islet cell coupling requires better insights into the intricate regulatory mechanisms of insulin release. All tested conditions can in some way be linked to events which are important for the establishment of an appropriate level of insulin secretion. The three pathways described above - modulation of potassium channel permeability, glucose metabolism, B-cell cAMP levels - are all involved in the initiation or modulation of hormone release. Investigation of such possible pathways is complicated by the fact that they interconnect. Glucose may affect potassium permeability [1], and changes in cellular cAMP content are often accompanied by changes in free calcium levels. Interesting parallels exist between the possible regulatory pathways described here and those suggested for insulin release [69]. Indeed, separate messenger systems may interact respectively with nutrients and hormones. cAMP may represent the hormone-induced messenger which plays a role in determining both gap junction quantity and connexon permeability, while glucose metabolism derived messengers may act primarily upon the latter characteristic. However, such model remains too speculative with the present data.

Insulin Release and Cell Junctions

The possible role of islet cell junctions in the process of hormone secretion appears from the observation that isolated single B-cells, respond much better to secretagogues when they are in direct contact with each other [4, 44, 68, 69]. Though an effect of adhesion itself cannot be excluded, gap junctions may be responsible for part of this phenomenon. In spite of their relatively small size - 10- to 100-fold smaller than the junctions between exocrine cells - the gap junctions create coupling domains for a variable number of B-cells. Such domains may well represent secretory units, consisting of electrically and metabolically coupled cells secreting insulin in a synchronized manner.

In this concept, pacemaker cells [52] could play an important role. Such cells, displaying a low stimulation threshold, would activate neighboring cells to hormone secretion through the gap junctional transfer of ions or small molecules like cAMP [41, 55].

Several observations point to a functional heterogeneity within the B-cell population. An increase in the percentage of mouse islet cells displaying electrical activity was reported when the concentration of glucose in the medium was gradually raised. The increase was greatest between 5.6 and 8.4 m*M* glucose and was interpreted as an indication for the existence of different populations of islet cells characterized by different glucose sensitivities [7]. A similar variation in B-cell stimulation thresholds was recently observed for glucose-stimulated insulin biosynthesis in cell-sorter-purified B-cells [75] and in the isolated perfused rat pancreas [32]. A functional heterogeneity was also reported for insulin release; when the insulin secretory activity of individual islet cells was assessed using a hemolytic plaque assay, it was shown that a rise in glucose concentration in the medium resulted in an increased number of active cells [73]. Taken together, these reports point to a heterogeneous B-cell mass in which individual B-cells require individual signal intensities to become active.

In the pacemaker-coupling domain model, the extent of B-cell coupling may determine what percentage of islet cells becomes active for a given signal [51, 52, 78]. The size of coupling domains has been shown to be variable and dependent both on the long-term metabolic history of the cells, changing the amount of gap junctions, and on short-term modulation of gap junction permeability.

Other possible functions of islet gap junctions, such as a role in islet growth have not been discussed. The observation that islets of Langerhans consist of a functionally heterogeneous B-cell population, may well represent the key to understanding the various implications of islet gap junctions.

Acknowledgements. We thank M. Berghmans and J. P. Pigeon for excellent technical assistance, H. Lox for secretarial work, and Drs. Pipeleers, Schuit, and Van Schravendijk for critical reading of the manuscript.

References

1. Ashcroft FM, Harrison DE, Ashcroft SJH (1984) Glucose induces closure of single potassium channels in isolated rat pancreatic B-cells. Nature 312: 446-448
2. Bonner-Weir S, Like AA (1980) A dual population of islets of Langerhans in bovine pancreas. Cell Tissue Res 206: 157-170
3. Bonner-Weir S, Orci L (1982) New perspectives on the microvasculature of the islets of Langerhans. Diabetes 31: 883-889
4. Chertow BS, Baranetsky NG, Sivitz WI, Meda P, Webb MD, Shih JC (1983) Cellular mechanisms of insulin release: effects of retinoids on rat islet cell-to-cell adhesion, reaggregation, and insulin release. Diabetes 32: 568-574
5. Cook DL, Hales CN (1984) Intracellular ATP directly blocks K^+ channels in pancreatic B-cells. Nature 311: 271-273
6. Dean PM, Matthews EK (1968) Electrical activity in pancreatic islet cells. Nature 219: 389-390
7. Dean PM, Matthews EK (1970) Glucose-induced electrical activity in pancreatic islet cells. J Physiol 210: 255-264
8. Dermietzel R, Leibstein A, Frixen U, Janssen-Timmen U, Traub O, Willecke K (1984) Gap junctions in several tissues share antigenic determinants with liver gap junctions. EMBO J 3: 2261-2270
9. Dragstein PR, Blumenthal R, Handler JS (1981) Membrane asymmetry in epithelia: is the tight junction a barrier to diffusion in the plasma membrane? Nature 294: 718-722
10. Eddlestone GT, Gonçalves A, Bangham JA, Rojas E (1984) Electrical coupling between cells in islets of Langerhans from mouse. J Membr Biol 77: 1-14

11. Edelman GM (1983) Cell adhesion molecules. Science 219: 450-457
12. Farquhar MG, Palade GE (1963) Junctional complexes in various epithelia. J Cell Biol 17: 375-412
13. Ferner H (1952) Das Inselsystem des Pankreas. Thieme, Stuttgart
14. Flagg-Newton JL, Dahl G, Loewenstein WR (1981) Cell junction and cyclic AMP: I. Upregulation of junctional membrane permeability and junctional membrane particles by administration of cyclic nucleotide or phosphodiesterase inhibitor. J Membr Biol 63: 105-121
15. Forssmann WG, Helmstaedter V, Metz J, Mühlmann G, Feurle GE (1978) Immunohistochemistry and ultrastructure of somatostatin cells with special reference to the gastroenteropancreatic (GEP) system. Metabolism 27 [Suppl 1]: 1179-1191
16. Fujita T (1973) Insulino-acinar portal system in the horse pancreas. Arch Histol Jpn 35: 161-171
17. Fujita T, Kobayashi S, Serizawa Y (1981) Intercellular canalicule system in pancreatic islet. Biomed Res 2 [Suppl 1]: 115-118
18. Goodenough DA (1976). In vitro formation of gap junction vesicles. J Cell Biol 68: 221-231
19. Gros DB, Nicholson BJ, Revel JP (1983) Comparative analysis of the gap junction protein from rat heart and liver: is there a tissue specificity of gap junctions? Cell 35: 539-549
20. Grube D, Bohn R (1983) The microanatomy of human islets of Langerhans with special reference to somatostatin (D-)cells. Arch Histol Jpn 46: 327-353
21. Grube D, Eckert I, Speck PT, Wagner HJ (1983) Immunohistochemistry and microanatomy of the islets of Langerhans. In: Fujita T, Kanno T, Yanaihara N (eds) Brain-gut axis. Biomed Res 4 [Suppl]: 25-36
22. Gumbiner B, Simons K (1986) A functional assay for proteins involved in establishing an epithelial occluding barrier: identification of a uvomorulin-like polypeptide. J Cell Biol 102: 457-468
23. Hax WMA, Van Venrooj GEPM, Vossenberg JBJ (1974) Cell communication: a cyclic-AMP mediated phenomenon. J Membr Biol 19: 253-266
24. Henquin JC (1979) Opposite effects of intracellular Ca^{2+} and glucose on K^+ permeability of pancreatic islet cells. Nature 280: 66-68
25. Hertzberg EL, Gilula NB (1979) Isolation and characterization of gap junctions from rat liver. J Biol Chem 254: 2138-2147
26. Hertzberg EL, Anderson DJ, Friedlander M, Gilula NB (1982) Comparative analysis of the major polypeptides from liver gap junctions and lens fiber junctions. J Cell Biol 92: 53-59
27. Hertzberg EL, Skibbens RV (1984) A protein homologous to the 27.000 Dalton liver gap junction protein is present in a wide variety of species and tissues. Cell 39: 61-69
28. Hertzberg EL, Spray DC, Bennett MVL (1985) Reduction of gap junctional conductance by microinjection of antibodies against the 27-kDa liver gap junction polypeptide. Proc. Natl Acad Sci (USA) 82: 2412-2416
29. In't Veld PA, Pipeleers DG, Gepts W (1984) Evidence against the presence of tight junctions in normal endocrine pancreas. Diabetes 33: 101-104
30. In't Veld PA, Schuit F, Pipeleers DG (1985) Gap junctions between pancreatic B-cells are modulated by cyclic AMP. Eur J Cell Biol 36: 269-276
31. In't Veld PA, Pipeleers DG, Gepts W (1986) Glucose alters configuration of gap junctions between pancreatic islet cells. Am J Physiol 251: C191-C196
32. In't Veld PA, Schuit F, Gepts W, Pipeleers DG (1987) Glucose recruits pancreatic B-cells to biosynthetic activity. Diabetologia 30: 535 A
33. Kachar B, Reese TS (1982). Evidence for the lipidic nature of tight junction strands. Nature 296: 464-466
34. Kataoka K, Yamamoto M, Yamamoto T, Ochi J (1982) Intercellular canalicular system and intercellular junctions in the pancreatic islet of the Mongolian gerbil. Biomed Res 3: 235-238
35. Kawai K, Ipp E, Orci L, Perrelet A, Unger RH (1982) Circulating somatostatin acts on the islets of Langerhans by way of a somatostatin-poor compartment. Science 218: 477-478
36. Kawai K, Chiba Y, Okuda Y, Yamashita K (1985) Hormone release from pancreatic islet cells perfused from the venous side. Diab Res Clin Pract [Suppl] 1: S293
37. Kohen E, Kohen C, Thorell B, Mintz DH, Rabinovitch A (1979) Intercellular communication in pancreatic islet monolayer cultures: a microfluorometric study. Science 204: 862-865

38. Kohen E, Kohen C, Rabinovitch A (1983) Cell-to-cell communication in rat pancreatic islet monolayer cultures is modulated by agents affecting islet-cell secretary activity. Diabetes 32: 95-98
39. Kumar NM, Gilula NB (1986) Cloning and characterization of human and rat liver cDNA's coding for a gap junction protein. J Cell Biol 103: 767-776
40. Larsen WJ (1983) Biological implications of gap junction structure, distribution and composition: review. Tissue Cell 15: 645-671
41. Lawrence TS, Beers WH, Gilula NB (1978) Transmission of hormonal stimulation by cell-to-cell communication. Nature 272: 501-506
42. Like AA (1970) The uptake of exogenous peroxidase by the Beta cells of the islets of Langerhans. Am J Pathol 59: 225-246
43. Loewenstein WR (1981) Junctional intercellular communication: the cell-to-cell membrane channel. Phys Rev 61: 829-913
44. Maes E, Pipeleers DG (1984). Effects of glucose and 3′, 5′-cyclic adenosine monophosphate upon reaggregation of single pancreatic B-cells. Endocrinology 114: 2205-2209
45. Makowski L (1985) Structural domains in gap junctions: implications for the control of intercellular communication. In: Bennet MVL, Spray DC (eds) Cold Spring Harbor Laboratory, Cold Spring Harbor, pp 5-12
46. Meda P, Perrelet A, Orci L (1979) Increase of gap junctions between pancreatic B-cells during stimulation of insulin secretion. J Cell Biol 82: 441-448
47. Meda P, Denef JF, Perrelet A, Orci L (1980) Nonrandom distribution of gap junctions between pancreatic B-cells. Am J Physiol 238: C114-C119
48. Meda P, Halban P, Perrelet A, Renold AE, Orci L (1980) Gap junction development is correlated with insulin content in the pancreatic B-cell. Science 209: 1026-1028
49. Meda P, Kohen E, Kohen C, Rabinovitch A, Orci L (1982) Direct communication of homologous and heterologous endocrine islet cells in culture. J Cell Biol 92: 221-226
50. Meda P, Michaels RL, Halban PA, Orci L, Sheridan JD (1983) In vivo modulation of gap junctions and dye coupling between B-cells of the intact pancreatic islet. Diabetes 32: 858-868
51. Meda P, Perrelet A, Orci L (1984) Gap junctions and cell-to-cell coupling in endocrine glands. In: Modern Cell Biology 3. Liss, New York, pp 131-196
52. Meissner HP (1976) Electrophysiological evidence for coupling between B-cells of pancreatic islets. Nature 262: 502-504
53. Michaels RL, Sheridan JD (1981) Islets of Langerhans: dye coupling among immunocytochemically distinct cell types. Science 214: 801-802
54. Montague W, Parkin EN (1980) Changes in membrane lipids of the B-cell during insulin secretion. Horm Metab Res [Suppl] 10: 153-157
55. Murray SA, Fletcher WH (1984) Hormone-induced intercellular signal transfer dissociates cyclic AMP-dependent protein kinase. J Cell Biol 98: 1710-1719
56. Neyton J, Trautman A (1985) Single-channel currents of an intercellular junction. Nature 317: 331-335
57. Nicholson BJ, Takemoto LJ, Hunkapiller MW, Hood LE, Revel JP (1983) Differences between liver gap junction protein and lens MIP26 from rat: implications for tissue specificity of gap junctions. Cell 32: 967-978
58. Orci L (1976) The microanatomy of the islets of Langerhans. Metabolism 25 [Suppl 1]: 1303-1313
59. Orci L, Unger RH (1975) Functional subdivision of islets of Langerhans and possible role of D-cells. Lancet 2: 1243-1244
60. Orci L, Perrelet A, Ravazzola M, Malaisse-Lagae F, Renold AE (1973) A specialized membrane junction between nerve endings and B-cells in islets of Langerhans. Eur J Clin Invest 3: 443-445
61. Orci L, Unger RH, Renold AE (1973) Structural coupling between pancreatic islet cells. Experientia 29: 1015-1018
62. Orci L, Amherdt M, Henquin JC, Lambert AE, Unger RH, Renold AE (1973) Pronase effect on pancreatic Beta cell secretion and morphology. Science 180: 647-649
63. Orci L, Malaisse-Lagae F, Amherdt M, Ravazzola M, Weisswange A, Dobbs R, Perrelet A, Unger R (1974) Cell contacts in human islets of Langerhans. J Clin Endocrinol Metab 41: 841-844

64. Orci L, Malaisse-Lagae F, Ravazzola F, Rouiller D, Renold AE, Perrelet A, Unger R (1975) A morphological basis for intercellular communication between Alpha- and Beta-cells in the endocrine pancreas. J Clin Invest 56: 1066-1070
65. Paul DL (1985) Antibody against liver gap junction 27-kD protein is tissue specific and cross-reacts with a 54-kD protein. In: Bennett MVL, Spray DC (eds) Gap junctions. Cold Spring Harbor Laboratory (old Spring Harbor), pp 107-122
66. Paul DL (1986) Molecular cloning of cDNA for rat liver gap junction protein. J Cell Biol 103: 123-134
67. Peracchia C (1977) Gap junctions: structural changes after uncoupling procedures. J Cell Biol 72: 628-641
68. Pipeleers DG, In't Veld PA, Maes E, Van de Winkel (1982) Glucose-induced insulin release depends on functional cooperation between islet cells. Proc Natl Acad Sci USA 79: 7322-7325
69. Pipeleers DG, Schuit FC, In't Veld PA, Maes E, Hooghe-Peters EL, Van De Winkel M, Gepts W (1985) Interplay of nutrients and hormones in the regulation of insulin release. Endocrinology 117: 824-833
70. Revel JP, Karrovsky MJ (1967) Hexagonal array of subunits in intercellular junctions of mouse heart and liver. J Cell Biol 33: C7-C12
71. Rose B, Loewenstein WR (1975) Permeability of cell junction depends on local cytoplasmic calcium activity. Nature 254: 250-252
72. Saez JC, Spray DC, Nairn AC, Hertzberg E, Greengard P, Bennett MVL (1986) cAMP increases junctional conductance and stimulates phosphorylation of the 27-kDa principal gap junction polypeptide. Proc Natl Acad Sci USA 83: 2473-2477
73. Salomon D, Meda P (1986) Heterogeneity and contact-dependent regulation of hormone secretion by individual B-cells. Exp Cell Res 162: 507-520
74. Schuit F, Pipeleers D (1986) Pancreatic A and B cells differ in their recognition of somatostatin. Diabetologia 29: 592A
75. Schuit F, In't Veld PA, Pipeleers DG (1988) Glucose recruits pancreatic B-cells to proinsulin biosynthesis Proc Natl Acad Sci USA (in press)
76. Schwarzmann G, Wiegandt H, Rose B, Zimmerman A, Ben-Haim D, Loewenstein WR (1981) Diameter of the cell-to-cell junctional membrane channels as probed with neutral molecules. Science 213: 551-553
77. Sheppard MS, Meda P (1981) Tetraethylammonium modifies gap junctions between pancreatic B-cells. Am J Physiol 240: C116-C120
78. Sheridan JD, Atkinson MM (1985) Physiological roles of permeable junctions: some possibilities. Ann Rev Physiol 47: 337-353
79. Simpson I, Rose B, Loewenstein WR (1977) Size limit of molecules permeating the junctional membrane channels. Science 195: 294-296
80. Sorenson RL, Michaels RL, Parsons JA, Sheridan JD (1983) Association of the glucose threshold of insulin release with gap junctional coupling of B-cells. Diabetes 32: 9A
81. Spray DC, Harris AL, Bennett MVL (1981) Gap junctional conductance is a simple and sensitive function of intracellular pH. Science 211: 712-715
82. Spray DC, Stern JH, Harris AL, Bennett MVL (1982) Gap junctional conductance: comparison of sensitivities to H and Ca ions. Proc Natl Acad Sci USA 79: 441-445
83. Staehelin LA (1973) Further observations on the structure of freeze cleaved tight junctions. J Cell Sci 13: 763-786
84. Sturges NC, Cook DL, Ashford MLJ, Hales CN (1985) The sulphonylurea receptor may be an ATP-sensitive potassium channel. Lancet 474-475
85. Turin L, Warner AE (1977) Carbon dioxide reversibly abolishes ionic communication between cells of early amphibian embryo. Nature 270: 56-57
86. Unwin PNT, Zampighi G (1980) Structure of the junction between communicating cells. Nature 283: 545-549
87. Unwin PNT, Ennis PD (1984) Two configurations of a channel-forming membrane protein. Nature 307: 609-613
88. Van Schravendijk CFH, Foriers A, Hooghe-Peters EL, Rogiers V, De Meyts P, Sodoyez JC, Pipeleers DG (1985) Pancreatic hormone receptors on islet cells. Endocrinology 117: 841-848

89. Veenstra RD, DeHaan RL (1986) Measurement of single channel currents from cardiac gap junctions. Science 233: 972-974
90. Verkleij AJ, Mombers C, Leunissen-Bijvelt J, Vervegaert PHJTh (1979) Lipidic intramembranous particles. Nature 279: 162-163
91. Wade MH, Trosko JE, Schindler M (1986) A fluorescence photobleaching assay of gap junction-mediated communication between human cells. Science 232: 525-528
92. Warner AE, Guthrie SC, Gilula NB (1984) Antibodies to gap-junctional protein selectively disrupt junctional communication in the early amphibian embryo. Nature 311: 127-131
93. Yamamoto M, Kataoka K (1984) A comparative study on the intercellular canalicular system and intercellular junctions in the pancreatic islets of some rodents. Arch Histol Jpn 47: 485-493

Calcium Transport and Deficient Insulin Release*

B. Hellman

Introduction

In his doctoral thesis PAUL LANGERHANS [55] demonstrated for the first time that the pancreas contains elements other than the exocrine acini. During the subsequent years there was only slow progress in the understanding of the pancreatic islets. The first international symposium on the pancreatic islets was held in Uppsala 1963, and 6 years later the centenary of PAUL LANGERHANS' discovery was celebrated in Umeå. On the latter occasion it was stated in the opening address [17] that more secrets had been revealed about the pancreatic islets since the first symposium than during the whole of the rest of the century since the discovery of the islets.

As is clear in the proceedings of the two islet symposia WILLY GEPTS should be regarded as one of the pioneers in the field of islet research. Since his fundamental studies of the human islets [25], I have had the privilege of sharing with him a common interest in both the morphology and enzymatic pattern of the islet cells. In recent decades WILLY GEPTS' major interest has been the immunological mechanisms evoking destruction of the pancreatic B-cells. In dedicating this chapter to WILLY I hope to convince him that disturbances in the B-cell handling of Ca^{2+} may be a decisive factor in the sequence of events precipitating diabetes.

Cytoplasmic Ca^{2+} as a Denominator of Insulin Release

Two decades ago it was observed that omission of extracellular Ca^{2+} results in a prompt inhibition of insulin release in response to glucose and other insulin secretagogues [26 63]. Such a requirement for extracellular Ca^{2+} may simply reflect that a certain concentration of the cation is essential for the proper functioning of the secretory machinery. However, in support of the concept of a direct regulatory role of Ca^{2+}, increase of its extracellular concentration was in itself sufficient for stimulating insulin release in the absence of glucose and other initiators of the secretory process [15, 32]. Indeed, the observed dependence on extracellular Ca^{2+} made

* The work reported from the author's laboratory was supported by the Swedish Medical Research Council (12X-562), the Swedish Diabetes Association, and the Nordic Insulin Foundation. The establishment of the patch clamp technique was made possible by donations from the Wallenberg Foundation and the Swedish Council for Planning and Coordination of Research.

it possible to postulate the existence of a regulatory pool of intracellular Ca^{2+} rapidly equilibrating with the exterior of the B-cells [40].

Studies of various types of cells have indicated that the secretory activity is closely related to their cytoplasmic concentration of free Ca^{2+}. The idea of cytoplasmic Ca^{2+} as the major denominator also for insulin secretion received ample support with the introduction of fluorescent indicators enabling direct measurements of this Ca^{2+} in the B-cells. Whereas the original studies were performed with clonal insulin-releasing cells of tumor origin [72, 83], later analyses have established a relationship between cytoplasmic Ca^{2+} and insulin release also in normal pancreatic B-cells [73]. The information obtained about the cytoplasmic Ca^{2+} activity is far from complete in that the existence of local variations is neglected; the high Ca^{2+} concentration of the secretory granules is also included. However, with the further development of methodology in combination with digital imaging microscopy of single B-cells it should be possible to pay particular attention to the part of the cytoplasm below the plasma membrane, as containing the Ca^{2+} supposed to initiate the exocytosis of the insulin secretory granules after binding to calmodulin.

Like other secretory processes, the release of insulin depends not only on the cytoplasmic Ca^{2+} activity but also on the sensitivity of the secretory machinery to this ion (Fig. 1). It is possible to determine this sensitivity by measuring insulin release at defined (submicromolar) concentrations of Ca^{2+} in B-cells made permeable to small molecules by electrical discharges or digitonin treatment. Such studies have indicated stimulation of insulin release after forskolin activation of adenylate cyclase [79]. Although it remains to be demonstrated that cyclic AMP has a similar effect, increase of the intracellular content of this nucleotide has been found to increase the insulin secretory response of intact cells without a concomitant rise of cytoplasmic Ca^{2+} [68, 85]. Other studies have demonstrated stimulated insulin release from permeabilized B-cells when activating protein kinase C with 12-*O*-tetradecanoylphorbol-13 acetate [52]. It is therefore tempting to postulate

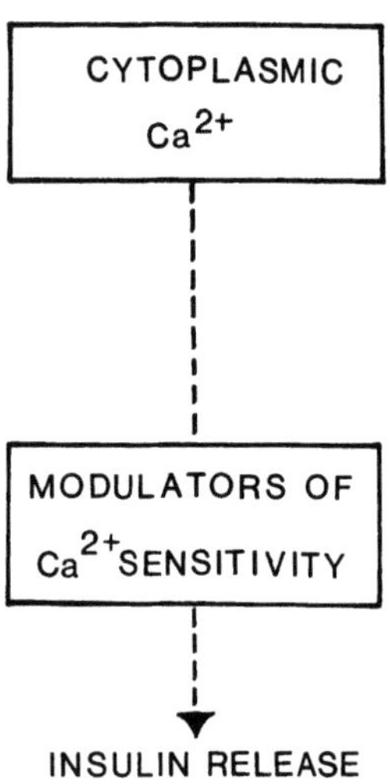

Fig. 1. Schematic presentation of insulin release as a Ca^{2-}-regulated process with different sensitivities to the Ca^{2+} stimulus

that phosphorylation processes other than those mediated by calmodulin can modify the sensitivity of the secretory machinery to the Ca^{2+} signal. When the temperature is reduced, the secretory machinery becomes less sensitive to the Ca^{2+} signal. Lowering of the temperature from 37 °C to 27 °C has been found to abolish glucose-stimulated insulin release without much affecting the electrical activity induced by the sugar [4].

Currents Responsible for the Opening of the Voltage-Dependent Ca^{2+} Channels

Studies with intracellular microelectrodes have indicated that insulin release in response to glucose and many other insulin secretagogues is associated with the appearance of electrical activity with action potentials superimposed on a depolarized plateau phase. The action potentials have been regarded as reflecting entry of Ca^{2+} into the B-cells through voltage-dependent channels, an idea supported by the effects of established blockers of such channels on the handling of Ca^{2+} and insulin release. Although both recordings of the membrane potential and measurements of tracer fluxes indicated that the depolarization involved a decrease in the membrane permeability to K^+, the detailed analyses of this process have been considerably aided with the introduction of the patch clamp technique. The latter approach has not only enabled the identification of the ionic currents responsible for the opening of the voltage-dependent Ca^{2+} channels but also made the B-cells accessible to voltage clamp experiments.

Table 1 summarizes the present knowledge of the different conductances in the plasma membrane based on the patch clamp observations made in various laboratories, including our own. In addition to describing the situation in normal and tumor-transformed B-cells, a comparison is made with the glucagon-producing A_2-cells. From observations made with conventional intracellular microelectrodes, Na^+ currents may be regarded as of minor importance for the membrane potential of the B-cells. Whereas the patch clamp technique has failed so far to demonstrate unequivocally the presence of inward Na^+ currents in normal B-cells, the glucagon-producing A_2-cells were characterized by large such currents (Table 1). The fact that also clonal lines of tumor-transformed B-cells possess distinct voltage-activated Na^+ currents is not surprising, when taking into account the fact that such cells are exceptional in releasing not only insulin but also glucagon and somatostatin [7].

As inferred from the studies with intracellular microelectrodes, the K^+ permeability is the major determinant for the resting potential of the B-cells. The patch clamp studies revealed at least three types of K^+ currents with the properties indicated in Table 1. In the B-cell the dominating K^+ channel is controlled by intracellular ATP and is insensitive to changes in the membrane potential. It is likely that this K^+ conductane has a major role in the depolarization of the B-cells, as indicated from its inhibition when the cells are stimulated by glucose or hypoglycemic sulfonylurea compounds. Although a Ca^{2+}-activated K^+ channel can be

Table 1. Ionic channels identified by the patch clamp technique in the pancreatic B-cells compared with those in insulin-producing tumor cells and glucagon-producing A_2-cells

Type of channel	B-cells	Insulin-producing tumor cells	A_2-cells
Na^+			
Species		RINm5F[13]	Rat[9], guinea pig[10]
Activation (mV)		−50	−50
Peak current (pA)		300	550
ATP-dependent K^+			
Species	Rat[1,2,6], mouse[11,12,16,17]	RINm5F[7], CRI-GI[15]	
Voltage dependence	No		
Conductance (pS)	50–70	60	
Ca^{2+}-dependent K^+			
Species	Rat[3,5,6], mouse[12]	RINm5F[7]	Rat[9]
Voltage dependence	Yes		
Conductance (pS)	250		
Delayed rectifying K^+			
Species	Mouse[12]		Guinea pig[10]
Voltage dependence	Yes		
Conductance (pS)	10		
Ordinary Ca^{2+}			
Species	Rat[14], mouse[8,12], guinea pig[10]	RINm5F[4,13]	Rat[9], guinea pig[10]
Activation (mV)	−40 to −50	−40	−40 to −50
Peak current (pA)	50–60	120	150–200
Low threshold Ca^{2+}			
Species			Guinea pig[10]
Activation (mV)			−60
Peak current (pA)			50–75

Whereas the maximal unit conductance is given for the K^+ currents, the Na^+ and Ca^{2+} channels are characterized by the peak currents for the whole cell

[1] Ashcroft et al. [3]
[2] Cook and Hales [13]
[3] Cook et al. [14]
[4] Findlay and Dunne [18]
[5] Findlay et al. [19]
[6] Findlay et al. [20]
[7] Findlay et al. [21]
[8] Hellman et al. [44]
[9] Marty and Neher [59]
[10] Rorsman and Hellman [69]
[11] Rorsman and Trube [70]
[12] Rorsman and Trube [71]
[13] Rorsman et al. [74]
[14] Satin and Cook [76]
[15] Sturgess et al. [78]
[16] Trube et al. [80]
[17] Trube et al. [81]

supposed to be involved in the feedback control of the Ca^{2+} uptake in the B-cells, assessment of its importance is difficult in view of controversial reports about its Ca^{2+}-dependence. It may well be that the Ca^{2+} sensitivity of these channels is modulated by cytoplasmic factors missing in the intracellular medium used for the patch clamp experiments. In addition to the two above-mentioned K^+ channels, others carrying minor currents have been described. Whereas some of these may represent subconductances of the established channels, available data suggest that the B-cells are equipped also with a delayed rectifying K^+ current. In analogy to what has been proposed for other cells, it is possible that these channels contribute to the repolarizing phase of the action potentials.

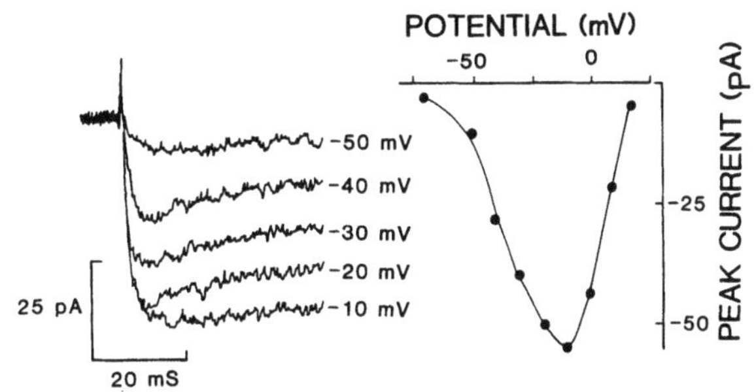

Fig. 2. Patch clamp analyses of the inward Ca^{2+} current during depolarizing voltage pulses from a holding potential of −70 mV. The studies were performed in the whole cell configuration mode with an extracellular Ca^{2+} concentration of 2.6 m*M* and intracellular K^+ replaced by *N*-methyl-glucamine. In addition to individual traces the corresponding current-voltage relationship is shown [44]

Movements of Ca^{2+} Across the B-Cell Membrane

Using the whole cell recording mode of the patch clamp technique under conditions of suppressed outward currents, it has been possible to analyze directly the voltage-dependent channels responsible for the entry of Ca^{2+} (Table 1). The specificity of the approach was demonstrated from the influence of the concentration of Ca^{2+} on the amplitude of the peak current and the inhibition obtained with established Ca^{2+} channel blockers. Both the B-cells and the glucagon-producing A_2-cells are equipped with voltage-dependent Ca^{2+} channels. Figure 2 shows the currents observed in a B-cell in the presence of 2.6 m*M* Ca^{2+} during depolarizing voltage pulses and the resulting current-voltage relationship. Being activated at voltages more positive than −50 mV and reaching a peak at about −10 mV, it is likely that the observed Ca^{2+} conductance is responsible for the inward current during the depolarizing phase of the action potential. In support of this idea the size of the inward current was consistent with the upstroke velocity of the action potentials recorded with intracellular electrodes. Although there was some inactivation of the Ca^{2+} channels with time, this effect was less pronounced than expected from previous studies of the release of insulin and the uptake of ^{45}Ca. It should be evaluated, in further whole cell experiments using a pipette medium with lower capacity of buffering Ca^{2+}, whether the inactivation of the Ca^{2+} channels can be accounted for by a rise in the intracellular concentration of this ion. By analogy to what has been described in various preparations, including clonal pituitary cells [61], two types of Ca^{2+} currents could be demonstrated in the glucagon-producing A_2-cells. In addition to the classical Ca^{2+} current, a smaller one appeared when the holding potential was lowered from −70 mV to −100 mV. It remains to be established whether application of depolarizing voltage steps from a lower holding potential may reveal another Ca^{2+} channel in the B-cells.

Knowing the inward current during the voltage step where the action potentials normally peak (about −20 mV), the amount of Ca^{2+} entering the B-cell during a single action potential was calculated as 10^{-18} mol. This figure compares favorably with estimates of the Ca^{2+} uptake based on measurements of the unidirectional

(15 s) influx of ^{45}Ca into B-cells subsequently centrifuged through oil into a solution of La^{3+}. When inducing continuous spike activity (5–10 action potentials/s^{-1}) with 20 mM glucose, the radioisotope approach indicated an increase in the influx rate of 0.9 $mmol \cdot kg^{-1} \cdot min^{-1}$ [82].

The extrusion of Ca^{2+} from the pancreatic B-cells is mediated both by Na^+-Ca^{2+} exchange diffusion [41, 48] and a calmodulin-activated transport system based on a high-affinity ATPase [64]. So far it has not been possible to measure the unidirectional efflux of Ca^{2+} under conditions of stimulated entry of the ion. Nevertheless it can be estimated how different agents affect the outward transport of Ca^{2+}, when influx data are compared with recordings of the total B-cell content of calcium. It was concluded from this approach that the opening of the voltage-dependent Ca^{2+} channels is accompanied by a stimulated efflux of the ion. Contrary to previous arguments for a direct inhibitory action of glucose on the outward transport [49, 84], the effect of the sugar is thus to stimulate the efflux of Ca^{2+} from the B-cells.

Regulation of Cytoplasmic Ca^{2+} by Cellular Organelles

Alteration of plasma membrane transport is by no means the only way of modulating the cytoplasmic Ca^{2+} concentration. Cytoplasmic Ca^{2+} is subject to complexation with anions and macromolecules, but more important it is also controlled by active uptake into, and passive leakage from, mitochondria, endoplasmic reticulum, and probably also the secretory granules. Since Ca^{2+} diffusion is restricted in the cytoplasm, the importance of the above-mentioned organelles should be assessed with regard to their contribution to the functionally important Ca^{2+} occurring in the immediate submembrane space. The Ca^{2+} concentration attained in this region following a single action potential has been estimated to be no less than 100 times the overall cytoplasmic concentration of this cation [60].

The secretory granules differ from other organelles in that they are involved in exocytosis. The granules may not only have local regulatory effects on the functionally important cytoplasmic Ca^{2+} in the cell periphery; it is also possible that a certain concentration of Ca^{2+} in the granule sac is a prerequisite for exocytosis. Various types of evidence indicate that the insulin secretory granules are rich in calcium. The granule content of calcium in the B-cell-rich pancreatic islets of *ob/ob* mice has been estimated at 50 $mmol \cdot kg^{-1}$ dry weight using graphite furnace atomic absorption spectroscopy [1]. Moreover, secretory granules obtained from a transplantable rat insulinoma were found to contain 229 mmol calcium/kg protein, implying that the secretory granules account for as much as 26% of the total cell calcium [51]. After simulating the ionic composition in the granules HUTTON et al. [51] estimated the free concentration of Ca^{2+} to be 10 mM in the granule sac. The concentration difference of Ca^{2+} across the granule sac may consequently be as high as 10^5.

The fact that the secretory granules contain large amounts of calcium does not necessarily mean, that these organelles participate in the regulation of the cytoplasmic Ca^{2+}. Even if the existence of the considerable concentration difference across the granule membrane reflects the existence of energy-linked Ca^{2+} transport, it has not been unequivocally demonstrated that such a mechanism operates after completion of granule formation. When studying the subcellular distribution of Ca^{2+}-stimulated ATPase in mouse pancreatic islets, FORMBY et al. [22] found the highest specific enzyme activity in the fraction rich in secretory granules. The data were compatible with the existence of two different forms of Ca^{2+}-ATPase with Km values for Ca^{2+} of 6.9×10^{-6} *M* and 1.9×10^{-7} *M*. As suggested by HELLMAN et al. [40] there is also the possibility of Ca^{2+} transport into the B-granules in exchange for protons. Using large amounts of insulin-secretory granules from a rat insulinoma, HUTTON and PESHAVARIA [50] were able to demonstrate the presence of a proton-translocating Mg^{2+}-dependent ATPase with properties similar to those found in chromaffin granules. Also, the presence of an Na^{+}-gradient across the granule membrane might be considered as an indirect way of providing the energy for the Ca^{2+} uptake, in analogy to what has been proposed for chromaffin granules [54].

The potential significance of the mitochondria for the regulation of cytoplasmic Ca^{2+} is apparent from the area of the Ca^{2+}-transporting inner membrane, which is almost 10 times that of the plasma membrane [8]. Experiments with in situ labeling of the organelles in the B-cell-rich pancreatic islets from *ob/ob* mice indicated that the mitochondria accounted for a considerable part of the ^{45}Ca taken up in response to glucose [1, 53]. In intact cells the mitochondrial net uptake of ^{45}Ca was activated by 4 m*M* glucose, a concentration insufficient to open the voltage-dependent Ca^{2+} channels in the plasma membrane. Moreover, the effect of glucose in retaining ^{45}Ca in the mitochondria could not be mimicked by introducing depolarizing concentrations of K^{+} in a medium deficient in Ca^{2+}. Sodium suppresses the net accumulation of Ca^{2+} in mitochondria isolated from normal islets [58] and a rat insulinoma [65, 66]. It is therefore important that indirect evidence has been provided that a major effect of glucose is to lower the B-cell content of Na^{+} [6] and that a rise of the intracellular concentration of this ion results in mobilization of calcium incorporated in response to glucose [37, 42].

In the attempts to elucidate how the mitochondria participate in the Ca^{2+} homeostasis of the B-cells it is essential to determine the set point for their buffering of cytoplasmic Ca^{2+}. So far such studies have been performed using well-coupled mitochondria isolated from a rat insulinoma [66]. These mitochondria maintained extramitochondrial Ca^{2+} at 0.9 μM, a concentration 5–10 times higher than the average cytoplasmic Ca^{2+} activity in the B-cells. Results obtained from isolated mitochondria are not necessarily representative for the situation in the intact cell. Moreover, the cytoplasmic Ca^{2+} activity can be expected to be considerably higher in the vicinity of the plasma membrane than in the remaining parts of the B-cell [60]. Even with these reservations in mind it seems likely that the mitochondria are active in buffering Ca^{2+} essentially under conditions of increased secretory activity of the B-cells.

The endoplasmic reticulum accounts for almost 20% of the volume of the pancreatic B-cell, providing a transport area for Ca^{2+} equivalent to about 9 times that of the plasma membrane. Using a fairly pure fraction of the endoplasmic reticulum from rat islets, COLCA et al. [11, 12] demonstrated accumulation of Ca^{2+}

against a concentration gradient. The characteristics of this uptake were similar to those described in other cell types with regard to the requirement for ATP, dependence on Mg^{2+}, and specific stimulation by K^+. The uptake process differed from that in mitochondria in not being inhibited by azide or ruthenium red and from that of plasma membrane vesicles in not being stimulated by calmodulin. In the experiments of COLCA et al. [11], estimates of the Ca^{2+} affinity in the uptake process indicated an apparent Km as high as 1.5 ± 0.3 μ*M*. The fact that this value considerably exceeds that supposed to exist in the B-cell cytoplasm might reflect the difficulties of mimicking the intracellular ionic milieu rather than being an argument against a role for the endoplasmic reticulum in the regulation of the B-cell calcium. Using rat insulinoma microsomes, PRENTKI and WOLLHEIM [65] observed lowering of the ambient $Ca^{2+}$to a value corresponding to that of the cytoplasm. However, so far no attempts seem have been made to determine the steady-state ambient Ca^{2+} concentration maintained by a preparation of endoplasmic reticulum devoid of contaminating plasma membrane fragments.

A major reason for postulating that the endoplasmic reticulum is important for controlling the cytoplasmic Ca^{2+} activity comes from its sensitivity to inositol 1,4,5-trisphosphate (IP_3). Comparing the effects of this metabolite on different subcellular fractions of rat insulinoma, PRENTKI and WOLLHEIM [65] observed selective mobilization of calcium from the microsomes. Addition of IP_3 was also found to increase rapidly the medium concentration of Ca^{2+}, when permeabilized B-cells had lowered the steady state concentration of ambient Ca^{2+} to 125 n*M* [44]. With the observation that some receptors in the plasma membrane mediate polyphosphoinositide breakdown also in a Ca^{2+}-deficient medium, the exploration of the IP_3 effect was considerably aided [29, 34, 35, 38, 45, 46]. Figure 3 illustrates schematically how interaction with plasma membrane muscarinic and P_2-purinergic receptors via activation of phospholipase C results in hydrolysis of phosphatidylinositol 4,5-bisphosphate with the formation of diacylglycerol and IP_3. Whereas diacylglycerol sensitizes the secretory machinery to the Ca^{2+} signal by stimulating protein kinase C, the water-soluble IP_3 serves an an intracellular messenger mobilizing calcium from the endoplasmic reticulum. The metabolism of glucose is essential for the effect of IP_3 in promoting accumulation of the calcium mobilized by this compound. Using IP_3 as a probe for the calcium present in the endoplasmic reticulum, it was evident that glucose stimulated the high affinity uptake of Ca^{2+} by this organelle in a way lowering the cytoplasmic concentration of the ion even below its resting level [46].

The Opposing Effects of Glucose on Cytoplasmic Ca^{2+} and Insulin Release

The exploration of how glucose affects the cytoplasmic Ca^{2+} activity in the panreatic B-cells was facilitated with the introduction of the fluorescence indicators quin-2 and fura-2. It is possible to introduce these compounds into the pancreatic B-cells using the membrane-permeable tetraacetoxymethyl esters, which are rapid-

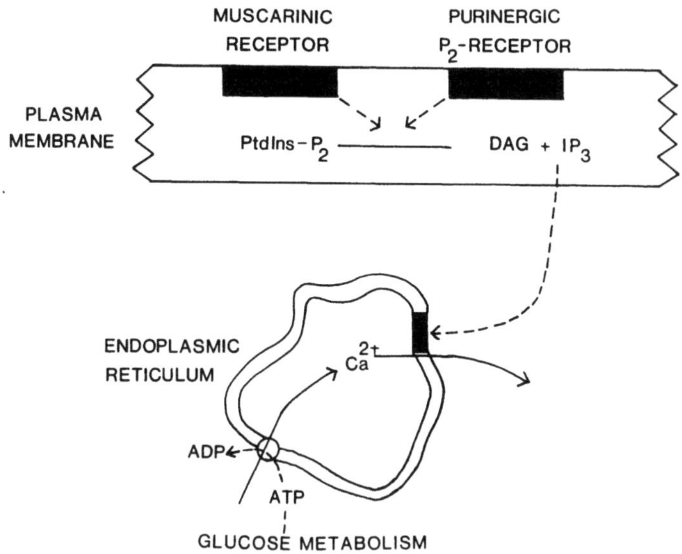

Fig. 3. Diagram illustrating hydrolysis of phosphatidylinositol 4,5-bisphosphate *(PtdIns-P_2)* accounted for by phospholipase C activation mediated by muscarinic and purinergic P_2 receptors. Whereas the resulting diacylglycerol *(DAG)* sensitizes the secretory machinery to the Ca^{2+} signal by activating protein kinase C, the 1, 4, 5 isomer of inositol trisphosphate (IP_3) is supposed to mobilize Ca^{2+} from the endoplasmic reticulum

ly hydrolyzed by intracellular esterases. The studies of RORSMAN et al. [73] represent the first demonstration using such a technique that glucose stimulation of insulin release is associated with a rise of cytoplasmic Ca^{2+}. However, it was also possible to demonstrate that the sugar decreased cytoplasmic Ca^{2+} in insulin-releasing cells, provided that the entry of Ca^{2+} was suppressed either by lowering its extracellular concentration or blocking the potential-dependent Ca^{2+} channels [73].

The observations described so far make it possible to summarize the principal actions of glucose on the cytoplasmic Ca^{2+} regulating insulin release as shown in Fig. 4. It is obvious that the available data call for a reconsideration of previous views of Ca^{2+} mobilization from intracellular stores as contributing to glucose-stimulated insulin release [65, 84] and that the sugar increases cytoplasmic Ca^{2+} in the B-cells by inhibiting the outward transport of the ion [49, 84]. Since glucose apparently has the opposite actions, the effect of the sugar on the cytoplasmic Ca^{2+} activity will instead reflect the balance between increased entry of Ca^{2+} and its enhanced removal from the cytoplasm by intracellular trapping and outward transport [34-37]. The glucose promotion of the three important Ca^{2+} movements differs with regard to both the sensitivity to the glucose stimulus and the latency of the effect (Table 2). As suggested from the studies of the ^{45}Ca efflux and confirmed from measurements of other variables including the cytoplasmic Ca^{2+} activity, the intracellular sequestration of Ca^{2+} can be expected to be manifested earlier and at lower concentrations of glucose than those facilitating the influx of Ca^{2+} with subsequently increased outward transport.

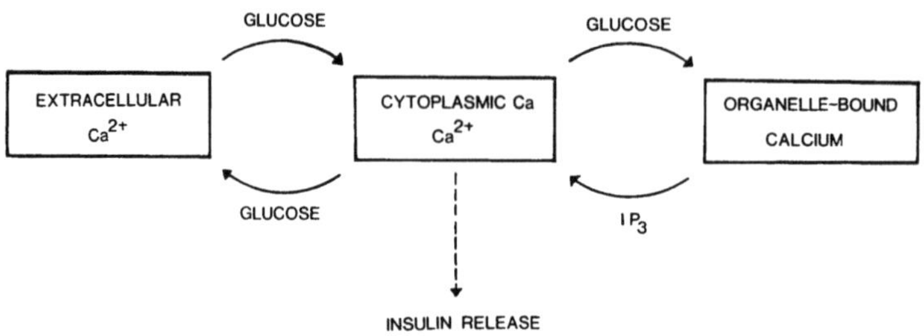

Fig. 4. Diagram illustrating the bidirectional glucose control of the cytoplasmic Ca^{2+} regulating insulin release. Glucose has the opposite action to inositol 1, 4, 5-trisphosphate (IP_3) in favoring sequestration of calcium in the organelles

Table 2. Principal actions of glucose on Ca^{2+} movements in the pancreatic B-cells

Property studied	Action of glucose	Latency of effect (min)	Threshold concentration for glucose (m*M*)	Alteration of cytoplasmic Ca^{2+} activity
Entry of Ca^{2+}	Stimulation	2	5	Increase
Intracellular sequestration of Ca^{2+}	Stimulation	0.5	0	Decrease
Outward transport of Ca^{2+}	Stimulation	2	5	Decrease

It follows from the observation that glucose lowers cytoplasmic Ca^{2+}, that situations might exist where the sugar even inhibits insulin release [36, 37, 42]. We have been able to demonstrate such a paradoxical effect under the following experimental conditions:

1. Use of a low concentration of glucose
2. Interference with the depolarizing action of glucose
3. Blockage of voltage-dependent Ca^{2+} channels in the plasma membrane

In view of the small effect of suppressing an already low cytoplasmic Ca^{2+} activity it is not surprising that the inhibitory component in the glucose action on insulin release has long been overlooked. In retrospect it became apparent that as much as 11 years ago we had data indicating glucose inhibition of insulin release from islets incubated in a Ca^{2+}-deficient medium [31]. In the search for experimental procedures to demonstrate the inhibitory component in the glucose action on insulin release, it has been considered important not only to counteract the glucose-mediated entry of Ca^{2+} but also to perform the studies under conditions of raised cytoplasmic Ca^{2+} activity. The existence of glucose inhibition was, for example, clearly demonstrated when increasing the Ca^{2+} permeability of the B-cells by previous culture of the islets in a Ca^{2+}-deficient medium. Under these circumstances 6 m*M* glucose clearly inhibited insulin release, whereas the maximally depolarizing concentration (20 m*M*) of the sugar was stimulatory [5]. The inhibitory component in the glucose action on insulin release was also unmasked when ex-

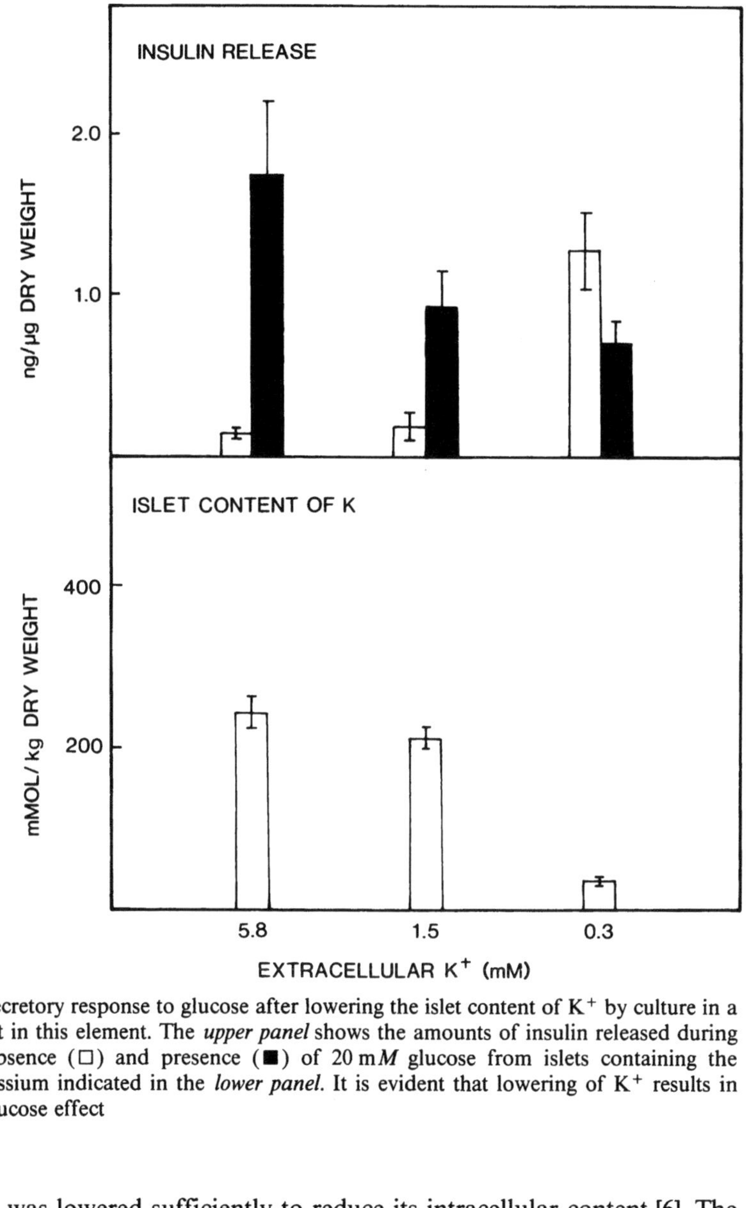

Fig. 5. Insulin secretory response to glucose after lowering the islet content of K^+ by culture in a medium deficient in this element. The *upper panel* shows the amounts of insulin released during 60 min in the absence (□) and presence (■) of 20 m*M* glucose from islets containing the amounts of potassium indicated in the *lower panel*. It is evident that lowering of K^+ results in reversal of the glucose effect

tracellular K^+ was lowered sufficiently to reduce its intracellular content [6]. The latter type of effect is exemplified in Fig. 5. A paradoxical glucose action with stimulation of insulin release as a result of reducing the concentration of the sugar has been observed during perfusion of the isolated rat pancreas. In the experiments of LEAHY and WEIR [56] and LEAHY et al. [57] this phenomenon became evident when the B-cell function was disturbed by pretreatment of the animals with streptozotocin or excessive amounts of glucose.

The discovery of the opposing actions of glucose on the cytoplasmic Ca^{2+} activity might aid in the understanding of several unresolved questions related to the function of the B-cells. Since Ca^{2+} is involved in the regulation of the K^+ permeability of the B-cells (see p. 252), the lowering of cytoplasmic Ca^{2+} may be part of the mechanism by which glucose induces electrical activity manifested as plateau potentials. The glucose stimulation of the intracellular Ca^{2+} buffering can be expected to become less pronounced with time. The concept of the dual action of glucose might consequently explain both its ability to induce an increasing second phase of insulin release and the fact that the secretory response is improved after priming with the sugar. Whereas glucose stimulation of the entry of Ca^{2+} can be regarded to be an effect fairly specific for the B-cells, the promotion of the intracellular sequestration may be a phenomenon of more general relevance. When rapidly metabolized, glucose can be expected to lower the cytoplasmic Ca^{2+} activity in other cells too. It is still an open question whether such a mechanism accounts for the inhibitory action of glucose on the release of glucagon from the A_2-cells.

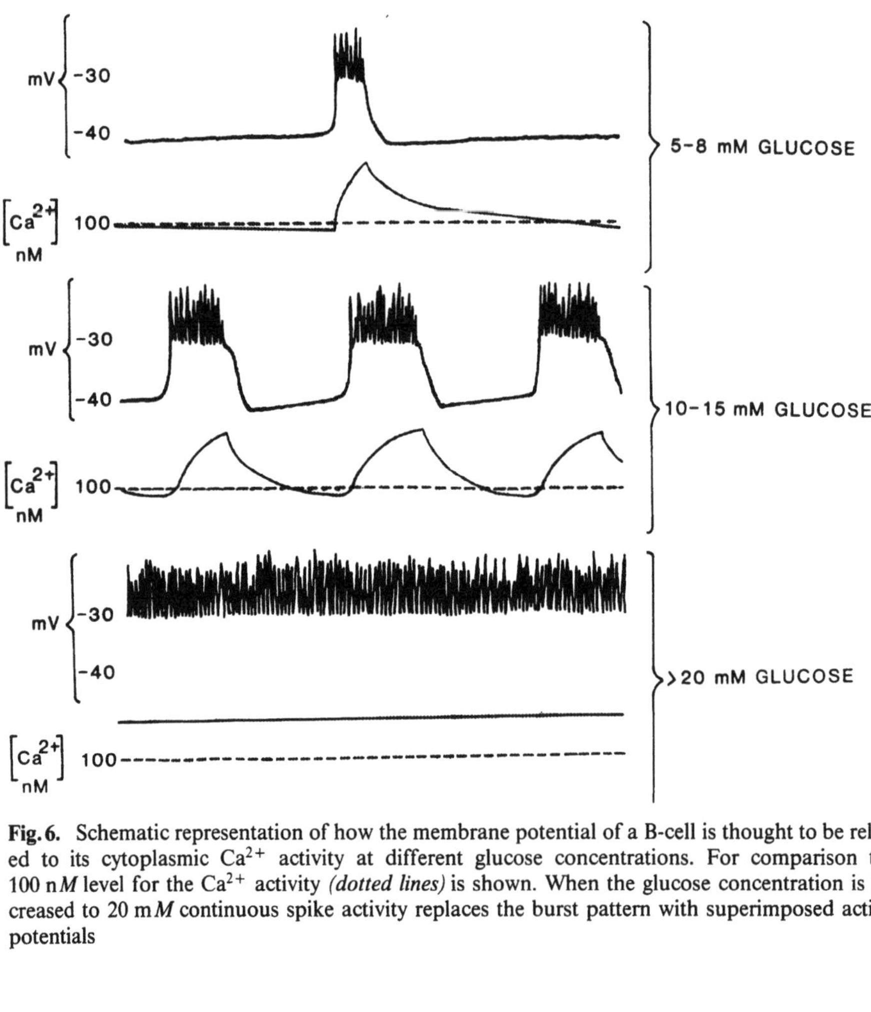

Fig. 6. Schematic representation of how the membrane potential of a B-cell is thought to be related to its cytoplasmic Ca^{2+} activity at different glucose concentrations. For comparison the 100 n*M* level for the Ca^{2+} activity *(dotted lines)* is shown. When the glucose concentration is increased to 20 m*M* continuous spike activity replaces the burst pattern with superimposed action potentials

The islet content of ATP has been found to increase with glucose concentration up to 5 m*M* [2, 39]. It is therefore likely that the slow depolarization obtained when raising glucose to this level involves closure not only of the K^+ channels dependent on Ca^{2+}, but also of those regulated by ATP. Figure 6 illustrates how the membrane potential of the B-cells is thought to be related to the cytoplasmic Ca^{2+} activity for concentrations of glucose above 5 m*M*. In this case depolarization reaches the threshold for opening of the voltage-dependent Ca^{2+} channels, resulting in a further rapid depolarization to a plateau phase, where bursts of action potentials appear. Whereas the entry of Ca^{2+} explains the initiation of the action potentials, their reversal is probably due to the activation of the delayed rectifying K^+ current. During each burst the uptake of Ca^{2+} outweighs its removal by intracellular sequestration and outward transport. The resulting increase of the cytoplasmic Ca^{2+} activity will eventually reach a level at which the Ca^2-dependent K^+ channels are activated. After subsequent repolarization, intracellular sequestration and outward transport will depress the Ca^{2+} activity to a level where the new cycle starts. With increase of the glucose concentration to 10–15 m*M*, there is a concomitant increase in the sequestration and outward transport of Ca^{2+}, resulting in a prolongation of the bursts. At maximally stimulating glucose concentrations the elimination of Ca^{2+} from the cytoplasm is rapid enough to balance its inflow across the voltage-dependent channels, resulting in a continous burst activity. It is evident from the model that when glucose is raised above 5 m*M*, lowering of Ca^{2+} below its resting activity occurs only during a short period preceding the burst. The time average effect of depolarizing concentrations of glucose is consequently to increase cytoplasmic Ca^{2+}, and this effect will be more pronounced with increasing glucose. Whereas the maximal average Ca^{2+} concentration is reached during the continous spike activity, the peak concentration of Ca^{2+} occurs at the end of the bursts, i.e. at concentrations of glucose inducing submaximal stimulation of insulin release.

Clinical Implications of a Disturbed B-Cell Handling of Ca^{2+}

Although movements of Ca^{2+} significant for insulin release have been analyzed mainly with islets isolated from experimental animals, various in vivo studies suggest that Ca^{2+} also has a key role in the insulin secretory process in man. Substances which were found during in vitro studies to promote the entry of Ca^{2+} after depolarization of the B-cells, such as glucose, sulfonylureas, and arginine, are known to increase the circulating levels of insulin in normal individuals. Moreover, after administration of the hyperpolarizing drug diazoxide the serum values of insulin are also depressed in man [77]. The presence of impaired insulin secretion during various syndromes characterized by hypokalemia [27] is not surprising in view of the decisive role of K^+ in stimulus-secretion coupling (see p. 251). In support of the idea that cyclic AMP sensitizes the human B-cells to Ca^{2+}, theophylline has been reported to correct the impaired insulin secretory response to glucose during hypocalcemia [24].

In the interpretation of how Ca^{2+} is involved in the process of insulin release from in vivo data, attention should be paid to the fact that Ca^{2+} also has effects on other variables significant for glucose homeostasis. Due to the hepatic extraction of insulin from the circulation, it is more informative to measure this hormone in the portal vein than in peripheral blood. The problem of insulin degradation is considerably reduced when estimations of the secretory activity of the B-cells are based on concomitant measurements of the C-peptide. When evaluating the role of Ca^{2+} in human B-cells, advantage has also been taken of islets isolated from kidney donors. Studying the washout of ^{45}Ca from such islets, indirect evidence has been obtained for bidirectional glucose control of cytoplasmic Ca^{2+} in human B-cells [47].

It follows from the concept of a dual action of glucose on the cytoplasmic Ca^{2+} that early stages of impaired B-cell function might be manifested as a paradoxical glucose suppression of the circulating insulin. Prompt reduction of serum insulin has actually been observed following intravenous glucose injections in diabetics [43, 62, 67]. It is not surprising that this phenomenon, usually representing a temporary depression of only 10%–15%, has been overlooked during conventional glucose infusion tests. Glucose-induced production of a nonadrenergic inhibitor should be considered as an alternative explanation for a reduction in serum insulin. It is, for example, well established that glucose stimulates the release of somatostatin, an islet product with inhibitory actions on adjacent B-cells. However, the effect of glucose in lowering the circulating insulin cannot be mimicked by sulfonylureas, although the release of somatostatin is stimulated also by these compounds [16]. So far the most impressive glucose suppression of the serum insulin has been observed in a mentally retarded girl with acanthosis nigricans and severe insulin resistance [43]. Figure 7 shows the results of intravenous infusions of glu-

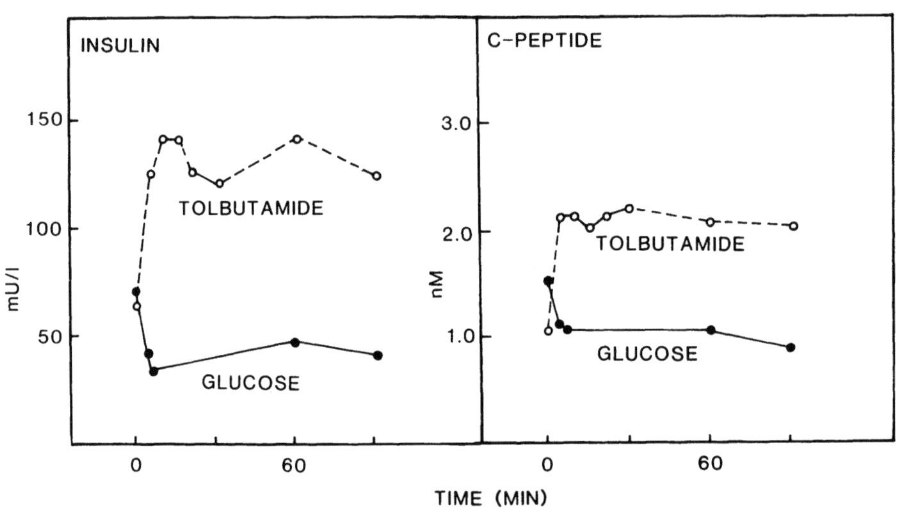

Fig. 7. Effects of glucose and tolbutamide on the serum values of insulin and C-peptide in a 14-year-old girl with mild diabetes. The curves indicate the changes obtained after intravenous injections of either 350 mg glucose/kg body weight (●) or 1 g tolbutamide (○). [43]

cose or the sulfonylurea compound tolbutamide in this patient. The falling serum concentrations of insulin and C-peptide obtained with glucose are compatible with half-lives for these hormones of only 4–5 min and 8–9 min respectively, suggesting an almost complete inhibition of the secretory activity of the B-cells during the initial phase. It is evident from Fig. 7 that tolbutamide has opposite effects to that of glucose in inducing a marked increase of circulating insulin and C-peptide. Previous studies have indicated that the insulin-releasing action of sulfonylureas can be attributed to Ca^{2+} influx into the B-cells after opening of voltage-dependent channels in the plasma membrane [30, 33]. The patient may therefore be taken as an example of a situation where the inhibitory component in the glucose action is unmasked due to interference with its depolarizing effect rather than to the absence of Ca^{2+} channels sensitive to voltage changes.

In Figure 8 an example is given of the progressive impairment of the insulin secretory response to glucose in a girl whose monozygotic twin has suffered for 3 years from type-1 diabetes. The curves are based on repeated intravenous glucose infusion tests performed by GANDA et al. [23]. At the time of the first investigation (October) she had cytoplasmic islet antibodies and impaired glucose tolerance despite a normal fasting blood glucose value. In December the same year the impairment of B-cell function had advanced to a stage where infusion of glucose resulted in an initial depression of circulating insulin. As shown in Figure 8, there

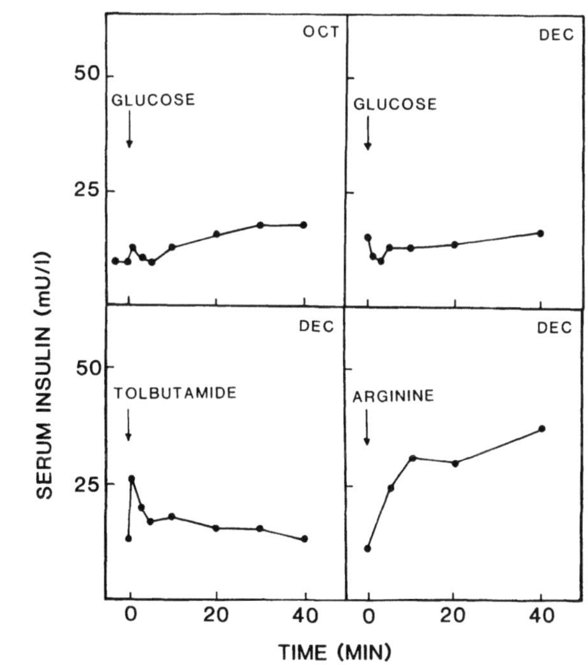

Fig. 8. Serum insulin levels in a 11-year-old girl whose monozygotic twin has suffered from diabetes for 3 years. The curves indicate the changes obtained after intravenous injection of 500 mg glucose/kg body weight, 460 mg arginine/kg body weight, or 1 g tolbutamide. The patient had a normal fasting blood glucose but circulating cytoplasmic islet antibodies [23]

Table 3. Possible defects in pancreatic B-cells revealed by measuring serum insulin after intravenous injections of glucose, sulfonylurea, and arginine

Deficient rise of serum insulin (+) in response to			Proposed defect
Glucose	Sulfonylurea	Arginine	
+			Deficient glucose metabolism or decreased sensitivity to the produced coupling factor (ATP?)
+	+		Impairment of the ATP-regulated K^+ channel or moderately reduced intracellular K^+
+	+	+	Reduced sensitivity to the Ca^{2+} signal or profound damage of the B-cells

was a defective insulin secretory response not only to glucose but also to tolbutamide. This might indicate a primary defect in the depolarization normally occurring with reduction of the K^+ permeability of the B-cells. Since infusion of arginine produced a substantial increase of serum insulin, there is reason to believe that the voltage-dependent Ca^{2+} channels are intact. Arginine has been considered to depolarize the B-cells in its capacity of a positively charged molecule and not by reducing the K^+ permeability of the plasma membrane [10].

As exemplified from the above-mentioned patients, a reduction of the insulin secretory response to glucose with resulting diabetes may arise from a diminished entry of Ca^{2+} into the B-cells. As suggested by the data presented in Table 3, a comparison of the insulin secretory response to glucose, sulfonylureas, and arginine might be useful in the elucidation of the defect resulting in impaired B-cell function in humans. So far there is no indication that diabetes results from a primary malfunction of the voltage-dependent Ca^{2+} channels. Although these channels appear to be relatively resistant to verapamil in the human B-cell [75], it has been reported that the blocker nifedipine interferes with insulin secretion [9, 28].

Acknowledgements. For permission to reproduce the data in Figure 8 I am indebted to Dr. George S. Eisenbarth, Joslin Diabetes Centre, Boston Mass., USA. For help in preparing the manuscript my thanks are due to Susanne Rydstedt.

References

1. Andersson T, Berggren P-O, Gylfe E, Hellman B (1982) Amounts and distribution of intracellular magnesium and calcium in pancreatic B-cells. Acta Physiol Scand 114: 235-241
2. Ashcroft SJH, Weerasinghe LCC, Randle PJ (1973) Interrelationship of islet metabolism, adenosine triphosphate content and insulin release. Biochem J 132: 223-231
3. Ashcroft FM, Harrison DE, Ashcroft SJH (1984) Glucose induces closure of single potassium channels in isolated rat pancreatic B-cells. Nature (London) 312: 446-448
4. Atwater I, Goncalves A, Herchuelz A, Lebrun P, Malaisse WJ, Rojas E, Scott A (1984) Cooling dissociates glucose-induced insulin release from electrical activity and cation fluxes in rodent pancreatic islets. J Physiol (Lond) 348: 615-627

5. Bergsten P, Hellman B (1984) Glucose inhibits insulin release when not promoting the entry of Ca^{2+} into the B-cells. Biochem Biophys Res Commun 125: 875-881
6. Bergsten P, Rorsman F, Hellman B (1986) Modifications of the pancreatic B-cell function after lowering their potassium content. Acta Physiol Scand 128: 619-628
7. Bhatena SJ, Awoke S, Voyles NR, Wilkins SD, Recant L, Oie HK, Gazdar AF (1984) Insulin, glucagon and somatostatin secretion by cultured rat islet cell tumor and its clones. Proc Soc Exp Biol Med 175: 35-38
8. Borg LAH, Andersson A (1981) Long-term effects of glibenclamide on the insulin production, oxidative metabolism and quantitative ultrastructure of mouse pancreatic islets maintained in tissue culture at different glucose concentrations. Acta Diabetol Lat 18: 65-83
9. Charles S, Ketelslegers JM, Buysschaert M, Lambert AE (1981) Hyperglycemic effect of nifedipine. Br Med J 283: 19-20
10. Charles S, Tamagawa T, Henquin JC (1982) A single mechanism for the stimulation of insulin release and ^{86}Rb efflux from rat islets by cationic amino acids. Biochem J 208: 301-308
11. Colca JR, McDonald JM, Kotagal N, Patke C, Fink J, Greider MH Lacy PE, McDaniel ML (1982) Active calcium uptake by islet-cell endoplasmic reticulum. J Biol Chem 257: 7223-7228
12. Colca JR, Kotagal N, Lacy PE, McDaniel ML (1983) Modulation of active Ca^{2+} uptake by the islet-cell endoplasmic reticulum. Biochem J 212: 113-121
13. Cook DL, Hales CN (1984) Intracellular ATP directly blocks K^+ channels in pancreatic B-cells. Nature (London) 311: 271-273
14. Cook DL, Ikeuchi M, Fujimoto WY (1984) Lowering of pH inhibits Ca^{2+}-activated K^+ channels in pancreatic B-cells. Nature (London) 311: 269-271
15. Devis G, Somers G, Malaisse WJ (1975) Stimulation of insulin release by calcium. Biochem Biophys Res Commun 67: 525-529
16. Efendić S, Enzmann F, Nylén A, Uvnäs-Wallensten K, Luft R (1979) Effect of glucose/sulfonylurea interaction on release of insulin, glucagon and somatostatin from isolated perfused rat pancreas. Proc Natl Acad Sci USA 76: 5901-5904
17. Falkmer S, Hellman B, Täljedal IB (1970) Opening address. In: Falkmer S, Hellman B and Täljedal IB (eds). The structure and metabolism of the pancreatic islets. A centennial of Paul Langerhans' discovery. Pergamon, Oxford, p 1
18. Findlay I, Dunne MJ (1985) Voltage-activated Ca^{2+} currents in insulin-secreting cells. FEBS Lett 189: 281-285
19. Findlay I, Dunne MJ, Petersen OH (1985) High-conductance K^+ channel in pancreatic islet cells can be activated and inactivated by internal calcium. J Membr Biol 83: 169-175
20. Findlay I, Dunne MJ, Petersen OH (1985) ATP-sensitive inward rectifier and voltage- and calcium-activated K^+ channels in cultured pancreatic islet cells. J Membr Biol 88: 165-172
21. Findlay I, Dunne MJ, Ullrich S, Wollheim CB, Petersen OH (1985) Quinine inhibits Ca^{2+}-independent K^+ channels whereas tetraethylammonium inhibits Ca^{2+}-activated K^+ channels in insulin-secreting cells. FEBS Lett 185: 4-8
22. Formby B, Capito K, Egeberg J, Hedeskov CJ (1976) Ca-activated ATPase activity in subcellular fractions of mouse pancreatic islets. Am J Physiol 230: 441-448
23. Ganda OP, Srikanta S, Brink SJ, Morris MA, Gleason RE, Soeldner SJ, Eisenbarth GS (1984) Differential sensitivity to β-cell secretagogues in "early" type 1 diabetes mellitus. Diabetes 33: 516-521
24. Gedik O, Zileli MS (1977) Effects of hypocalcemia and theophylline on glucose tolerance and insulin release in human beings. Diabetes 26: 813-819
25. Gepts W (1957) Contributions à l'étude morphologique des ilots de Langerhans au cours du diabète. Thesis. Editions Acta Med Belg, Bruxelles, pp 1-108
26. Grodsky GM, Bennett LL (1966) Cation requirements for insulin secretion in the isolated perfused pancreas. Diabetes 15: 910-912
27. Grunfeld C, Chappell DA (1983) Hypokalemia and diabetes mellitus. Am J Med 75: 553-554
28. Giugliano D, Torella R, Cacciapuoti F, Gentile S, Verza M, Varriechio M (1980) Impairment of insulin secretion in man by nifedipine. Eur J Clin Pharmacol 18: 395-398
29. Gylfe E, Hellman B (1986) Glucose-stimulated sequestration of Ca^{2+} in clonal insulin-releasing cells. Biochem J 233: 865-870
30. Gylfe E, Hellman B, Sehlin J, Täljedal IB (1984) Interaction of sulfonylurea with the pancreatic β-cell. Experientia 40: 1126-1134

31. Hellman B (1975) The significance of calcium for glucose stimulation of insulin release. Endocrinology 97: 392-398
32. Hellman B (1976) Stimulation of insulin release after raising extracellular calcium. FEBS Lett 63: 125-128
33. Hellman B (1982) The mechanism of sulfonylurea stimulation of insulin release. Acta Biol Med Germ 41: 1211-1219
34. Hellman B (1985) β-cell cytoplasmic Ca^{2+} balance as a determinant for glucose-stimulated insulin release. Diabetologia 28: 494-501
35. Hellman B (1986) Calcium transport in pancreatic β-cells: implications for glucose regulation of insulin release. Diabetes Metab Rev 2: 215-241
36. Hellman B, Gylfe E (1985) Glucose regulation of insulin release involves intracellular sequestration of calcium. In: Rubin RP, Weiss GB and Putney Jr JW (eds) Calcium in biological systems. Plenum, New York, pp 93-99
37. Hellman B, Gylfe E (1986) Calcium and the control of insulin secretion. In: Cheung WY (ed) Calcium and cell function, vol 6. Academic, New York, pp 253-326
38. Hellman B, Gylfe E (1986) Mobilization of different intracellular calcium pools after activation of muscarinic receptors in pancreatic beta-cells. Pharmacology 32: 257-267
39. Hellman B, Idahl L-Å, Danielsson Å (1969) Adenosine trisphosphate levels in mammalian pancreatic β-cells after stimulation with glucose and hypoglycemic sulfonylureas. Diabetes 18: 509-516
40. Hellman B Andersson T, Berggren P-O, Flatt P, Gylfe E, Kohnert K-D (1979) The role of calcium in insulin secretion. In: Dumont J, Nunez J (eds) Hormone and cell regulation, vol 3. Elsevier, Amsterdam, pp 69-96
41. Hellman B, Andersson T, Berggren P-O, Rorsman P (1980) Calcium and pancreatic β-cell function. II Modification of ^{45}Ca fluxes by Na^+ removal. Biochem Med 24: 143-152
42. Hellman B, Honkanen T, Gylfe E (1982) Glucose inhibits insulin release induced by Na^+ mobilization of intracellular calcium. FEBS Lett 148: 289-292
43. Hellman B, Hällgren R, Abrahamsson H, Bergsten P, Berne C, Gylfe E, Rorsman P, Wide L (1985) The dual action of glucose on the cytosolic Ca^{2+} activity in pancreatic β-cells. Demonstration of an inhibitory effect of glucose on insulin release in the mouse and man. Biomed Biochim Acta 44: 63-70
44. Hellman B, Arkhammar P, Berggren P-O, Bergsten P, Gylfe E, Nilsson T, Rorsman F, Rorsman P, Trube G, Wesslén N (1986) Evidence for bidirectional glucose control of the cytoplasmic calcium regulating insulin release. In: Serrano-Rios M, Lefèbvre PJ (eds) Diabetes 1985. Elsevier, Amsterdam, pp 177-180
45. Hellman B, Gylfe E, Wesslén N (1986) Inositol 1,4,5-trisphosphate mobilizes glucose-incorporated calcium from pancreatic islets. Biochem Int 13: 383-389
46. Hellman B, Gylfe E, Bergsten P (1987) Mobilization of different pools of glucose-incorporated calcium in pancreatic β-cells after muscarinic receptor activation. In: Atwater I, Rojas E, Soria B (eds), Biophysics of the pancreatic β-cell. Plenum, New York, pp 325-341
47. Henriksson C, Claes G, Gylfe E, Hellman B, Zettergren L (1978) Collagenase isolation and ^{45}Ca efflux studies of human islets of Langerhans. Eur Surg Res 10: 343-351
48. Herchuelz A, Malaisse WJ (1980) Regulation of calcium fluxes in rat pancreatic islets: dissimilar effects of glucose and of sodium ion accumulation. J Physiol (Lond) 302: 263-280
49. Herchuelz A, Malaisse WJ (1981) Calcium movements and insulin release in pancreatic islet cells. Diabète Métab 7: 283-288
50. Hutton JC, Peskavaria M (1982) Proton-translocating Mg^{2+}-dependent ATPase activity in insulin-secretory granules. Biochem J 204: 161-170
51. Hutton JC, Penn EJ, Peskavaria M (1983) Low-molecular weight constituents of isolated insulin-secretory granules. Bivalent cations, adenine nucleotides and inorganic phosphate. Biochem J 210: 297-305
52. Jones PM, Stuchfield J, Howell SL (1985) Effects of Ca^{2+} and a phorbol ester on insulin secretion from islets of Langerhans permeabilized by high voltage discharge. FEBS Lett 191: 102-106
53. Kohnert KD, Hahn HJ, Gylfe E, Borg H, Hellman B (1979) Calcium and pancreatic β-cell function. 6. Glucose and intracellular ^{45}Ca distribution. Mol Cell Endocrinol 16: 205-220

54. Krieger-Brauer H, Gratzl M (1982) Uptake of Ca^{2+} by isolated secretory vesicles from adrenal medulla. Biochim Biophys Acta 691: 61-70
55. Langerhans P (1869) Beiträge zur mikroskopischen Anatomie der Bauchspeicheldrüse. Thesis, Lange, Berlin, pp 1-32
56. Leahy JL, Weir GC (1985) Unresponsiveness to glucose in a streptozocin model of diabetes. Inappropriate insulin and glucagon responses to a reduction of glucose concentration. Diabetes 34: 653-659
57. Leahy JL, Cooper HE, Deal DA, Weir GC (1986) Chronic hyperglycemia is associated with impaired glucose influence on insulin secretion. A study in normal rats using chronic in vivo glucose infusions. J Clin Invest 77: 908-915
58. MacDonald MJ (1984) The use of calcium uptake by small amounts of mitochondria from pancreatic islets to study mitochondrial respirations. The effects of diazoxide and sodium. Biochem Int 8: 771-778
59. Marty A, Neher E (1982) Ionic channels in cultured rat pancreatic islet cells. J Physiol (Lond) 326: 36-37P
60. Matthews EK (1979) Calcium translocation and control mechanisms for endocrine secretion. Symp Soc Exp Biol 33: 225-249
61. Matteson DR, Armstrong CM (1986) Properties of two types of calcium channels in clonal pituitary cells. J Gen Physiol 87: 161-182
62. Metz SA, Halter JB, Robertson RP (1979) Paradoxical inhibition of insulin secretion by glucose in human diabetes mellitus. J Clin Endocrinol Metab 48: 827-835
63. Milner RDG, Hales CN (1967) The role of calcium and magnesium in insulin secretion from rabbit panreas studied in vitro. Diabetologia 3: 47-49
64. Pershadsingh HA, McDaniel ML, Landt M, Bry CG, Lacy PE, McDonald JM (1980) Ca^{2+}-activated ATPase and ATP-dependent calmodulin-stimulated Ca^{2+}transport in islet cell plasma membrane. Nature (London) 288: 492-495
65. Prentki M, Wollheim CB (1984) Cytosolic free Ca^{2+}in insulin secreting cells and its regulation by isolated organelles. Experientia 40: 1052-1060
66. Prentki M, Janjic D, Wollheim CB (1983) The regulation of extramitochondrial steady state free Ca^{2+} concentration by rat insulinoma mitochondria. J Biol Chem 258: 7597-7602
67. Robertson RP, Brunzell JD, Hazzard WR, Lerner RL, Porte D Jr (1972) Paradoxical hypoinsulinaemia: an alpha-adrenergic-mediated response to glucose. Lancet 2: 787-789
68. Rorsman P, Abrahamsson H (1985) Cyclic AMP potentiates glucose-induced insulin release from mouse pancreatic islets without increasing cytosolic free Ca^{2+}. Acta Physiol Scand 125: 639-647
69. Rorsman P, Hellman B (1987) Voltage-activated currents in guinea-pig pancreatic α_2-cells. Evidence for Ca^{2+}-dependent action potentials. J Gen Physiol (in press)
70. Rorsman P, Trube G (1985) Glucose-dependent K^+-channels in panreatic β-cells are regulated by intracellular ATP. Pflugers Arch 405: 305-309
71. Rorsman P, Trube G (1986) Calcium and delayed potassium currents in mouse pancreatic β-cells under voltage-clamp conditions. J Physiol (Lond) 374: 531:-550
72. Rorsman P, Berggren P-O, Gylfe E, Hellman B (1983) Reduction of the cytosolic calcium activity in clonal insulin-releasing cells exposed to glucose. Biosci Rep 3: 939-946
73. Rorsman P, Abrahamsson H, Gylfe E, Hellman B (1984) Dual effects of glucose on the cytosolic Ca^{2+} activity of mouse pancreatic B-cells. FEBS Lett 170: 196-200
74. Rorsman P, Arkhammar P, Berggren P-O (1986) Voltage-activated Na^+ currents and their suppression by phorbol ester in the clonal insulin-producing cell line RINm5F. Am J Physiol 251, C912-C919
75. Röjdmark S, Andersson DEH (1984) Influence of verapamil on glucose tolerance. Acta Med Scand [Suppl] 681: 37-42
76. Satin LS, Cook DL (1985) Voltage-gated Ca^{2+} current in pancreatic β-cells. Pflugers Arch 404: 385-387
77. Seltzer HS, Crout JR (1968) Insulin secretory blockade by benzothiadiazines and catecholamines: reversal by sulfonylureas. Ann NY Acad Sci 150: 309-321
78. Sturgess NC, Ashford MLJ, Cook DL, Hales CN (1985) The sulphonylurea receptor may be an ATP-sensitive potassium channel. Lancet 8453: 474-475
79. Tamagawa T, Niki H, Niki A (1985) Insulin release independent of a rise in cytosolic free Ca^{2+} by forskolin and phorbol ester. FEBS Lett 183: 430-432

80. Trube G, Ohno-Shosaku T, Rorsman P, Zünkler BJ (1986) Hypoglycemic sulfonylureas inhibit ATP-dependent K channels in pancreatic B-cells. Pflugers Arch 406: R63
81. Trube G, Rorsman P, Ohno-Shosaku T (1986) Opposite effects of tolbutamide and diazoxide on the ATP-dependent K^+ channel in mouse pancreatic β-cells. Pflugers Arch 407: 493-499
82. Wesslén N, Hellman B (1986) The influx of Ca^{2+} into pancreatic β-cells and its regulation by glucose. Biomed Res 7: 339-344
83. Wollheim CB, Pozzan T (1984) Correlation between cytosolic free Ca^{2+} and insulin release in an insulin-secreting cell line. J Biol Chem 259: 2262-2267
84. Wollheim CB, Sharp GWG (1981) Regulation of insulin release by calcium. Physiol Rev 61: 914-973
85. Wollheim CB, Ullrich S, Pozzan T (1984) Glyceraldehyde but not cyclic AMP-stimulated insulin release is preceded by a rise in cytosolic free Ca^{2+}. FEBS Lett 177: 17-22

Autoimmune Diabetes in the BioBreeding/Worcester Rat*

A. A. Like and E. J. Weringer

Introduction

The BioBreeding rat develops a spontaneous diabetic syndrome resembling human type 1 diabetes mellitus. The salient features include: abrupt onset of insulin-dependent, ketosis-prone diabetes between 60-120 days of age [1]; lymphocytic insulitis with virtually complete destruction of the pancreatic B-cells [2, 3]; genetic predisposition and the occurrence of hyperglycemia in approximately 40%-80% of the inbred BioBreeding/Worcester (BB/Wor) colony [4].

Support for the hypothesis that BB/Wor diabetes is the result of autoimmune destruction of the insulin-synthesizing pancreatic B-cells is derived from the following lines of evidence: (1) Lymphocytic insulitis occurs prior to and during the acute phase of hyperglycemia [1-3]. (2) Susceptibility to diabetes is linked to the major histocompatability complex (MHC) $RT1^u$ of the rat [4]. (3) Prevention and amelioration of the diabetic syndrome is accomplished by neonatal thymectomy [5] and a variety of immune suppressive agents [6-10]. (4) Prevention of diabetes follows immune enhancement measures such as neonatal bone marrow, peripheral blood, and splenic lymphocyte transfusions [11-14]. (5) Adoptive transfer of diabetes to young diabetes-prone and diabetes-resistant animals is possible with transfusions of concanavalin-A (Con-A)-stimulated diabetic spleen cells [15-17].

Other features of the BB/Wor syndrome which also give credence to an immune pathogenesis include: the presence of lifelong genetically transmitted lymphopenia (18-23) and the virtual absence of cytotoxic/suppressor T-lymphocyte subsets in peripheral blood and lymphoid tissues (24, 25); the presence of circulating (auto)-antibodies to smooth muscle, thyroid colloid, and gastric parietal cell antigens [26, 27] and to lymphocytes [21, 28]; the evidence that diabetic and diabetes-prone rat sera frequently contain immunoglobulins that bind to insulinoma cells, mediate lysis of radioactively labeled islet cells and suppress islet insulin secretion [28-33].

While most investigators are in agreement with the above description of the syndrome's (auto)immune characteristics, there is no general agreement concerning the precise mechanism of B-cell destruction. Nor is there a true understanding of the significance of the syndrome's several apparently contradictory characteristics.

* Supported in part by USPHS Grant # NIDDK-19155 and Contract # NO1-DK-4-2254

The BB Rat Dilemma

Although many laboratories have reported the existence of profound T-cell lymphopenia among DB-PRN rats and its association with increased susceptibility to infection, impaired in vitro T-lymphocyte function and depressed alloreactivity, it is not clear whether the association of T-lymphocyte lymphopenia and diabetes is obligatory, with the implication of a mechanistic cause and effect relationship of lymphopenia and B-cell destruction. An obligatory relationship between lymphopenia and diabetes was favored by the reports that transfusions of bone marrow [12] and peripheral lymphocytes [13] both corrected lymphopenia and prevented diabetes. Yet immunosuppressive measures such as neonatal thymectomy, antilymphocyte serum, and cyclosporin also protected against diabetes [5-9]. It is not understood why the lymphocytes of an animal which mount so sluggish an allograft response should evidence striking autoaggression against self. Nor is it understood why neonatal infusions of bone marrow or adult transfusions of T-lymphocytes should enhance lymphocyte competence yet interfere with immune destruction of B-cells. Why should further reductions in the number and function of an already depressed lymphocyte population protect against diabetes? The lymphopenia/diabetes dilemma may have been resolved or complicated further, now that diabetes has appeared among the family lines of nonlymphopenic BB/Wor rats that remained free of diabetes for approximately 12 generations of inbreeding ($n > 1000$) [34]. It is worth recalling that lymphocyte transfusions from non-lymphopenic diabetes-resistant BB/Wor rats corrected T-lymphocyte lymphopenia and prevented diabetes among BB/Wor diabetes-prone animals [14]. The appearance of diabetes among nonlymphopenic BB/Wor rats should end speculation concerning the obligatory role of T-lymphocyte lymphopenia in the pathogenesis of diabetes. It should also emphasize the importance of identifying the effector and protector cells and the regulation of their activity. Obviously the diabetes-resistant nonlymphopenic BB/Wor rats still harbor beta-cytolytic effector cells. What are those cells? What cells keep them in check?

The BB/Wor dilemma concerning the mechanism of B-cell destruction was also brought into focus by islet and adrenal transplantation studies which suggested that BB/Wor B-cell destruction may not be MHC-restricted [35]. Prowse and Lafferty also concluded that BB/W B-cell destruction may not be MHC-restricted after experiments where cultured PVG ($RT1^c$) islets but not pituitary tissues were destroyed in diabetic BB rats [36]. Prowse and Lafferty's suggestion that antibodies (Abs) play a role in BB diabetes is supported by the presence of islet cell surface Abs (ICSA) in prediabetic and diabetic animals [28]. It has also been suggested that natural killer (NK)-cells are increased in number and activity in diabetic and diabetes-prone rats and play a role in B-cell destruction [25, 37]. Perhaps NK-cells are the effector cells responsible for B-cell destruction in DB-PRN rats. This hypothesis is consistent with non-MHC-restricted cell killing and with ICSA providing specificity. An NK hypothesis might also be consistent with the inability to detect phenotypic cytotoxic T-lymphocytes ($OX8^+/OX19^+$) in diabetes-prone and diabetic BB/Wor rats [24] and the reduction in diabetes frequency after treatment with OX8 monoclonal antibodies (MoAbs) which bind to and reduce the number of NK-cells as well as cytotoxic-suppressor cells [25]. An

NK mechanism would explain the lack of MHC restriction in transplantation experiments and raises the possibility of an Ab-dependent cell-mediated cytotoxicity (ADCC) reaction.

Nonlymphopenic diabetic (NLD) rats are however not depleted of phenotypic cytotoxic T-lymphocytes (CTL), nor do they have increased NK-cells [34]. Are we, then, to believe that the effector cells responsible for B-cell destruction are NK-cells among diabetes-prone rats and CTL among NLD rats?

In conflict with the evidence of MHC-unrestricted killing are the data derived from the experiments of NAJI et al., where LEWIS ($RT1^{l}$) and WISTAR-FURTH ($RT1^{u}$) isolated islets were transplanted into diabetic BB rats [38]. Although both groups of transplants revealed a lymphocytic infiltrate, only $RT1^{u}$ rats sustained sufficient B-cell injury to become diabetic again. Perhaps NK-cells require "help" from lymphokine-synthesizing helper cells, which in turn require self class II antigens to become fully activated. Is it possible that helper cells provide this assistance to NK-cells in diabetes-prone rats (directly or indirectly by B-lymphocyte synthesis of ICSA), and provide help to CTL in nonlymphopenic diabetic rats? Will each type of diabetic animals commit autoaggression with whatever cells available? The importance of non-$OX8^+$ (i.e., helper) T-lymphocytes is emphasized in our experiments, where OX8 MoAb injections reduced the frequency of diabetes but did not prevent insulitis [25]. OX19 injections, however, completely prevented diabetes and insulitis, without reducing the number of $OX8^+$ cells. These data contribute to the "BB dilemma" because they suggest an important role for non-$OX8^+$ cells, i.e., phenotypic $W3/25^+$ helper T-lymphocytes, which presumably must act in association with class II antigens.

Is there a role for delayed-type hypersensitivity, with macrophages primarily responsible for B-cell loss? Although theoretically a nonspecific mechanism of immunologic injury, is it conceivable that "informational molecules" (Roitt) confer specificity for a macrophage-induced B-cell attack? The reports of interleukin-1-mediated rat islet cytotoxicity [39] and of protection by silica injections against BB diabetes [40] emphasize the possible importance of this mechanism of cell injury.

A final speculative reflection on the results of our transplantation experiments [35, 41]: If BB/Wor-induced B-cell killing is not MHC-restricted, is it possible that genetically abnormal BB/Wor effector cells recognize nonpolymorphic B-cell antigens as similar to class I antigens, in a cross-reactive manner similar to an alloreactive response? If so, $OX8^+$ effector cells could initiate insulitis and B-cell injury, with a contribution from $W3/25^+$ cells.

All of the above experimental data appear to direct our attention to the immune effector and regulatory cells, to the virtual exclusion of other factors, such as hormonal, environmental (infectious agents), and nutritional. Previous reports discounted the possible roles of infection [42] and hormonal [43] agents and were mixed concerning dietary factors [43, 44]. We are not aware of prior studies designed to determine whether the metabolic status of the target (B-)cells influences their susceptibility to immune attack in this animal model of diabetes.

The immunopathologic studies described below were designed to:

1. Identify the effector cells responsible for B-cell destruction and diabetes, and the mechanism of their action

2. Examine the role of donor MHC upon the fate of islets transplanted into diabetic or diabetes-prone BB/Wor rats
3. Determine whether the metabolic biosynthetic state of the pancreatic B-cells influences the initiation/outcome of the immune attack

Effector Cells Responsible for Pancreatic B-cell Destruction in BB/Wor Rats

In a series of experiments that extended over a 2-year period of time, we injected a series of mouse anti-rat MoAbs into BB/Wor diabetes-prone rats. Animals were injected with MoAb-containing tissue culture supernatants (TCS) 3 times weekly for 14-16 weeks (from 35-40 days until 120 days of age). We injected the following MoAbs which react with distinct antigenic moieties on the surfaces of: cytotoxic/suppressor (C/S) T-lymphocytes and NK-cells (OX8); all T-lymphocytes (OX19); helper/inducer (H/I) T-lymphocytes (W3/25); and Ia^+ cells (OX6, IaA; OX17, IaE).

OX8 TCS injections reduced the number of $OX8^+$ splenic and peripheral blood lymphocytes and OX19 TCS injections reduced splenic and peripheral blood $OX19^+$ cells (Tables 1, 2). Analysis of two-color flow cytometry data, in which peripheral blood lymphocytes were incubated sequentially with OX8 and OX19 MoAbs, also revealed that OX19 TCS-injected rats evidenced reductions in circulating H/I T-lymphocytes which are, by definition, $OX8^-/OX19^+$ (Table 2). This technique also revealed that DB-PRN BB/Wor rats, which lack the C/S T-lymphocytes ($OX8^+/OX19^+$) were selectively depleted of peripheral blood NK-cells ($OX8^+/OX19^-$) after injection with OX8 TCS (Table 2). In contrast, DB-PRN animals injected with the other MoAbs revealed no reductions in splenic lymphocyte subsets (Table 1).

The accumulated data clearly indicate that OX19 and OX8 MoAb injections significantly reduced the frequency of diabetes. The apparent marginal protection afforded by W3/25 and OX17 injections did not withstand the statistical (Bonferroni) adjustment used to correct for type I additive errors (Table 3).

The magnitude of the protection afforded by OX19 injections became apparent when pancreatic sections of injected nondiabetic animals were examined microscopically. None of 43 of the nondiabetic OX19-treated and 40 of 53 (75%) of the nondiabetic OX8-treated rats evidenced pancreatic insulitis (Table 4). Since OX8 injections did not reduce the number of helper T-lymphocytes, we speculated that $OX8^+$ cells (NK-cells) may be the effector cells responsible for diabetes in the BB/Wor rat. OX19 injections, however, were more protective than OX8 treatment (0/49 vs 9/72). These data, taken together with the marginal protection following W3/25 MoAb injections, suggested an important participatory role for the helper T-lymphocyte in the pathogenesis of BB/Wor diabetes. Additional data favoring the functional significance of reduced numbers of NK and H/I cells in treated rats were derived from two additional studies. Assays of in vitro NK-cell killing of Yac-1 target cells document that Yac-1 lysis was unchanged in OX19-treated ani-

Table 1. Effects of monoclonal antibody injections on splenic lymphocyte subsets

Injections	OX19	W3/13	W3/25	OX8	OX6
None ($n=12$)	7.3±0.8	12.3±1.3	7.2±0.9	7.1±0.8	59.2±5.8
OX19 ($n=14$)	1.9±0.3[a]	10.9±1.6	5.2±0.6	6.8±1.3	56.0±6.6
OX8 ($n=13$)	8.5±0.7	14.6±2.9	9.2±0.7	1.3±0.2[b]	61.9±5.2
W3/25 ($n=4$)	6.8±1.0	22.5±5.8	9.0±1.3	9.3±2.4	67.5±9.2
OX6 ($n=6$)	7.6±0.9	8.7±1.1	8.3±1.1	7.0±0.4	72.7±4.0

The data are expressed as mean ± SEM (%) of positively stained cells and were derived from algycosuric animals sacrificed after 5, 9, and 14 weeks of TCS injections. The splenic lymphocyte subsets were similar at each time point and were pooled

[a] $p<0.05$ OX19 treatment vs all other groups; $p<0.001$ OX19 treatment vs all other groups (except W3/25)

[b] $p<0.05$ OX8 treatment vs all other groups; $p<0.01$ OX8 treatment vs no treatment and 0X19 treatment

Table 2. Two-color flow cytometry of peripheral blood lymphocytes

Injections	$OX8^+/OX19^-$ (NK)	$OX8^-/OX19^+$ (H/I)	$OX8^+/OX19^+$ (C/S)	$OX52^+/OX19^+$ (all T)
None ($n=7$)	5.3 ±1.1	6.2 ±0.8	0.51±0.1[c]	6.4 ±0.8
OX19 ($n=12$)	9.03±1.2	1.08±0.4[b]	0.16±0.04	0.82±0.3[d]
OX8 ($n=9$)	0.56±0.4[a]	7.79±1.1	0.21±0.04	NE

Data expressed as mean ± SEM (%) of positively stained cells

[a] $p<0.05$ OX8 treatment vs no treatment and OX19 treatment

[b] $p<0.001$ OX19 treatment vs no treatment and OX8 treatment

[c] $p<0.01$ No treatment vs OX19 treatment and OX8 treatment

[d] $p<0.001$ OX 19 treatment vs no treatment

Table 3. Frequency of diabetes after monoclonal antibody injections

Injections	Diabetes (%)	Fisher
None	43/70 (61)	NS
RPMI	17/27 (63)	NS
OX19	0/49 (0)	$p<0.001$[a, b]
OX8	11/90 (12)	$p<0.001$[a, b]
W3/25	12/35 (34)	$p<0.02$[a] $p<0.05$[b]
OX6	28/56 (50)	NS
OX17	7/22 (32)	$p<0.03$[a] $p<0.05$[b]

[a] Compared with no injections

[b] Compared with RPMI injections

The data included in Tables 3 and 4 are the combined results of eight separate experiments. Three of the eight experiments included RPMI-injected rats as controls and the remaining five included uninjected controls. After correction of stand alone p values with a Bonferroni adjustment, only OX8- and OX19-injected rats were protected against diabetes ($p<0.01$)

Table 4. Frequency of diabetes and insulitis

Injections	Diabetes (%)	Insulitis[a] (%)
None	43/70 (61)	10/18 (56)
RPMI	17/27 (63)	NE
OX19	0/49 (0)	0/43 (0)[b]
OX8	11/90 (12)	44/57 (77)
W3/25	12/35 (34)	12/15 (80)
OX6	28/56 (50)	3/10 (30)

[a] Frequency of insulitis in the absence of hyperglycemia
[b] $p < 0.001$ OX19 treatment vs all other groups

mals, but significantly reduced in rats after OX8 injections [25]. Finally, OX19-injected animals revealed significant reductions in the frequencies and titers of autoantibodies to smooth muscle and thyroid colloid. OX8-treated rats did not evidence reductions in autoantibodies. In fact the frequency and intensity of smooth muscle and thyroid colloid autoantibodies may be increased after OX8 injections (data not illustrated). Taken together, these results were interpreted as providing additional support for the conclusion that impaired B-lymphocyte synthesis of autoantibodies is the result of helper cell reduction and the reduced level of NK-cell killing is related to $OX8^+$ cell reduction.

In our first series of transplantation experiments [35], it was observed that transplants comprised of isolated pancreatic islets, treated and cultured to preclude allograft rejection, were the target of immune attack in diabetic BB/Wor rats and in normoglycemic BB/Wor recipients with lymphocytic insulitis of endogenous pancreatic islets. Our results also indicated that islets from inbred MHC-discordant rats, as well as islet grafts from DB-RES BB/Wor rats, will be the target of BB insulitis. We concluded that: (1) collagenase-isolated, cultured islets retained antigenic specificity for autoimmune attack in BB/Wor rats; (2) effector cells responsible for induction of insulitis need not share the MHC of their target cells; (3) the immune attack on pancreatic B-cells was directed against nonpolymorphic B-cell-specific antigen(s) common to BB/Wor and non-BB/Wor rat strains and not necessarily recognized in association with self MHC ($RT1^u$); (4) B-cells may be but need not be antigenically abnormal or geographically located within the pancreas as a prerequisite for immune attack; and (5) donor Ia^+ cells are not required to initiate BB/Wor insulitis. Since our experiments did not address the possible MHC restriction of the induction phase (afferent limb) of BB/Wor insulitis, it is possible that host macrophages invade the islet grafts before antigen presentation and activation of host effector cells.

Our transplantation experiments permitted the distinction between specific BB/Wor immune insulitis and inflammation associated with an allograft response. By transplanting islets into normoglycemic DB-PRN rats, we predicted that although a majority of graft recipients would become diabetic or evidence lymphocytic insulitis without hyperglycemia, a significant number would be free of both insulitis and diabetes. Therefore, if our islet preparation techniques prevented allograft rejection, we anticipated that there would be no appreciable evidence of graft insulitis in recipients without endogenous insulitis. This was true in the majority of transplant recipients. Because graft insulitis was almost exclusively limited to recipients with diabetes or insulitis, we concluded that graft insulitis was the result of the BB/Wor immune attack on the transplanted B-cells rather than an allograft reaction. This conclusion was supported by experiments where cultured megaislets and adrenal cortex were simultaneously transplanted under the kidney capsule of DB-PRN or diabetic BB/Wor rats. In all of these animals, lymphocytic insulitis was observed in the recipient's endogenous islets and the islet graft; the adrenal grafts, however, were free of inflammation. These results supported the islet cell specificity of the BB/Wor immune attack and rendered less likely the possibility that graft insulitis in diabetic recipients was the result of enhanced alloreactivity coincident with the onset of BB/Wor insulitis and diabetes.

In a sequel to our first transplant manuscript, we reported [41] that islet grafts derived from DB-RES rats became the target of immune attack when transplanted into recipients with variable durations of diabetes, with and without persistent insulitis within host pancreatic islets. Islet grafts were attacked even when transplanted into rats with diabetes of long-term duration (30-150 days). We interpreted these results to suggest that: (1) abnormal B-cell antigens are not a prerequisite for the *re*currence of BB/Wor insulitis within islet grafts; (2) there is no requirement for ongoing host pancreatic insulitis for the initiation of insulitis within the transplant; (3) the presence of intense graft insulitis in recipients with end-stage islets, without residual insulitis, and with few surviving B-cells suggests that sufficient numbers of memory effector cells persist in long-term diabetics and are capable of renewing the immune attack on the newly introduced (graft) B-cells. The manuscript also reported that simultaneously transplanted cultured adrenal grafts were not immunologically attacked. These findings provide additional support for the islet specificity of the BB/Wor immune attack and are consistent with the conclusion that the inflammatory response to the islet grafts was not an allograft reaction.

Possible Role of B-Cell Ia Expression

Another important hypothesis which attempts to explain the B-cell specificity of the BB/Wor immune attack is the suggestion that pancreatic B-cells which are normally negative for Ia antigens [45, 46] can be induced to express these antigens. It is proposed that this (pathological) expression of Ia may then become an important initiating event leading to immune destruction of the B-cell [47, 48].

In preliminary studies conducted on pancreatic islet lesions in acutely diabetic and prediabetic animals we noted the presence of numerous infiltrating cells (? macrophages, dendritic cells) which were intensely positive for Ia antigens. The pancreatic islet cells were, however, negative for Ia [49].

An analysis of our results indicated that once an islet is heavily infiltrated with inflammatory cells, it is impossible to differentiate Ia^+ infiltrating macrophages from residual islet cells. Firstly, it is difficult or impossible to delineate the borders of individual cells within the 5-μm cryostat sections of pancreas. Secondly, the heavily infiltrated islet reveals (by electron microscopy) many examples of macrophages with intracellular phagocytosed B-cell debris (Fig. 1) [50]. Thus, the strategy employed by DEAN and BOTTAZZO [47, 48] to demonstrate the presence of B-cell Ia expression, by double-staining tissue sections for both insulin and Ia, might detect macrophages (Ia^+) which are also positive for insulin because of ingested fragments of dead B-cells. These images might be (and have been) incorrectly interpreted. By studying early islet lesions with a sparse inflammatory cell infiltrate and with confluent aggregates of surviving islet cells, it is possible to delineate inflammatory cells from the residual islet epithelial cells. Under these circumstances, B-cells are clearly not Ia^+ (Fig. 2).

More recently, we tested the hypothesis that the metabolic activity of the pancreatic B-cell plays a role in determining whether or not it will be the target of BB/

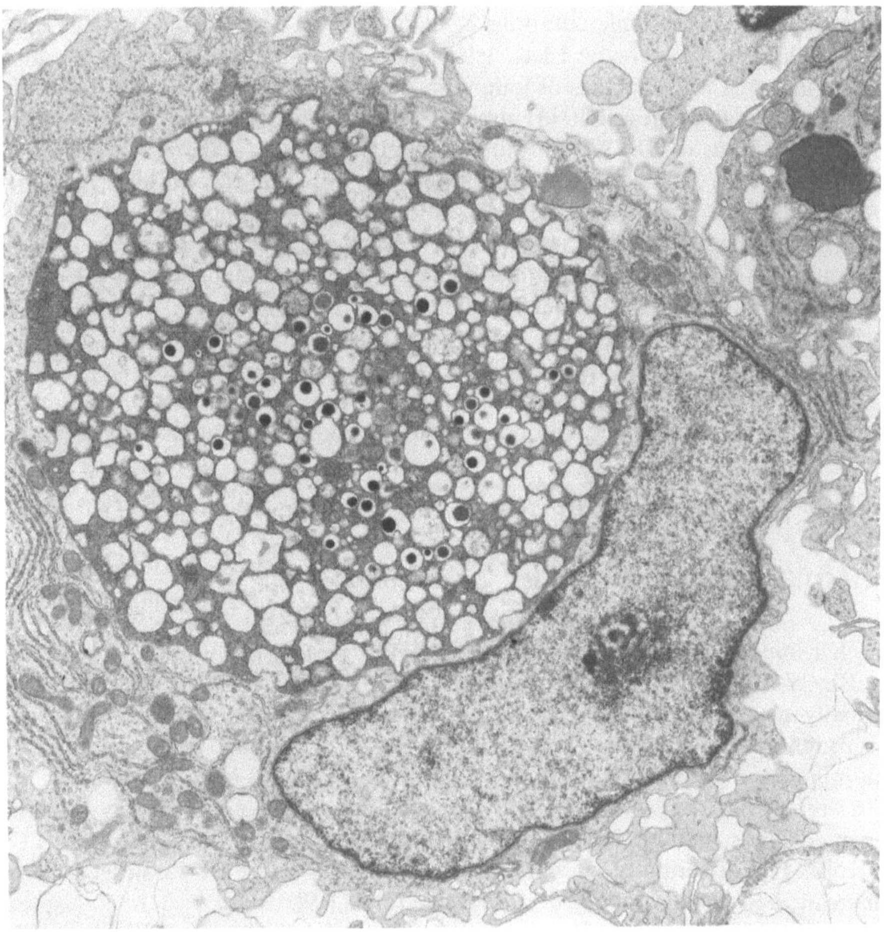

Fig. 1. This micrograph shows an example of B-cell degeneration and necrosis in acutely diabetic BB/Wor rats. The centrally located B-cell in this micrograph is more electron-dense than one would expect for a normal cell and evidences scattered dense bodies within the cytoplasm, as well as a general disarray of the cytoplasmic organelles. The cell is surrounded by the slender processes of a macrophage which is in close contact with two activated lymphocytes. ×10000

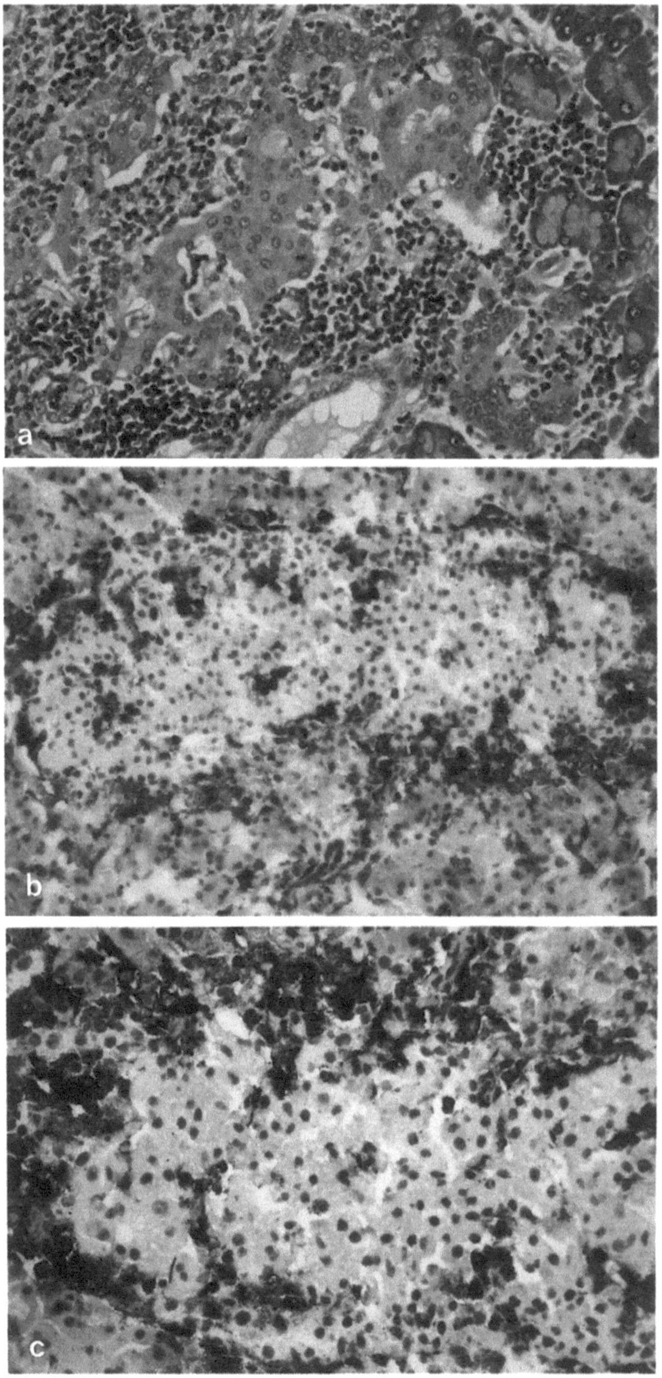

Fig. 2a–c. Photomicrographs of three early BB/Wor insulitis lesions. Section **a** is stained with HE and reveals a prominent lymphocytic infiltrate. Sections **b** and **c** are stained immunocytochemically for the presence of Ia antigen with MoAb OX6. The islets, from different rats, reveal variable degrees of inflammation but display recognizable surviving islet cells. Sections **b** and **c** reveal a predominantly peri-insular infiltrate with a less pronounced intraislet component. Ia^{+} cells are *dark brown* in this immunoperoxidase stain. The centrally located aggregates of islet cells are negative for Ia antigen. **a** ×170; **b** ×170; **c** ×264

Wor immune attack. More specifically we asked whether BB/Wor B-cells with decreased insulin biosynthesis would be protected from immune destruction. There was precedent for this hypothesis. It is known that mice genetically resistant to the diabetogenic effects of encephalomyocarditis (EMC) virus become susceptible to viral injury after the induction of obesity by gold thioglucose [51]. Furthermore, genetically obese mice (ObOb) are also more susceptible to EMC-induced diabetes [52]. Since the pancreatic B-cells of mice with spontaneous and induced obesity evidence increased insulin biosynthesis and mitotic activity, Craighead suggested that increased B-cell metabolic activity and replication may be responsible for enhanced susceptibility to viral injury [51, 52]. It has also been reported that the metabolic state of certain target cells influences their susceptibility to T-lymphocyte or NK-cell injury, presumably by inhibiting membrane repair processes and/or influencing effector-target cell binding [53]. It is also suspected that mitogenic stimuli may alter the expression of surface differentiation antigens. Stimulation of insulin secretion increases B-cell cytoplasmic calcium and potassium and is associated with B-cell membrane depolarization [54]. Stimulation of insulin secretion by glucose and glyburide decreases the number of intramembranous particles, increases the number and size of gap junctions, and may alter membrane lipid content [55]. Chronic hypoglycemia induced by exogenous insulin (or insulin-producing neoplasms) leads to inhibition of insulin biosynthesis, decreased B-cell size, insulin stores, and mitotic activity [56-59]. Finally, hypoglycemia-induced B-cell suppression inhibits alloxan-induced B-cell necrosis [60].

We therefore hypothesized that protracted hypoglycemia might prevent BB/Wor diabetes by decreasing B-cell antigenicity, or enhancing the B-cell's ability to withstand immunologic injury after effector cells have been attracted to the islet.

In preliminary experiments [61], DB-PRN rats were either uninjected or received increasing quantities of insulin (1.0-2.5 units protamine zine insulin subcutaneously/100 g body weight), from 35-45 to 120 days of age. Insulin was administered daily from Monday through Friday of each week. Body weights were recorded weekly and plasma glucose levels measured twice weekly. The results of the insulin injections are graphically recorded in Figs. 3 and 4. Figure 3 illustrates the mean body weights of the male rats and documents the more rapid weight gain of the insulin-treated animals. Mean plasma glucose (PG) levels are illustrated in Fig. 4. The lower PG levels of the insulin-treated rats are consistent and significant. Among untreated rats, 16 of 25 (64%) became diabetic. Of the insulin-treated animals, only one of 45 (2.2%) became diabetic ($p < 0.0001$). We examined the pancreatic islets of *five* nondiabetic rats during the course of insulin injections and *none* evidenced insulitis. Among 18 *non*diabetic rats followed for 30 days after the cessation of insulin treatment, none became diabetic. At autopsy, however, 11 of 18 revealed insulitis, although in five of these 11, the degree of insulitis was considered mild. WBC and differential counts were performed on 10 injected and uninjected rats (110-115 days of age) and flow cytometry performed on splenic lymphocytes of two injected and two uninjected rats (110-115 days of age). The injected and uninjected animals could not be differentiated on the basis of lymphocyte subsets, total white cell numbers, or differential counts (Tables 5, 6). Morphologically the pancreatic islets of insulin-treated hypoglycemic rats appeared to

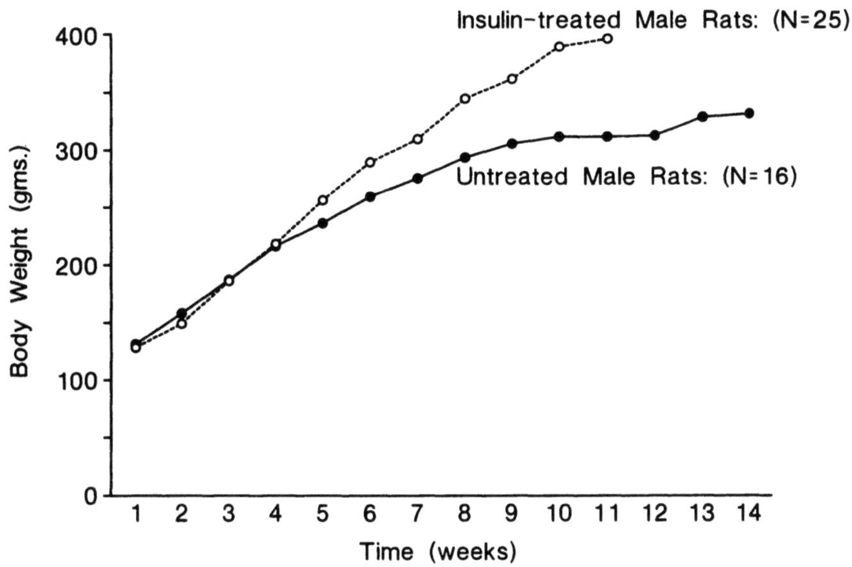

Fig. 3. Mean body weights of untreated and insulin treated BB/Wor rats. The differences were significant after 6 weeks of insulin injections ($p < 0.01$)

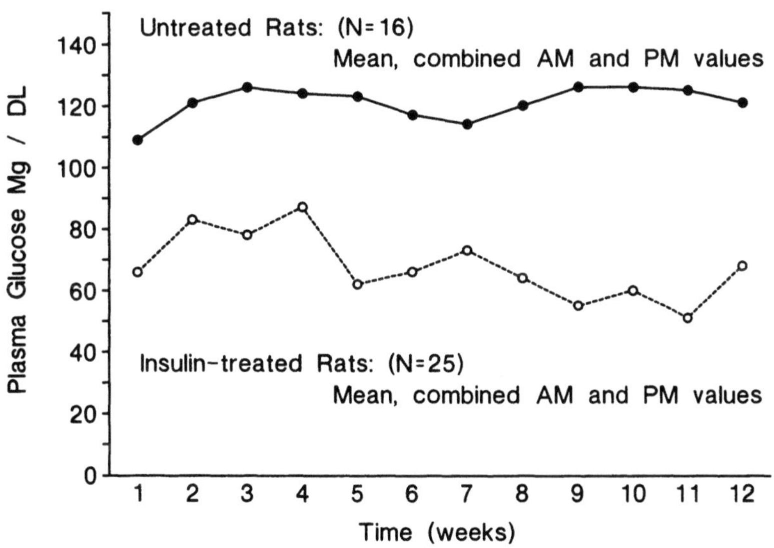

Fig. 4. Mean plasma glucose of untreated and insulin-treated rats. Mean values for insulin-injected rats were always significantly lower than those for uninjected rats ($p < 0.001$)

Table 5. Effects of insulin injections on peripheral white blood cells

Injections	WBC	Lymphocytes (%)	Polynuclears (%)	Eosinophils (%)	Total Lymphocytes
None ($n=12$)	9371 ± 881	62.3 ± 4.2	33.5 ± 3.8	4.2 ± 1.0	5381 ± 603
Insulin ($n=12$)	7070 ± 476*	68.9 ± 2.5	28.8 ± 2.3	2.3 ± 0.8	4842 ± 341

Data expressed as mean ± SEM
* $p<0.05$ insulin vs no injections

Table 6. Effects of insulin injections on peripheral blood lymphocyte subsets

Injections	$OX8^+/OX19^-$ (NK)	$OX8^-/OX19^+$ (H/I)	$OX8^+/OX19^+$ (C/S)	OX6
None ($n=7$)	7.5 ± 1.0	8.4 ± 0.5	0.6 ± .06	69.3 ± 2.6
Insulin ($n=7$)	9.9 ± 0.7	6.5 ± 0.3*	0.5 ± .03	63.6 ± 1.7

Data expressed as mean ± SEM (%) of positively stained cells
* $p<0.05$ insulin vs no injections

be biosynthetically suppressed. They were uniformly smaller and contained reduced stainable insulin, by immunocytochemistry, compared with uninjected normoglycemic rats (Fig. 5).

Conclusions

Although many of the uncertainties concerning the pathogenesis of diabetes among BB/Wor rats remain unresolved, the following conclusions are supported by the data presented above:

1. MoAb-induced reductions of NK-cells or helper T-lymphocytes protect against diabetes among lymphopenic diabetes-prone BB/Wor rats.
2. Although Ia^+ dendritic cells and macrophages infiltrate the islets during the early stages of the BB/Wor immune attack, pancreatic B-cells do not express Ia antigens. Hence, the explanation for the specificity of B-cell destruction remains to be established with certainty.
3. Exogenous insulin injections with resulting hypoglycemia reduce B-cell biosynthetic activity and protect against insulitis and diabetes. Although we suspect that suppression of B-cell insulin synthesis and storage alters effector cell activation and attraction for target B-cells and/or the susceptibility of B-cells to immunologic injury, it is possible that hypoglycemia per se generally and nonspecifically perturbs or suppresses the BB/Wor immune response.

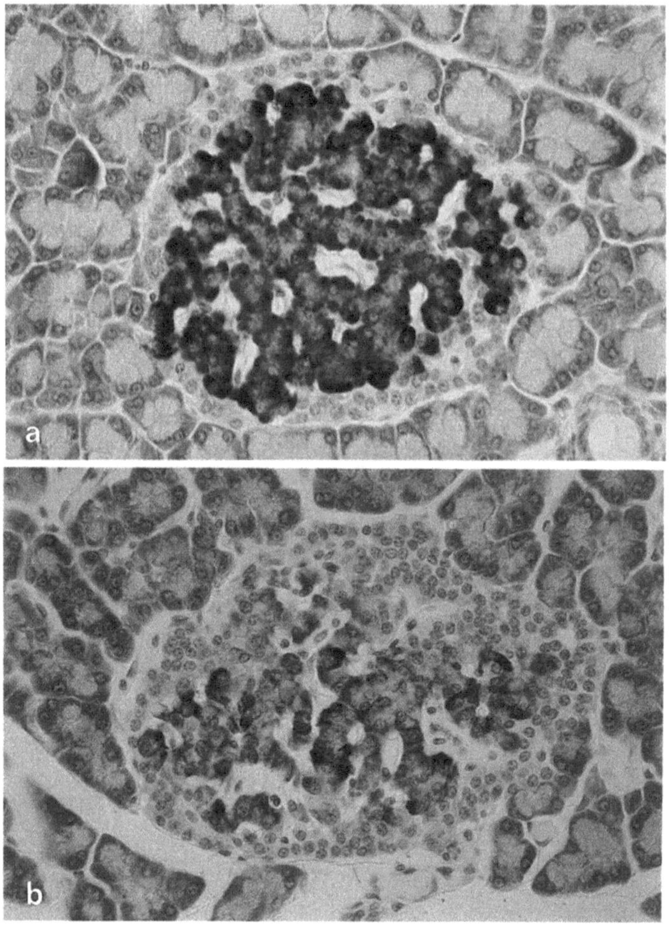

Fig. 5 a, b. Photomicrographs of pancreatic islets from untreated and insulin-injected hypoglycemic BB/Wor rats. Sections were stained immunocytochemically for insulin. **a** The islet from an uninjected normoglycemic rat depicts the expected size and insulin content *(brown cytoplasmic stain)* of normal B-cells. **b** The islet from an insulin-injected, hypoglycemic animal is comprised of smaller B-cells with decreased staining *(brown)* for stored insulin. The reduced size and insulin content of these B-cells is characteristic of animals with prolonged hypoglycemia. **a, b** × 264

References

1. Nakhooda AF, Like AA, Chappel CI, Murray FT, Marliss EB (1977) The spontaneously diabetic Wistar rat. Metabolic and morphologic studies. Diabetes 26: 100
2. Seemayer TA, Tannenbaum GS, Goldman H, Colle E (1982) Dynamic time course studies of the spontaneously diabetic BB Wistar rat. III. Light microscopic and ultrastructural observations of pancreatic islets of Langerhans. Am J Pathol 106: 237
3. Logothetopoulos J, Valiquette N, Madura E, Cvet D (1984) Onset and progression of pancreatic insulitis in the overt, spontaneously diabetic young adult BB rat studied by pancreatic biopsy. Diabetes 33: 33

4. Colle E, Guttmann RD, Seemayer T (1981) Spontaneous diabetes mellitus in the rat. I. Association with the major histocompatibility complex. J Exp Med 154: 1237
5. Like AA, Kislauskis E, Williams RM, Rossini AA (1982) Neonatal thymectomy prevents spontaneous diabetes in the BB/W rat. Science 216: 644
6. Like AA, Rossini AA, Guberski DL, Williams RM (1979) Spontaneous diabetes mellitus: reversal and prevention in the BB/W rat with antiserum to rat lymphocytes. Science 206: 1421
7. Like AA, Anthony M, Guberski DL, Rossini AA (1983) Spontaneous diabetes mellitus in the BB/W rat. Effects of glucocorticoids, Cyclosporin-A, and antiserum to rat lymphocytes. Diabetes 32: 326
8. Laupacis A, Stiller CR, Gardell G, Keown P, Dupre J, Wallace AC, Thibert P (1983) Cyclosporin prevents diabetes in BB Wistar rats. Lancet 1: 10
9. Like AA, DiRodi V, Thomas S, Guberski DL, Rossini AA (1984) Prevention of diabetes mellitus in the BB/W rat with Cyclosporin-A. Am J Pathol 117: 92
10. Rossini AA, Slavin S, Woda BA, Geisberg M, Like AA Mordes JP (1984) Total lymphoid irradiation prevents diabetes mellitus in the BioBreeding/Worcester (BB/W) rat. Diabetes 33: 543
11. Naji A, Silvers WK, Bellgrau D, Barker CF (1981) Spontaneous diabetes in rats: destruction of islets is prevented by immunological tolerance. Science 213: 1390
12. Naji A, Silvers WK, Bellgrau D, Anderson AO, Plotkins S, Barker CF (1981) Prevention of diabetes in rats by bone marrow transplantation. Ann. Surg 194: 328
13. Rossini AA, Mordes JP, Pelletier A, Like AA (1983) Transfusions of whole blood prevent spontaneous diabetes mellitus in the BB/W rat. Science 219: 975
14. Rossini AA, Faustman D, Woda BA, Like AA, Szymanski I Mordes JP (1984) Lymphocyte transfusions prevent diabetes in the BioBreeding/Worcester rat. J Clin Invest 74: 39
15. Koevary S, Rossini AA, Stoller W, Chick WL, Williams RM (1983) Passive transfer of diabetes in the BB/W rat. Science 220: 727
16. Like AA, Weringer EJ, Holdash A, McGill P, Atkinson D, Rossini AA (1985) Adoptive transfer of autoimmune diabetes mellitus in BioBreeding/Worcester (BB/W) inbred and hybrid rats. J Immunol 134: 1583
17. Koevary SB, Williams DE, Williams RM, Chick WL (1985) Passive transfer of diabetes from BB/W to Wistar-Furth rats. J Clin Invest 75: 1904
18. Jackson R, Rassi N, Crump T, Haynes B, Eisenbarth GS (1981) The BB diabetic rat. Profound T-cell lymphocytopenia. Diabetes 30: 887
19. Poussier P, Nakhooda AF, Falk JA, Lee C, Marliss EB (1982) Lymphopenia and abnormal lymphocyte subsets in the "BB" rat: relationship to the diabetic syndrome. Endocrinology 110: 1825
20. Bellgrau D, Naji A, Silvers WK, Markmann JF, Barker CF (1982) Spontaneous diabetes in BB rats: evidence for a T-cell dependent immune response defect. Diabetologia 23: 359
21. Elder ME, Maclaren NK (1983) Identification of profound peripheral T lymphocyte immunodeficiencies in the spontaneously diabetic BB rat. J Immunol 130: 1723
22. Guttman RD, Colle E, Michel F, Seemayer T (1983) Spontaneous diabetes mellitus syndrome in the rat. II. T-lymphopenia and its association with clinical disease and pancreatic lymphocytic infiltration. J Immunol 130: 1732
23. Naji A, Silvers WK, Kimura H, Bellgrau D, Markmann JF, Barker CF (1983) Analytical and functional studies on the T cells of untreated and immunologically tolerant diabetes-prone BB rats. J Immunol 130: 2168
24. Woda BA, Like AA, Padden C, McFadden M (1986) Deficiency of phenotypic cytotoxic-suppressor T lymphocytes in the BB/W rat. J Immunol 136: 856
25. Like AA, Biron CA, Weringer EJ, Byman K, Sroczynski E, Guberski DL (1986) Prevention of diabetes in BioBreeding/Worcester rats with monoclonal antibodies that recognize T lymphocytes or natural killer cells. J Exp Med 164: 1145
26. Elder M, Maclaren N, Riley W, McConnell T (1982) Gastric parietal and other autoantibodies in the BB rat. Diabetes 31: 313
27. Like AA, Appel MC, Rossini AA (1982) Autoantibodies in the BB/W rat. Diabetes 31: 816
28. Dyrberg T, Nakhooda AF, Baekkesov S, Lernmark A, Poussier P, Marliss EB (1982) Islet cell surface antibodies and lymphocytic antibodies in the spontaneously diabetic BB Wistar rat. Diabetes 31: 278

29. Pollard DR, Gupta K, Mancino L, Hynie I (1983) An immunofluorescence study of anti-pancreatic islet cell antibodies in the spontaneously diabetic BB Wistar rat. Diabetologia 25: 56
30. Dyrberg T, Poussier P, Nakhooda AF, Baekkeskov S, Marliss EB, Lernmark A (1984) Time course of islet cell surface antibodies in the diabetic syndrome of the "BB" Wistar rat. Diabetologia 26: 159
31. Baekkeskov S, Dyrberg T, Lernmark A (1984) Autoantibodies to a 64-Kilodalton islet cell protein precede the onset of spontaneous diabetes in the BB rat. Science 224: 1348
32. Martin DR, Logothetopoulos J (1984) Complement-fixing islet cell antibodies in the spontaneously diabetic BB rat. Diabetes 33: 93
33. Laborie C, Sai P, Feutren G, Debray-Sachs M, Poussier P, Marliss EB, Assan R (1985) Time course of cytotoxic islet-cell antibodies in diabetic and nondiabetic BB rats. Diabetes 34: 904
34. Like AA, Guberski DL, Butler L (1986) Diabetic BioBreeding/Worcester (BB/Wor) rats need not be lymphopenic. J Immunol 136: 3254
35. Weringer EJ, Like AA (1985) Immune attack on pancreatic islet transplants in the spontaneously diabetic BioBreeding/Worcester (BB/W) is not MHC restricted. J Immunol 134: 2383
36. Prowse SJ, Bellgrau D, Lafferty KJ (1986) Islet allografts are destroyed by disease occurrence in the spontaneously diabetic BB rat. Diabetes 35: 110
37. MacKay P, Jacobson J, Rabinovitch A (1986) Spontaneous diabetes mellitus in the BB/W rat: evidence in vitro for natural killer cell lysis of islet cells. J Clin Invest 77: 916
38. Woehrle M, Markmann JF, Silvers WK, Barker CF, Naji A (1986) Transplantation of cultured pancreatic islets to BB rats. Surgery 100: 334
39. Mandrup-Poulsen T, Bendtzen K, Nerup J, Dinarello CA, Svenson M, Nielson JH (1986) Affinity-purified human interleukin I is cytotoxic to isolated islets of Langerhans. Diabetologia 29: 63
40. Kiesel U, Oschilewski M, Kantwerk G, Maruta M, Hanenberg H, Triechel U, Kolb-Bachofen V, Hartung HP, Kolb H (1986) Essential role of macrophages in the development of type I diabetes in BB rats. Trans Proc 18: 1525
41. Weringer EJ, Like AA (1986) Diabetes mellitus in the BB/W rat. Insulitis in pancreatic islet grafts after transplantation in diabetic recipients. Am J Pathol 125: 107
42. Rossini AA, Williams RM, Mordes JP, Appel MC, Like AA (1979) Spontaneous diabetes in the gnotobiotic BB/W rat. Diabetes 28: 1031
43. Rossini AA, Mordes JP, Gallina DL, Like AA (1983) Hormonal and environmental factors in the pathogenesis of BB rat diabetes. Metabolism 32 [Suppl 1]: 33
44. Elliott RB, Martin JM (1984) Dietary protein: a trigger of insulin-dependent diabetes in the BB rat. Diabetologia 26: 297
45. Faustman D, Hauptfeld V, Davie JM, Lacy PE, Shreffler DC (1980) J Exp Med 151: 1563
46. Hart DNJ, Fabre JW (1981) Demonstration and characterization of Ia-positive dendritic cells in the interstitial connective tissues of rat heart and other tissues, but not brain. J Exp Med 153: 347
47. Dean BM, Walker R, Bone AJ, Cooke A, Bottazzo GF, Baird JD (1984) Development of diabetes in the BB/E rat: expression of class II molecules (Ia) in islet cells. Diabetologia 27: 269A
48. Bottazzo GF, Dean BM, McNally JM, MacKay EH, Swift MA, Gamble DR (1985) In situ characterization of autoimmune phenomena and expression of HLA molecules in the pancreas in diabetic insulitis. N Engl J Med 313: 353
49. Like AA, Forster RM, Woda BA, Rossini AA (1983) T cell subsets in islets and lymph nodes of BioBreeding/Worcester (BB/W) rats. Diabetes 32: 201A
50. Like AA (1985) Spontaneous diabetes in animals. In: Volk BW, Arquilla ER (eds) The diabetic pancreas. Plenum, 2nd ed. p 385
51. Craighead JE (1982) Viral islet injury. In: Mechanisms of beta cell injury. A state of the art workshop. Juvenile Diabetes Foundation International, p 37
52. D'Andrea BJ, Wilson GL, Craighead JE (1981) Effect of genetic obesity in mice on the induction of diabetes by encephalomyocarditis virus. Diabetes 30: 451
53. Kunkel LA, Welsh RM (1981) Metabolic inhibitors render resistant target cells sensitive to natural killer cell-mediated lysis. Int J Cancer 27: 73
54. McDaniel ML, Colca JR, Kotagal N, Lacy PE (1985) Regulation and role of intracellular

Ca^{2+} in insulin secretion by the beta cell. In: Volk BW, Arquilla ER (eds) The diabetic pancreas, Plenum, 2nd ed. p 213
55. Orci L, Perrelet A (1985) Morphology of membrane systems in pancreatic islets. In: Volk BW, Arquilla ER (eds) The diabetic pancreas. Plenum, 2nd ed. p 171
56. Logothetopoulos J, Kaneko M, Wrenshall GA, Best CH (1964) Zinc, granulation and extractable insulin of islet cells following hyperglycemia or prolonged treatment with insulin. In: Brolin SE, Hellman B, Knutson H (eds) The structure and metabolism of the pancreatic islets, eds. Pergamon, Oxford, p 333
57. Turner RC, Johnson PC (1973) Suppression of insulin release by fish insulin induced hypoglycemia. Lancet I: 1483
58. Horowitz DC, Rubenstein AH, Reynolds C, Molnar GD, Yanaihara N (1975) Prolonged suppression of insulin release by insulin-induced hypoglycemia: demonstration by C-peptide assay. Horm. Metab. Res. 7: 449
59. Chick WL, Warren S, Chute RN, Like AA, Lauris V, Kitchen KC (1977) A transplantable insulinoma in the rat. Proc Natl Acad Sci 74: 628
60. Appel MC, Chick WL, Rossini AA (1981) Sensitivity of suppressed islet B-cells to alloxan. Diabetologia 21: 243
61. Like AA (1986) Insulin injections prevent diabetes (DB) in BioBreeding/Worcester (BB/Wor) rats. Diabetes 35: 74a

Rat Models of Non-Insulin-Dependent Diabetes Mellitus: Evidence that Mild Increases in Plasma Glucose Play an Important Role in Pathogenesis*

J. L. Leahy, S. Bonner-Weir and G. C. Weir

Introduction

The pathogenesis of non-insulin-dependent diabetes mellitus (NIDDM) has been the subject of debate for many years, and it still remains poorly understood [55, 82]. Current dogma states that it is a heterogeneous disorder; indeed, several patients have now been identified with mutant insulins [63, 69] or one of a variety of syndromes characterized by abnormal insulin receptors, extreme insulin resistance, and acanthosis nigricans [16, 17, 29]. Also, in some series, up to 10% are islet cell antibody-positive [14]. However, these groups together represent only a small minority of those with NIDDM, and while new syndromes will probably be described in the future, it seems reasonable to assume that the bulk of patients share a common etiology.

It has been known for years that defects in insulin secretion and action are both present in NIDDM, but no consensus yet exists as to which occurs first, or how the two are related. Moreover, this issue will likely not be resolved in the near future, for both defects are well established by the time glucose tolerance is impaired, and at present there is no way to identify an earlier stage of the disease.

Animal models, then, play an important role in our efforts at reconstructing the events which culminate in NIDDM. We have found in rats that if one reduces the B-cell mass, defects in insulin secretion and action develop which in many ways resemble those described in human diabetes. This review will provide support for our contention that an absolute or relative reduction in B-cell mass and/or function is a critical element in the pathogenesis of NIDDM.

NIDDM: Background Considerations

Abnormalities of Insulin Secretion

The insulin secretion abnormalities which have been described in NIDDM include the following:

* This work has been supported by grant AM-35449 (formerly AM-20349) from the National Institutes of Health, and 185296 from the Juvenile Diabetes Foundation. Dr. Leahy is the recipient of a Research and Development Award from the American Diabetes Association.

1. Fasting insulin levels are sometimes reported to be elevated, especially when subjects with mild glucose intolerance are studied [3]. However, when their hyperglycemia is taken into account, it becomes clear that the insulin levels are really inappropriately low [27, 74]. On the other hand, absolute fasting hypoinsulinemia has not been convincingly described [31].
2. The most characteristic B-cell defect is loss of the first-phase insulin response to an intravenous glucose challenge [11, 62]. Second-phase release, on the other hand, tends to be preserved, but cannot be considered truly normal [78].
3. In contrast to the glucose insensitivity, B-cell responsiveness to nonglucose secretagogues such as arginine, isoproterenol, secretin, and glucagon remains relatively intact [13, 27, 48].
4. Glucose potentiation of the response to nonglucose secretagogues is impaired. Normally, an agent like arginine causes a much larger release of insulin when it is given at a high versus low glucose concentration; in NIDDM, this effect is considerably reduced [27, 78].

In summary, the ability of glucose to influence insulin secretion is selectively impaired in NIDDM, similar to what has been described in the early stages of IDDM [20].

Islet Pathology in NIDDM

The B-cell mass in NIDDM becomes a fundamental question, for if one believes that insulin resistance is the initial defect in this disease, then a compensatory increase in B-cell mass would be expected. The ideal study to address this question would determine the B-cell mass in many subjects with various degrees of glucose intolerance; this is a formidable task which probably awaits development of a noninvasive procedure which can be used antemortem. On the other hand, several small studies using established techniques have been published which together comprise a sizeable number of patients, and all but one of these reached the same conclusion, namely that in NIDDM islets are smaller and the B-cell mass is about 60% of that in nondiabetic control subjects [22, 43, 60, 67, 84]. In addition, the lone dissenting paper which found no difference in B-cell mass between NIDDM and nondiabetics is called into question because of its small number of subjects and failure to control for the effects of obesity [53]. Interestingly, although not a lot of data are available, it seems that this reduction may be specific for B-cells in that the other islet cells appear relatively preserved [60]. The cause of the B-cell loss is not known, but we suspect that it plays a central role in the development of NIDDM.

Other morphologic findings have been described including islet fibrosis and amyloid deposition along the capillaries, but their significance is not clear [23].

Insulin Resistance in NIDDM

Over the past 15 years, so much work has focused on insulin resistance in NIDDM that many believe this is the primary defect. In fact, fundamental gaps still remain in our understanding of it.

Obesity is a well-known cause of insulin resistance [47], and this clearly plays a role for most patients. On the other hand, the majority of obese individuals never develop glucose intolerance, which suggests that their B-cells have the capacity to fully compensate. One can argue therefore that obesity in NIDDM simply acts to unmask an underlying B-cell inadequacy.

Clearly, insulin resistance also occurs in nonobese NIDDM patients, and it is generally accepted that the most important cause is a so-called postbinding defect in insulin action [73]. A fundamental issue then is could this be secondary to B-cell dysfunction? This question has been addressed in man by trying to determine if it reverses when the diabetic state is normalized with insulin treatment; indeed, partial reversal has now been demonstrated in several studies [1, 21, 61] although complete return to normal sensitivity is rare. This suggests that B-cell failure does play an important role in the insulin resistance, but other factors must also be involved.

Definitions of the Animal Models

The first two models were designed to study the consequences of a reduced B-cell mass. More recently, a third has been added in which hyperglycemia can be produced in normal rats using chronic glucose infusions.

Neonatal Streptozotocin Rat

Two-day-old male Sprague-Dawley rats are injected with 90 mg/kg streptozotocin intraperitoneally [4] which causes marked B-cell destruction such that their plasma glucose concentration at 4 days of age averages 345 ± 15 mg/dl (Fig. 1); we always check it at this time and only follow those pups with values greater than 275 mg/dl. Partial B-cell regeneration then occurs, presumably accompanied by increased insulin release so that by 10 days of age their plasma glucose has returned to a value that usually can't be differentiated from controls. At 4 weeks of age, one is hard pressed to identify individual neonatal streptozotocin (NSZ) rats from control rats based on body weight or random plasma glucose or insulin measurements, but small differences are demonstrable when large populations are compared [72]. On the other hand, overt glucose intolerance to a meal challenge and an intraperitoneal glucose tolerance test is present. By 6 weeks of age, unequivocal hyperglycemia in the fed state has developed which is then chronically maintained at about 200 mg/dl. Mild hypoinsulinemia also becomes established by this time, with fed values that average 30%–70% of controls [4].

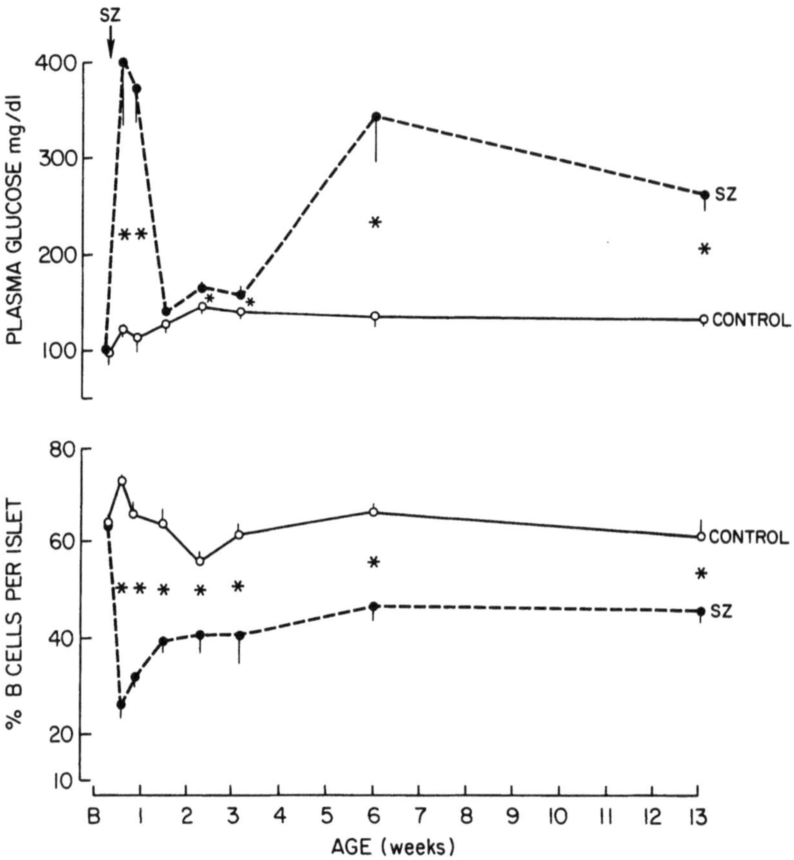

Fig. 1. A time course of fed plasma glucose values and the percentage of B-cells per islet in the NSZ model *(SZ)*. The *top panel* shows the plasma glucose values as determined from blood sampled by cardiac puncture up to 16 days of age, and then by tail snipping. The same animals were used in the morphometric quantitation shown in the *bottom panel*. As a reflection of the B-cell mass, the percentage of B-cells was counted in the first 12 islets in immunoperoxidase-stained, random paraffin sections. As in all the following figures, data points are mean ± SEM. *Top panel $2p \leq 0.05$, *bottom panel $2p \leq 0.02$. (Reproduced with permission of *Diabetes* and the American Diabetes Association, Inc. [4])

A variation of this model has been described by PORTHA and coworkers in which 100 mg/kg streptozotocin is given intravenously to pups of both sex on the day of birth [51]. Their level of hyperglycemia in adulthood is somewhat less than that described above, but otherwise these rats show similar defects in glucose tolerance and glucose-induced insulin release [52].

Both of these models suffer from the drawback of using streptozotocin. Although we believe that its dominant effect is to lower the B-cell mass, questions persist about other possible long-term effects, since it has been associated with DNA damage [85] and is also known to inhibit insulin release acutely through an unknown mechanism [70]. To get around these concerns, we studied another model in which the B-cell mass is reduced surgically.

90% Pancreatectomy Rat

Foglia [18] described a method for pancreatectomy in the rat in which the tissue is removed by gentle abrasion. We modified this technique to perform a 90% pancreatectomy in 4- to 5-week-old male Sprague-Dawley rats by removing all of the pancreas except for an anatomically defined remnant bordered by the common bile duct and the first duodenal loop [6]. This portion contains 12.0% ± 0.5% of the pancreatic weight and 9.7% ± 1.0% of the insulin content.

Four days later, mild hyperglycemia is present which then rises over the next few days to reach 160-180 mg/dl as compared to 140 mg/dl in the controls; the plasma glucose concentration is then chronically maintained at this level. At no time have we found any difference in body weight or plasma insulin measurements between the 90% pancreatectomy (Px) rats and the sham-operated controls. Six weeks postoperatively, glucose tolerance to a meal challenge and an intraperitoneal glucose tolerance test are both markedly impaired.

The Px model allows one to lower the B-cell mass without having to worry about lingering effects from a chemical toxin. In addition, the anatomical definition of the remnant insures that the degree of pancreatectomy is constant from rat to rat so that variability within the model is minimal. Finally, the method can presumably be adapted fairly easily in the future to allow other levels of subtotal pancreatectomy.

Chronic Glucose Infusions

A long-term aim of this work is to identify factors that contribute to the insulin secretion defects which follow a reduction in B-cell mass. One hypothesis is that hyperglycemia initially occurs, and that chronic exposure of the remaining cells to it eventually results in changes in function which are characterized by loss of glucose responsiveness. Therefore, to examine the effects of chronic hyperglycemia on insulin secretion in normal rats, we adapted the glucose infusion method of Cole and Logothetopoulos [12]. Male Sprague-Dawley rats weighing 200-250 g are infused intravenously using a syringe pump and an infusion device consisting of a swivel above the cage and a hollow metal cable attached to the rat by way of a metal neck ring and velcro vest such that the rats are unrestrained and have free access to food and water [38]. To date, we have infused 20%, 30%, 35%, and 50% glucose at 2 ml/h for up to 96 h; controls get 0.45% NaCl in the same way. The plasma glucose concentration in glucose-infused rats tends to rise quickly and peak within 24 h, but then falls such that rats given 50% glucose average 447 ± 36 mg/dl at 24 h vs only 166 ± 7 mg/dl after 96 h infusion [39]. A similar pattern is seen in rats given 35% glucose with a rise to 305 ± 16 mg/dl after 24 h, but then return to a value not different from that of controls by 72 h. The plasma insulin concentration also rises quickly, averaging 12.1 ± 1.28 ng/ml after 24 h in rats given

50% glucose and 11.3 ± 0.01 ng/ml in those given 35% glucose, in contrast to a value of 1.16 ± 0.25 ng/ml seen in the controls. It also falls, but more slowly, so that at 96 h plasma insulin levels are still 7 times normal in the 50% group and 4 times normal in 35% animals.

This model offers several advantages. One can address an issue which is fundamental in diabetes research: what are the consequences of chronic hyperglycemia? Also, one can easily vary the level of hyperglycemia and length of infusion period, making it possible to control the experimental conditions precisely. Moreover, the infusion can be turned off so that recovery from the effects of chronic hyperglycemia can be studied.

Morphology and B-Cell-Mass

Neonatal Streptozotocin Rat

B-cell mass was estimated at numerous time points after the streptozotocin injection by counting B- and non-B-cells in the first 12 islets encountered on slides stained by immunoperoxidase techniques [4]. We believe that this method gives a reasonable estimate of B-cell mass, since data for 4 days and 6 weeks were similar when comparing this method and the more rigorous point-counting method of Weibel [80].

At 4 days of age (48 h following streptozotocin) the rise in plasma glucose to 345 ± 15 mg/dl was accompanied by a fall in B-cell percentage per islet to a nadir of 27%, compared to 73% in controls (Figure 1). By 10 days of age, the plasma glucose returned to normal and the B-cell proportion per islet reached 40%. Mitotic figures were frequent in the NSZ islets at this time. Since all the islets had reduced B-cell cores, the replenishment of B-cells seems to be mainly from replication of existing B-cells rather than from neogenesis or new formation of islets. Following 10 days of age, the B-cell percentage per islet remained at about 40% (compared to 60% in controls). With the more rigorous morphometric protocol, the B-cell mass was 49% of the controls at 6 weeks of age and 34% of controls at 10 weeks of age, while the non-B-cell mass did not differ from controls at either age.

In the adult NSZ rats (6 weeks and older), the islets are smaller than in controls; the non-B-cell mantle is several cells thick and without gaps, in contrast to the control islets, which have a discontinuous mantle one to two cells thick. In these older rats, there is an increase in the number of B-cells with hypertrophied nuclei [83].

After the marked destruction of B-cells by streptozotocin, there is partial replenishment of the B-cell mass but it does not return to normal. In fact, as the control animals double their B-cell mass (from 6 to 10 weeks of age), the NSZ rats fall further behind, even though their B-cell mass continues to increase in that time period. When 10-week-old animals are treated with dexamethasone (0.125 mg/kg intramuscularly) for 13 days, there are increases in islet size, B-cell number per islet, and pancreatic insulin concentration in control rats; however, there are no such increases when dexamethasone-treated and untreated NSZ rats are compared [5]. This lack of further increase in the NSZ animals may be a result of an alteration in growth capacity or simply another manifestation of glucose blindness.

B-cell destruction has been documented ultrastructurally in the variation used by PORTHA and coworkers [15]. They report little or no replication of remaining B-cells but significant formation of islets budding from ducts [10]. They may have missed dividing B-cells due to the scoring of mitotic figures only in immunofluorescent B-cells, for many B-cells may be degranulated and hence not scored. Nevertheless, an important fact becomes clear when viewing the two variations: the timing of the streptozotocin injection and how it coincides with the normal development of the islets may influence not only the extent of regeneration but also its mode.

90% Pancreatectomy Rat

At 8-12 weeks postoperatively the portion of the control pancreas which corresponds to the remnant left in the Px rats still averages 10.5% ± 1.0% of the pancreatic weight and 10.3% ± 0.9% of the insulin content [6]. On the other hand, the pancreatic tissue in Px rats has attained 26% of the pancreatic weight and 32% of the insulin content of controls, showing that pancreatic growth has accelerated in this model. This finding is further reflected in the B-cell mass (measured by point-counting morphometrics) which now averages 42% of control, and the non-B-cell mass which is 47%. Morphologically, the islet tissue is more heterogeneous than controls, with four distinct configurations seen: (1) normal-appearing islets making up the bulk, (2) enlarged islets with a seemingly lowered ratio of non-B-cells to B-cells, (3) small islets which contain almost exclusively B-cells, and (4) enlarged fibrotic islets that show disorganization of the usual mantle-core relationship. This fibrosis is found only in the islet and perinsular region, none being seen in the exocrine acini.

There is massive regeneration of exocrine and endocrine tissue after the partial pancreatectomy. In Px animals, the accumulated mitotic frequency of B-cells after colchicine treatment is increased fourfold at 3 and 7 days as compared to sham-operated controls, and it is still increased twofold at 21 days [7]. At 7 days, even though there is only mild hyperglycemia (166 ± 7 vs 143 ± 4 mg/dl), the cell birth rate (number of new cells per hundred cells per 24 h) of the Px animals is 10-fold higher than the shams and comparable to that of fetal rat pancreas [68].

To study if additional manipulations could further enhance this growth of B-cells, pancreatectomized animals (Px + 2 weeks) were given ventromedial hypothalamic (VMH) lesions [8], which are known to increase islet size and cause hyperinsulinemia and hyperphagia [19, 26]. Four weeks after the VMH lesions, the B-cell mass was increased almost twofold in both control and Px rats. Thus, the already extensive growth of islet tissue in the Px model can be further enhanced by a neural mechanism, even though the increase is quantitatively less than in the controls.

Chronic Glucose Infusions

The glucose infusion model was introduced in our laboratory only recently, so few morphological studies have been done as yet. After 4 days of 50% glucose infusion, the accumulated mitotic frequency of B-cells has increased fivefold compared to that of B-cells from saline-infused rats (BONNER-WEIR, unpublished observation) even though the plasma glucose levels are only slightly elevated. Interestingly, animals with a normal B-cell mass before the infusion now had a 50% increase after 4 days of 50% glucose infusion when compared to those that received saline, showing that the B-cells in 7- to 8-week-old rats have a tremendous capacity for growth.

Other morphological studies using a similar model have been reported by LOGOTHETOPOULOS and colleagues. They reported in rats whose plasma glucose levels averaged 300-500 mg/dl that B-cell degranulation is evident after 7 h infusion and even more marked at 24 h [41]. Furthermore, they found that mitotic activity of B-cells peaked at 3 days with a 14-fold increase over that seen in controls [9]. Unfortunately, most of their histologic data focused on isolated islets, so that it is difficult to obtain a complete picture.

Insulin Secretion

Neonatal Streptozotocin Rat

B-Cell Responsiveness to Glucose and Nonglucose Secretagogues

Insulin secretion studies have been carried out primarily in 8- to 14-week-old rats using a modification of the in vitro perfused pancreas technique of PENHOS et al. [49] in which the pancreas is perfused in situ with Krebs-Ringer bicarbonate buffer containing 4% dextran and 0.1% bovine serum albumin.

In the first protocol, the insulin response to a glucose increase from 7.8 to 21 m*M* (140 to 375 mg/dl) was compared with that to 10 m*M* arginine (Fig. 2). The control rats showed typical biphasic release to both; in contrast, an insulin response was seen only with arginine in the NSZ group. We attempted to overcome the glucose insensitivity with higher glucose levels (41.9 m*M*) and repeated glucose challenges (priming) but saw no increase in insulin release. On the other hand, a glucose increase from 4.5 to 41.9 m*M* in the presence of 5 m*M* theophylline did cause a definite increase in insulin output in NSZ rats, although its magnitude was much less than that in controls, showing that B-cells in this model are not completely glucose-blind [81].

In contrast to the glucose insensitivity, insulin responses have been described to many of the classical nonglucose agents, including arginine, leucine, isoproterenol, tolbutamide, and 3-isobutyl-1-methylxanthine (IBMX) [24, 25, 81], and while some disagreement exists about quantitative results, there is universal agreement that the B-cells in this model retain their responsiveness to nonglucose secretagogues.

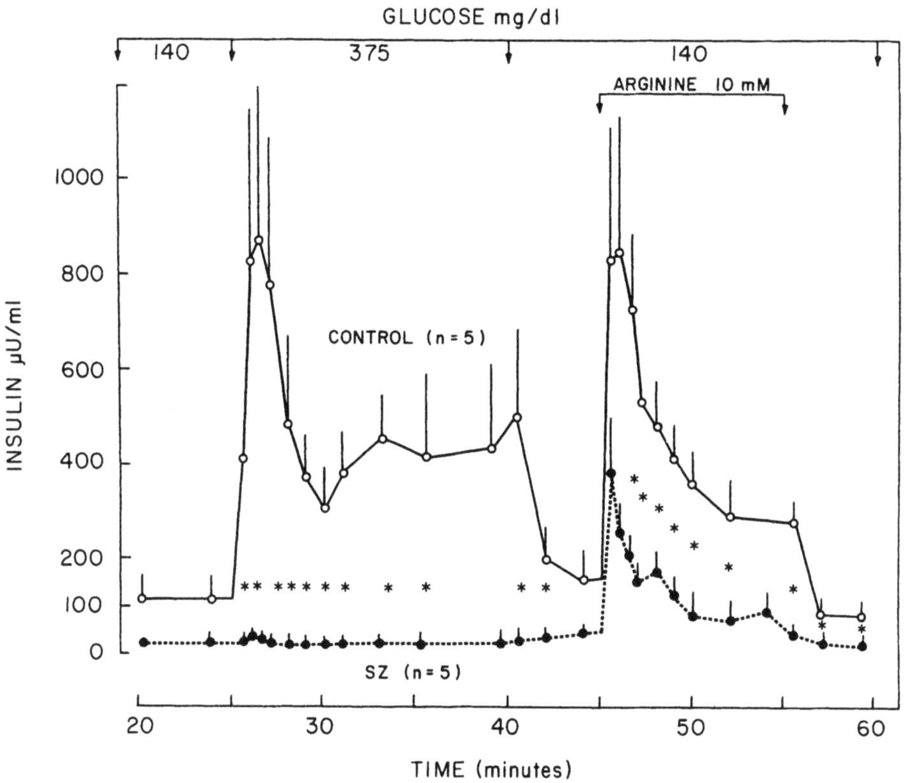

Fig. 2. Effects of glucose and 10 m*M* arginine on insulin secretion in NSZ rats *(SZ)* and control rats assessed using the in vitro isolated perfused pancreas. *2$p \leq 0.05$. (Reproduced with permission of *Diabetes* and the American Diabetes Association, Inc. [81])

An interesting parallel to these results has been the discovery that insulin release in NSZ rats also fails to fall appropriately when the glucose concentration is reduced [35]. A decrease in the perfusate glucose concentration from 11.1 to 2.8 m*M* caused the insulin secretory rate in control rats to fall rapidly to a level that approached the sensitivity of the assay; in the NSZ rats, a paradoxical stimulation was seen. On the other hand, epinephrine and somatostatin, normally potent inhibitors of insulin release, caused similar qualitative suppression in both groups.

Taken together, these results show that the B-cells in the NSZ model are essentially blind to changes in the glucose concentration, while nonglucose responses are preserved. This sounds very similar to what has been described in human diabetes; however, differences do exist. In Fig. 2, for instance, it is clear that both first- and second-phase release to the high glucose challenge are absent, while only first-phase defects are classically described in NIDDM. The reason for this disparity is not clear, nor is its significance. As the human studies were carried out in vivo, one possibility may be that second-phase glucose-induced insulin release is differently expressed in this environment. It may also simply reflect a species difference. The discrepancy does seem important and requires further attention.

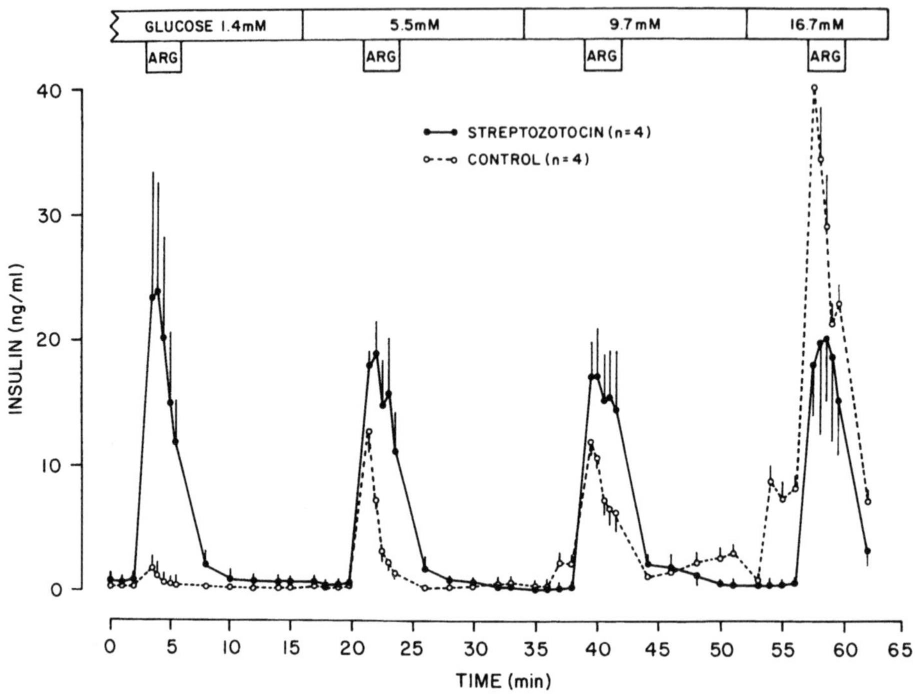

Fig. 3. Effects of varying glucose concentrations on the insulin response to a 10 m*M* arginine stimulus in NSZ and control rats assessed using the in vitro isolated perfused pancreas. (Reproduced with permission of *Diabetes* and the American Diabetes Association, Inc. [36])

Glucose Potentiation of the B-Cell Response to Nonglucose Secretagogues

Glucose normally modulates the insulin response to most nonglucose secretagogues so that the amount of insulin released increases in a linear fashion over a glucose range from 2.8 to 16.7 m*M*. We studied glucose modulation of arginine-stimulated insulin release in the NSZ model by giving 10 m*M* arginine at 1.4, 5.5, 9.7, and 16.7 m*M* glucose (Fig. 3). As expected, the insulin response in controls increased as the level of background glucose rose; in contrast, all of the responses in the NSZ group were brisk and essentially equal [36]. We have found similar results with another nonglucose agent, IBMX, so that in addition to loss of glucose-induced insulin release in this model, glucose modulation of non-glucose-mediated insulin secretion is also severely impaired.

Reversibility of B-Cell Defects

We hypothesized that chronic exposure of the remaining B-cells to abnormally high glucose levels had caused their glucose insensitivity. Indeed, the link seemed most obvious with the inability of glucose to potentiate arginine-stimulated insulin secretion, for the B-cells responded to arginine as if the glucose level were high, no matter what it truly was. We tested this hypothesis by lowering the plasma glucose for 24 h with insulin injections, and then studied glucose potentiation with the perfused pancreas [37]. NSZ and control rats received 20 U/kg ultralente insulin subcutaneously at 9 a.m. and 10 U/kg at 5 p.m. The next morning, the plasma glucose concentration in the NSZ group averaged 101 ± 9 mg/dl and in controls 99 ± 8 mg/dl, considerably less than the 131 ± 44 mg/dl measured in the untreated control rats. The perfused pancreas protocol and results are shown in Fig. 4. As previously described, arginine caused marked insulin responses in the untreated NSZ rats at both glucose concentrations; in contrast, the results in the insulin-treated NSZ rats were very similar to those of both control groups, so that glucose potentiation was returned virtually to normal. This provides strong evidence in support of the hypothesis that chronic hyperglycemia was responsible for this secretory defect.

It is equally clear from Fig. 4 that the response to 16.7 m*M* glucose alone was not improved in the treated NSZ rats. One possibility, which we favor, is that chronic hypoglycemia produced by the insulin treatment had a suppressive effect. Consistent with this possibility was the finding that glucose-induced insulin release was reduced 80% in control rats given insulin. We therefore cannot conclude from this study whether hyperglycemia is playing any role in this secretory defect or, whether once established, it is reversible.

B-Cell Responsiveness in 4-Week-Old NSZ Rats

We wondered if the modest level of hyperglycemia in 4-week-old NSZ rats (151 ± 6 vs 133 ± 4 mg/dl in controls) would also be associated with abnormal insulin secretion. No measurable insulin response was seen to an intraperitoneal glucose tolerance test; in contrast, a meal challenge caused equivalent rises in both the NSZ and control groups [72]. Paralleling these results, glucose-induced insulin release assessed with the perfused pancreas was absent, while that to arginine persisted. Portha and Kergoat [50] have demonstrated in their model that an unequivocal insulin response to glucose is present at 3 weeks of age. Taken together, these results suggest that this secretory defect becomes fully established during the time when the plasma glucose is only very modestly elevated.

90% Pancreatectomy Rat

Although the B-cell abnormalities in the NSZ model were reminiscent of what has been described in human diabetes, the possibility that they resulted from some long-term effect of streptozotocin remained. We therefore studied the B-cell responsiveness in a second model in which B-cell mass was reduced surgically with a 90% partial pancreatectomy. The results were in fact quite similar.

The insulin response caused by a glucose increase from 6.7 to 16.7 m*M* (120 to 300 mg/dl) was compared to that from 10 m*M* arginine (Fig. 5) [6]. The controls showed the typical biphasic response to both stimuli; in contrast, no response to the high glucose was seen in Px rats as opposed to that from arginine which was similar in both groups when the B-cell mass was taken into account. In a second

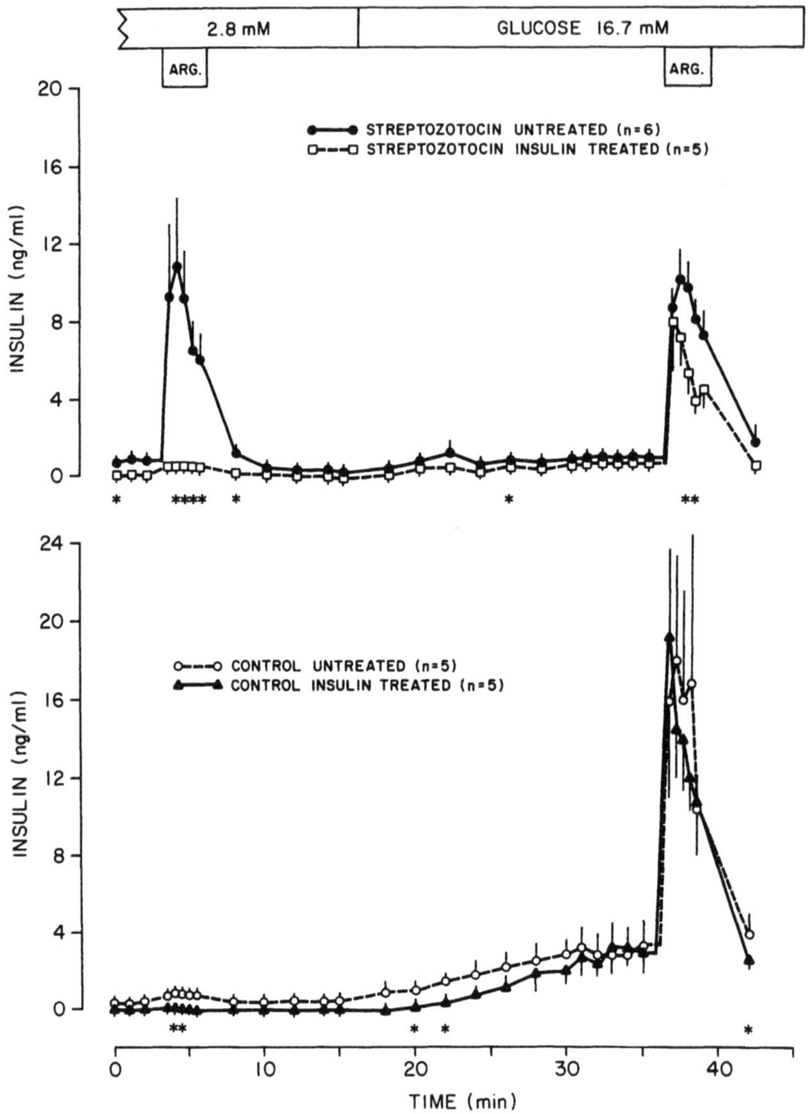

Fig. 4. Effects of 24 h insulin treatment on the insulin response to 16.7 m*M* glucose and glucose potentiation of arginine-stimulated insulin release in NSZ and control rats assessed using the in vitro isolated perfused pancreas. $*2p < 0.05$. (Reproduced with permission of *Diabetes* and the American Diabetes Association, Inc. [37])

protocol, glucose potentiation of arginine-stimulated insulin release was tested by giving 10 m*M* arginine at 2.8 and 16.7 m*M* glucose [36]. The response at the low glucose background was similar in both groups (0.5 ± 0.2 ng/ml in Px rats vs 0.4 ± 0.2 ng/ml in controls). On the other hand, the ability of glucose to potentiate release was markedly reduced in the Px rats, where the response averaged only 3.2 ± 2.6 ng/ml vs 17.3 ± 1.9 ng/ml in controls. Therefore, although impaired, a

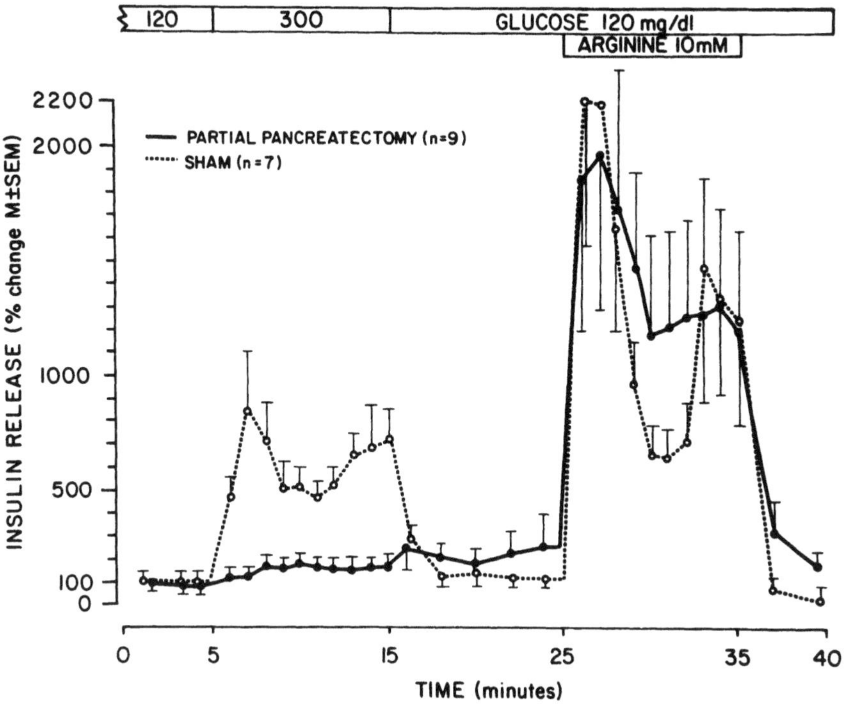

Fig. 5. Effects of glucose and 10 m*M* arginine on insulin secretion in Px and sham-operated control rats assessed using the in vitro isolated perfused pancreas. For ease in comparing the groups, the data are expressed as percent change from baseline rather than as the absolute quantity of insulin released. (Reproduced with permission of *Journal of Clinical Investigation*. [6])

potentiating effect of glucose was still demonstrable. This pattern more closely resembles that described in NIDDM [27, 78] rather than the total absence noted in the NSZ model.

Therefore, a selective glucose insensitivity is also present in Px rats. On the other hand, the absence of a marked response to arginine when given at a low glucose concentration, coupled with the fact that Px rats are less hyperglycemic than the NSZ model, leads us to hypothesize that perhaps two kinds of B-cell defects occur with chronic hyperglycemia: a loss of glucose-stimulated insulin release with barely detectable levels of hyperglycemia, and a defect in potentiation which only becomes severe with greater degrees of glycemia.

Chronic Glucose Infusions

B-Cell Responsiveness to Glucose

The findings in the NSZ and Px models provided strong evidence for an association between a reduction in B-cell mass and subsequent abnormalities in the function of the remaining B-cells, and it was decided to test further the hypothesis that chronic hyperglycemia was the link between the two, employing another approach. We therefore developed a way of causing varying levels of hyperglycemia in normal rats, using an adaption of the glucose infusion method of COLE and LOGOTHETOPOULOS [12].

Initially rats were infused for 48 h with various glucose concentrations; 20% glucose caused no discernable hyperglycemia at the end of the infusion period, but the plasma glucose was raised 18 mg/dl in the 30% group, 37 mg/dl in the 35% group, and 224 mg/dl in the 50% group. On the other hand, plasma insulin levels were similar in all the glucose-infused rats [38].

In the first perfusion protocol, the direct effect of glucose on insulin secretion was studied by decreasing the concentration in the perfusate from 16.7 to 2.8 mM

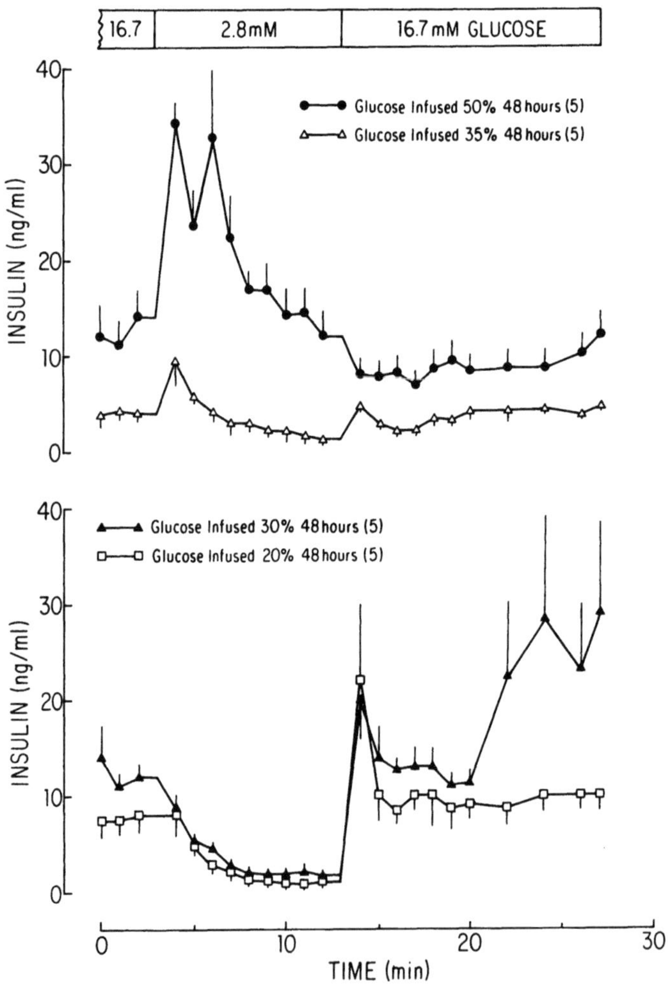

Fig. 6. Effects of an acute reduction and then increase in perfusate glucose concentration on insulin secretion in rats infused with 20%, 30%, 35%, or 50% glucose for 48 h assessed using the in vitro isolated perfused pancreas. (Reproduced with permission of *Journal of Clinical Investigation.* [38])

for 10 min, and then returning it to 16.7 m*M* (Fig. 6). The insulin release pattern in the 20% rats was essentially identical to that of saline-infused controls (not shown), showing rapid suppression following the glucose reduction and a biphasic response when the high glucose was returned. In the 30% rats, the response to the high glucose was potentiated. In the 35% group, in contrast, it was severely blunted, and in the most hyperglycemic 50% rats, return of the high glucose had no effect at all on insulin release. Therefore, glucose-induced insulin secretion was strikingly impaired in the rats with the greatest hyperglycemia, which provides strong evidence in support of our hypothesis. It is also apparent from Fig. 6 that the 50% rats had a marked, transient, paradoxical insulin response following the glucose reduction. We have previously seen this phenomenon in the NSZ model [35], and although the mechanism is not known, its appearance suggests that the pathophysiologic events in the two groups are identical.

We then examined the effects of a longer infusion period, 96 h, to see if the secretory defects evolved further in any of the groups [39]. These studies were complicated by the interesting finding that a constant level of hyperglycemia was not maintained in the glucose-infused rats. Instead, plasma glucose levels decreased with time, so that in the 50% group, for instance, it averaged 166 ± 7 mg/dl after 96 h as opposed to 361 ± 24 mg/dl at 48 h. Moreover, in the 30% and 35% rats, the value fell back to normal by 72 h. Nonetheless, the same protocol as shown in Fig. 6 was repeated, and the results in all groups were remarkably similar at both time points. Several possibilities come to mind to explain these findings. For instance, once established, perhaps the B-cell defects are not reversible, or reverse very slowly. Experiments have been done to address this question and will be discussed below.

Glucose Potentiation of Arginine–Stimulated Insulin Secretion

In a second protocol, glucose potentiation was studied in animals infused for 48 h, with 10 m*M* arginine given at 2.8 and 16.7 m*M* glucose (Fig. 7) [38]. The results in the 20% rats were identical to those of the saline controls (not shown) at all time points, as were those of the 30% group except for increased release to the 16.7 m*M* glucose alone. In contrast, arginine-stimulated insulin release at 2.8 m*M* glucose was markedly increased in the 35% rats and an even greater rise was seen in the 50% rats, while that at 16.7 m*M* glucose was equal in all groups. Therefore, paralleling the impaired effect of glucose to directly alter insulin secretion, glucose modulation of arginine-stimulated insulin release was also markedly altered in the most hyperglycemic groups. A similar series of experiments was carried out after 96-h infusions, and the results were essentially identical [39]. It should be noted that the pattern of release in the most hyperglycemic rats is very reminiscent of what we found in the NSZ rats (Fig. 3), which lends further credence to our belief that the pathophysiology is similar in both models.

An interesting finding is that the quantitative response to arginine at 2.8 m*M* glucose in the 50% group far exceeded that in the controls at 16.7 m*M* glucose, even though pancreatic insulin content was reduced by more than 60%. This strongly suggests that under most circumstances the quantitative response to a stimulus is not limited by reduced insulin stores.

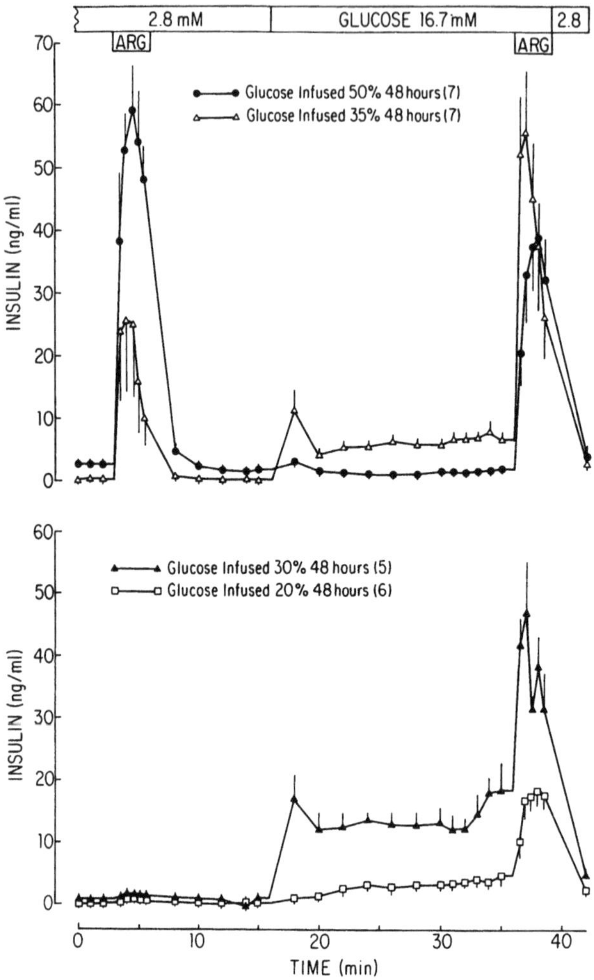

Fig. 7. Effects of glucose and 10 m*M* arginine on insulin secretion in rats infused with 20%, 30%, 35%, or 50% glucose for 48 h assessed using the in vitro isolated perfused pancreas. (Reproduced with permission of *Journal of Clinical Investigation*. [38])

Reversibility of B-Cell Defects

The glucose infusion model allows a unique opportunity to study reversibility of secretory defects, for the infusion can simply be stopped and the pancreas perfused some time later. We infused a group of rats for 48 h with 50% glucose and then removed them from the infusion devices and studied them 72 h later with the perfusion protocol shown in Fig. 6 [38]. Glucose-induced insulin secretion was now identical to that of noninfused control rats in that the paradoxical stimulation following the glucose reduction and the failure to respond to the high glucose were no longer present. Therefore, these defects were fully reversible.

In a second set of experiments, we wished to determine whether the abnormal B-cell responses might take up to 72 h to reverse, which could explain why they persisted with 96 h infusions even though plasma glucose was considerably lower. We infused rats with 50% glucose for 48 h and then added 4.6 m*M* phloridzin to the syringes during the next 48 h [39]. Phloridzin inhibits renal tubular reabsorption of glucose, thereby causing glycosuria [66], this effect being most pronounced in animals with preexisting hyperglycemia, so that in these animals plasma glucose tends to fall, while in normal animals it usually does not change. Indeed, plasma glucose levels in the 50% rats given phloridzin at the end of the 96-h infusion period now averaged 140 ± 10 mg/dl vs 151 ± 5 mg/dl in the saline-infused control rats given phloridzin (P = NS). A study with the perfused pancreas using the protocol of Fig. 6 then showed that B-cell responsiveness to glucose was restored to normal in the 50% group. Moreover, the secretory pattern in the saline rats given phloridzin remained similar to that of rats given 0.45% NaCl alone, which argues against a direct effect of the drug to alter B-cell function when used at this dose.

These results therefore suggest that during a period of overt hyperglycemia in the rat, B-cell secretory defects completely evolve within 48 h, and their severity depends on the level of glycemia reached. Once established, they are then maintained by some effect of the infusion even as plasma glucose levels fall. One might wonder if a metabolic consequence of hyperinsulinemia is the cause at this time, but this seems unlikely, for we have found similar secretory defects in the NSZ model which is hypoinsulinemic. Instead, the results with phloridzin strengthen the likelihood that the abnormal secretion is maintained because of persistent although less severe hyperglycemia during the later parts of the 96-h infusion period. Indeed, the fact that 35% rats have plasma insulin levels at 96 h that are 4 times normal even though their plasma glucose concentration is not obviously abnormal seems consistent with this view. These experiments raise the possibility that chronic increases in plasma glucose that are so small as to be hard to measure with established techniques may still be perceived by B-cells as a toxic environment.

Insulin Resistance

Neonatal Streptozotocin Rat

It has been known for years that a severe reduction in B-cell mass results in insulin resistance [33, 57], but the more pertinent question for our studies was whether a more modest decrease such as that seen in the NSZ model would be associated with a similar impairment. We examined conversion of ^{14}C-glucose to ^{14}Co^{2} in isolated adipocytes from 6-week-old NSZ rats, and found that insulin's effect to stimulate it was impaired, and that the dose-response curve suggested a so-called post-binding defect [72]. These results were later confirmed by LEVY et al. [40] who found using an in vivo technique that glucose disposal was markedly reduced in the presence of a high circulating plasma insulin level. A critical question, then, is: when does the insulin resistance develop in this model? Studies have been carried out with adipocytes in 4-week-old NSZ rats and the results were essentially identical, so that the resistance seems to evolve at a time when the level of glycemia is barely abnormal, averaging 151 ± 6 mg/dl in fed NSZ rats vs 133 ± 4 mg/dl in controls [72].

Our results, however, have been called into question by the observations of KERGOAT and PORTHA [30], who did not find insulin resistance in their model using the glucose clamp technique. Specifically, they found that the suppressive effect of insulin on hepatic glucose production was increased, and peripheral glucose uptake when measured at their usual glucose level was comparable to that of controls. The reason for this disparity is not known, but the fact that KERGOAT and PORTHA's model is less hyperglycemic may be an important variable. In support of this idea, BEVILACQUA et al. [2] have recently described a model in which mild hyperglycemia and hypoinsulinemia is caused by streptozotocin in dogs such that fasting plasma glucose levels averaged 200 ± 34 mg/dl vs 104 ± 2 in controls, and plasma insulin was 15 ± 2 μU/ml as opposed to 21 ± 2 in the controls. They found defects in hepatic glucose production and peripheral glucose uptake when assessed with the glucose clamp technique that in many ways mirror those described in NIDDM, so that the bulk of evidence would seem to suggest that mild hyperglycemia and hypoinsulinemia is associated with insulin resistance.

90% Pancreatectomy Rat

ROSSETTI et al. [59], have reported preliminary data in which insulin resistance has been found in the Px model using the glucose clamp technique. Moreover, they showed that insulin sensitivity returned to normal following treatment with phloridzin, which normalized the plasma glucose level without changing the plasma insulin. These results implicate chronic hyperglycemia as the cause of the insulin resistance in this model. Indeed, it is clear that glucose transport into brain, a non-insulin-mediated process, decreases as the plasma glucose is raised [45], and it certainly seems plausible that insulin-mediated glucose transport such as that into muscle may similarly be involved.

The bulk of evidence, then, suggests that insulin resistance does result from a modest B-cell reduction, and that it can occur even when the level of glycemia is mild and plasma insulin values are relatively preserved. These findings are reminiscent of what has been described in mild NIDDM. Relative hypoinsulinemia is present at this time, although absolute hypoinsulinemia is rare, and we suspect that some metabolic consequence of this deficiency, such as hyperglycemia [75], or another factor, such as elevated free fatty acid levels [54], causes the insulin resistance.

Discussion

The studies in this review have attempted to define the functional consequences of a reduced B-cell mass, hoping that this would provide insight into the pathophysiologic disturbances which characterize diabetes mellitus in man. We have found results which closely resemble what has been described in NIDDM, including abnormal patterns of insulin secretion and insulin resistance. Also, a substantial body of information has been accumulated which indicates that chronic exposure of cells to modest elevations of plasma glucose (such as that seen in 4-week-old NSZ rats) is a critical factor in the development of each of these.

It seems reasonable to hypothesize that similar events occur in man, and that chronic hyperglycemia is an important pathogenic factor in human diabetes. Consistent with this possibility, both insulin secretion [74, 76] and insulin resistance [1, 21, 61] have been shown to improve in many subjects with NIDDM after a period of close diabetic control. However, B-cell secretory defects have also been described in IDDM at a time when plasma glucose seems to be normal [20, 65]. How could a normal or imperceptibly raised plasma glucose level alter B-cell function? A thermostat analogy seems relevant. An air-conditioned room in either Texas or Vermont can be maintained at 72° F, but the work of the Texas air conditioner must be far higher than the one in Vermont. Likewise, in IDDM as the B-cell mass shrinks, but before the onset of clinical disease, the work required of the remaining cells in order to maintain euglycemia must include increased release from each functioning cell. What this continued stress does to B-cell function is not known; we continue to wonder whether, in the absence of hyperglycemia, it of itself is sufficient to eventually cause B-cell dysfunction.

Another possibility could be that the plasma glucose is actually not normal, but raised to a degree so small as to be imperceptible. Implicit in this idea is the notion that fasting plasma glucose in normal individuals is very tightly controlled even though physiologic oscillations are seen [34], so that a rise in this value by as little as 5 mg/dl, an amount generally regarded as trivial, represents a major derangement of the homeostatic control mechanisms. Our results in the 4-week-old NSZ rats suggest that major alterations in B-cell function can be associated with very minor degrees of hyperglycemia [72]. One might also envisage other ways in which subtle abnormalities in glucose homeostasis could act, such as through an alteration in the amplitude or duration of the plasma glucose oscillation cycle.

Following the B-cell reduction in both the NSZ and Px models, a period of accelerated B-cell growth is seen such that partial replenishment occurs. This observation raises many important questions. What is the signal that tells the original B-cells to replicate, or new islets to form, and why isn't it sustained such that full restoration occurs? What is the functional capacity of the newly regenerated B-cells with regard to insulin secretion and biosynthesis? Is a similar regenerative process present in man, and is it influenced by age? Clearly, much needs to be learned about the processes which influence B-cell growth.

Insulin resistance also occurs in the NSZ and Px models, and the data from the 4-week-old NSZ rats suggests that it develops when plasma glucose is barely abnormal. It is probably metabolic in origin, with some of the potential mechanisms already having been discussed. It is clear that mild glucose intolerance in man is also associated with insulin resistance [3], and it is hoped that investigation into the molecular abnormalities in our models will provide valuable clues to help unravel the cause of the defects in human diabetes.

Based on these results, we can construct a model that predicts the sequence of events that may occur during the development of both NIDDM and IDDM

(Fig. 8). Initially, the original B-cell pool is reduced. This may result from autoimmune destruction such as presumably occurs in the earliest stages of IDDM, or by a gradual decline which might occur with aging in NIDDM. Perhaps an abnormal gene in NIDDM somehow leads to an inability to maintain normal B-cell mass. Some individuals may have a genetically predetermined mild reduction in mass that usually would not be sufficient to cause any overt abnormality, but if insulin resistance such as occurs with obesity is superimposed, then hyperglycemia develops with its attendant effects on insulin secretion. In any event, as the original pool declines, regeneration presumably takes place and the mass remains near-normal even in the face of a substantial depletion of the original pool. Eventually, however, the total mass of B-cells would be reduced in an absolute or relative sense, and we suggest that a mass of 70%-80% of normal is likely to be associated with a rise in blood glucose that may appear trivial, but, as discussed earlier,

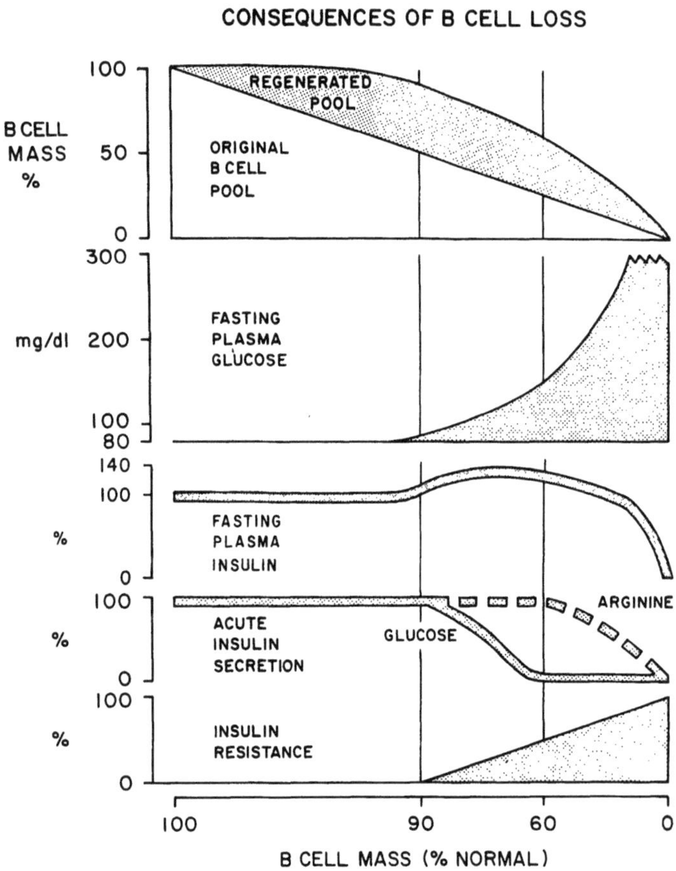

Fig. 8. A hypothetical scheme as to how a progressive decline in B-cell mass might lead to the sequential appearance of the known abnormalities found in human diabetes. It is based on data obtained from animal models, the results of studies carried out in man, and our own best guesses. Elaboration upon this pathogenic progression can be found in the text. (Reproduced with permission of *Diabetes/Metabolism Reviews.* [83])

means that the normal compensatory mechanisms of the B-cell have been overcome.

In this early stage, the plasma insulin level may actually increase, a characteristic termed the "horseshoe phenomenon" [3, 56], which probably means that each unit of B-cell mass, or perhaps each individual cell, is chronically secreting much more insulin than normal. The cause of this hyperinsulinemia is not completely known, but the most attractive explanation is that insulin resistance is present. Another possibility is that some of the secreted immunoreactive material has reduced biologic activity. Consistent with this idea, some investigators have reported that the ratio of proinsulin to insulin is increased in NIDDM [44].

Altered B-cell secretory function also occurs early and is characterized by failure to respond to an acute glucose challenge. During these early stages, the insulin response to a variety of nonglucose agents remains relatively preserved, but the ability of glucose to potentiate these is also abnormal. Recently, a great deal of interest has focused on the possibility that glucose potentiation may become abnormal prior to glucose-induced insulin release, and it has been suggested that quantifying it may represent the most sensitive test for picking up early B-cell damage and/or loss [46, 79]. As the B-cell mass continues to fall to the point where severe hyperglycemia develops, the response to nonglucose secretagogues is also diminished and eventually disappears. Fasting plasma insulin levels also fall in these advanced stages.

Insulin resistance occurs early and probably contributes substantially to the rise in glucose level that occurs as the functional capacity of the dwindling B-cells fails. Once overt hyperglycemia becomes established, insulin resistance as determined by an increase in hepatic glucose output seems to play the dominant role in determining the level of glycemia reached [3, 58, 64].

How does B-cell exhaustion fit into this picture? The word "exhaustion" has many meanings and implications, so that its use in this context needs to be carefully defined. Exhaustion could be either functional or structural. Certainly, insulin secretion is very abnormal in diabetes, and one could consider the loss of glucose-induced insulin secretion to be an example of functional exhaustion. Indeed, there is good evidence in man for functional exhaustion - assumed to be functional because there is no reason to evoke a structural explanation - for several studies show an enhanced insulin response to oral glucose in NIDDM following a sustained reduction in plasma glucose achieved with various treatments [21, 28, 32]. Other evidence supporting the exhaustion concept was generated decades ago with the observation that partially pancreatectomized cats given injections of anterior pituitary extract developed diabetes, and if the injections were continued long enough, the diabetes persisted after the injections were stopped [42].

Evidence for the existence of structural exhaustion is more difficult to find. The term "hydropic degeneration" was used for many years, but modern techniques have shown that it represents an artifact which results from extraction of B-cell glycogen by the histological methods used [71]. We are not aware of any convincing evidence showing that B-cell mass is reduced by the presence of chronic hyperglycemic "stress", but must admit that we have not yet rigorously looked for it in our models. We do have the impression that the B-cell mass of NSZ rats is not substantially lower at 12 months than it is at 2 months. It is possible that structural exhaustion does occur in diabetic Chinese hamsters and *db/db* mice, for the B-cell mass of these models does become severely reduced with time [77]. However, it is not clear whether these changes are due to hyperglycemia or some unknown genetic mechanism.

In summary, we suggest that a reduction in B-cell mass which is sufficient to cause alterations in glucose homeostasis eventually results in defects in B-cell function and insulin sensitivity that closely resemble those described in human diabetes. The available evidence points to chronic exposure of cells to very modest elevations in plasma glucose as being an important pathogenic factor in human diabetes.

Acknowledgements. The authors thank A. ROSENSTEIN and S. SKVORAK for preparation of this manuscript.

References

1. Andrews WJ, Vasquez B, Nagulesparan M, Klimes I, Foley J, Unger R, Reaven GM (1984) Insulin therapy in obese, non-insulin-dependent diabetes induces improvements in insulin action and secretion that are maintained for two weeks after insulin withdrawal. Diabetes 33: 634-642
2. Bevilacqua S, Barrett EJ, Smith D, Simonson DC, Olsson M, Bratusch-Marrain P, Ferrannini E, DeFronzo RA (1985) Hepatic and peripheral insulin resistance following streptozotocin-induced insulin deficiency in the dog. Metabolism 34: 817-825
3. Bogardus C, Lillioja S, Howard BV, Reaven G, Mott D (1984) Relationships between insulin secretion, insulin action, and fasting plasma glucose concentration in nondiabetic and noninsulin-dependent diabetic subjects. J Clin Invest 74: 1238-1246
4. Bonner-Weir S, Trent DF, Honey RN, Weir GC (1981) Responses of neonatal rat islets to streptozotocin: limited B-cell regeneration and hyperglycemia. Diabetes 30: 64-69
5. Bonner-Weir S, Trent DF, Zmachinski CJ, Clore ET, Weir GC (1981) Limited B-cell regeneration in a B-cell deficient rat model: studies with dexamethasone. Metabolism 30: 914-918
6. Bonner-Weir S, Trent DF, Weir GC (1983) Partial pancreatectomy in the rat and subsequent defect in glucose-induced insulin release. J Clin Invest 71: 1544-1554
7. Bonner-Weir S, Brockenbrough JS, Weir GC (1985) Discordance of exocrine and B cell growth following partial pancreatectomy. Diabetes 34: 169 A
8. Bonner-Weir S, Deery D, Weir GC (1986) Growth of regenerating islet tissue is enhanced by VMH lesions. Diabetes 35: 97 A
9. Brodsky GM, Kern HF, Logothetopoulos J (1972) Ultrastructure, mitotic activity and insulin biosynthesis of pancreatic beta cells stimulated by glucose infusions. Fed Proc 31: 250
10. Cantenys D, Portha B, Dutrillaux MC, Hollande E, Roze C, Picon L (1981) Histogenesis of the endocrine pancreas in newborn rats after destruction by streptozotocin: an immunocytochemical study. Virchows Arch B 35: 109-122
11. Cerasi E, Luft R (1967) The plasma insulin response to glucose infusion in healthy subjects and in diabetes mellitus. Acta Endocrinol 55: 278-304
12. Cole E, Logothetopoulos J (1974) Glucose oxidation ($^{14}CO_2$ production) and insulin secretion by pancreatic islets isolated from hyperglycemic and normoglycemic rats. Diabetes 23: 469-473
13. Deckert T, Lauritsen UB, Madsen SN, Morgensen P (1972) Insulin response to glucose, tolbutamide, secretin, and isoprenaline in maturity-onset diabetes mellitus. Dan Med Bull 19: 222-226
14. DiMario U, Irvine WJ, Borsey DQ, Kyner JL, Weston J, Galfo C (1983) Immune abnormalities in diabetic patients not requiring insulin at diagnosis. Diabetologia 25: 392-395

15. Dutrillaux MC, Portha B, Roze C, Hollande E (1982) Ultrastructural study of pancreatic B-cell regeneration in newborn rats after desctruction by streptozotocin. Virchows Arch B 39: 173-185
16. Flier JS, Young JB, Landberg L (1980) Familial insulin resistance with acanthosis nigricans, acral hypertrophy and muscle cramps. N Engl J Med 303: 970-973
17. Flier JS, Eastman RC, Minaker KL, Matteson D, Rowe JW (1985) Acanthosis nigricans in obese women with hyperandrogenism: characterization of an insulin-resistant state distinct from the type A and B syndromes. Diabetes 34: 101-107
18. Foglia VG (1944) Caracteristicas de la diabetes en la rata. Rev Soc Argent Biol 20: 21-37
19. Frohman LA, Bernardis LL, Schnatz JD, Burek L (1969) Plasma insulin and triglyceride levels after hypothalamic lesions in weanling rats. Am J Physiol 216: 1496-1501
20. Ganda OP, Srikanta S, Brink SJ, Morris MA, Gleason RE, Soeldner JS, Eisenbarth GS (1984) Differential sensitivity to beta cell secretagogues in "early" type I diabetes mellitus. Diabetes 33: 516-521
21. Garvey WT, Olefsky JM, Griffin J, Hamman RF, Kolterman OG (1985) The effect of insulin treatment on insulin secretion and insulin action in type II diabetes mellitus. Diabetes 34: 222-234
22. Gepts W (1957) Contribution à l'étude morphologique des ilots de Langerhans au cours du diabète. Ann Soc R Sci Med Natur Brux 10: 5-108
23. Gepts W, LeCompte PM (1981) The pancreatic islets in diabetes. Am J Med 70: 105-115
24. Giroix MH, Portha B, Kergoat M, Balbe D, Picon L (1983) Glucose insensitivity and amino acid hypersensitivity of insulin release in rats with non-insulin-dependent diabetes: a study with the perfused pancreas. Diabetes 32: 445-451
25. Grill V, Rundfeldt M (1986) Abnormalities of insulin response after ambient and previous exposure to glucose in streptozotocin-diabetic and dexamethasone-treated rats. Role of hyperglycemia and increased B-cell demands. Diabetes 35: 44-51
26. Hales CN, Kennedy GC (1964) Plasma glucose, non-esterified fatty acid and insulin concentrations in hypothalamic-hyperphagic rats. Biochem J 90: 620-624
27. Halter JB, Graf RJ, Porte D Jr (1979) Potentiation of insulin secretory responses by plasma glucose levels in man: evidence that hyperglycemia in diabetes compensates for impaired glucose potentiation. J Clin Endocrinol Metab 48: 946-954
28. Hidaka H, Nagulesparan M, Klimes I, Clark R, Sasaki H, Aronoff SL, Vasquez B, Rubenstein AH, Unger RH (1982) Improvement of insulin secretion but not insulin resistance after short term control of plasma glucose in obese type II diabetes. J Clin Endocrinol Metab 54: 217-222.
29. Kahn CR, Flier JS, Bar RS, Archer JA, Gorden P, Martin MM, Roth J (1976) The syndrome of insulin resistance and acanthosis nigricans: insulin receptor disorders in man. N Engl J Med 294: 739-745
30. Kergoat M, Portha B (1985) In vivo hepatic and peripheral insulin sensitivity in rats with non-insulin-dependent diabetes induced by streptozotocin. Assessment with the insulin-glucose clamp technique. Diabetes 34: 1120-1126
31. Kingston ME, Skoog WC (1986) Maintenance of basal insulin secretion in severe non-insulin-dependent diabetes. Diabetes Care 9: 232-235
32. Kosaka K, Kuzuya T, Akanuma Y, Hagura R (1980) Increase in insulin response after treatment of overt maturity-onset diabetes is independent of the mode of treatment. Diabetologia 18: 23-28
33. Kosuga M, Akanuma Y, Iwamoto Y, Kosaka K (1978) Insulin binding and glucose metabolism in adipocytes of streptozotocin-diabetic rats. Am J Physiol 235: E175-E182
34. Lang DA, Matthews DR, Peto J, Turner RC (1979) Cyclic oscillations of basal plasma glucose and insulin concentration in human beings. N Engl J Med 301: 1023-1027
35. Leahy JL, Weir GC (1985) Unresponsiveness to glucose in a streptozotocin model of diabetes: inappropriate insulin and glucagon responses to a reduction of glucose concentration. Diabetes 34: 653-659
36. Leahy JL, Bonner-Weir S, Weir GC (1984) Abnormal glucose regulation of insulin secretion in models of reduced B-cell mass. Diabetes 33: 667-673
37. Leahy JL, Bonner-Weir S, Weir GC (1985) Abnormal insulin secretion in a streptozotocin model of diabetes: effects of insulin treatment. Diabetes 34: 660-666

38. Leahy JL, Cooper HE, Deal DA, Weir GC (1986) Chronic hyperglycemia is associated with impaired glucose influence on insulin secretion. A study in normal rats using chronic in vivo glucose infusions. J Clin Invest 77: 908-915
39. Leahy JL, Cooper HE, Weir GC (1987) Impaired insulin secretion associated with near-normoglycemia. A study in normal rats using 96 hour in vivo glucose infusions. Diabetes 36: 459-464
40. Levy J, Gavin JR, Fausto A, Gingerich RL, Avioli LV (1984) Impaired insulin-action in rats with non-insulin-dependent diabetes. Diabetes 33: 901-906
41. Logothetopoulos J, Kaneko M, Wrenshall GA, Best CH (1964) Zinc, granulation and extractable insulin of islet cells following hyperglycemia or prolonged treatment with insulin. In: Brolin SE, Kellman B, Knutson K (eds) The structure and metabolism of the pancreatic islets. Pergamon, Oxford
42. Lukens FDW, Dohan FC (1942) Pituitary-diabetes in the cat: recovery following insulin or dietary treatment. Endocrinology 30: 175-202
43. Maclean N, Ogilvie RF (1955) Quantitative estimation of the pancreatic islet tissue in diabetic subjects. Diabetes 4: 367-376
44. Mako ME, Starr JI, Rubenstein AH (1977) Circulating proinsulin in patients with maturity onset diabetes. Am J Med 63: 865-869
45. Matthaei S, Horuk R, Olefsky JM (1986) Blood-brain glucose transfer in diabetes mellitus: decreased number of glucose transporters at blood-brain barrier. Diabetes 35: 1181-1184
46. McCulloch DK, Raghu PK, Klaff LJ, Koerker DJ, Palmer PJ (1985) Impaired glucose potentiation of arginine-stimulated insulin release is a sensitive and reliable marker of B-cell damage. Diabetes 34: 85A
47. Olefsky JM, Kolterman OG (1981) Mechanisms of insulin resistance in obesity and noninsulin-dependent (type II) diabetes. Am J Med 70: 151-168
48. Palmer JP, Benson JW, Walter RM, Ensinck JW (1976) Arginine-stimulated acute phase of insulin and glucagon secretion in diabetic subjects. J Clin Invest 58: 565-570
49. Penhos JC, Wu CH, Basabe JC, Lopez N, Wolff FW (1969) A rat pancreas-small gut preparation for the study of intestinal factor(s) and insulin release. Diabetes 18: 733-738
50. Portha B, Kergoat M (1985) Dynamics of glucose-induced insulin release during the spontaneous remission of streptozotocin diabetes induced in the newborn rat. Diabetes 34: 574-579
51. Portha B, Levacher C, Picon L, Rosselin G (1974) Diabetogenic effect of streptozotocin in the rat during perinatal period. Diabetes 23: 889-895
52. Portha B, Levacher C, Picon L, Rosselin G (1974) Diabetogenic effect of streptozotocin in the rat during perinatal period. Diabetes 23: 889-895
52a. Portha B, Picon L, Rosselin G (1979) Chemical diabetes in the adult rat as the spontaneous evolution of neonatal diabetes. Diabetologia 17: 371-377
53. Rahier J, Goebbels RM, Henquin JC (1983) Cellular composition of human diabetic pancreas. Diabetologia 24: 366-371
54. Randle PJ, Garland PB, Hales CN, Newholne EA (1963) The glucose fatty-acid cycle: its role in insulin sensitivity and the metabolic disturbances of diabetes mellitus. Lancet 1: 785-789
55. Reaven GM (1984) Insulin secretion and insulin action in non-insulin-dependent diabetes mellitus: which defect is primary? Diabetes Care 7 [Suppl 1]: 17-24
56. Reaven G, Miller R (1968) Study of the relationship between glucose and insulin responses to an oral glucose load in man. Diabetes 17: 560-569
57. Reaven GM, Sageman WS, Swenson RS (1977) Development of insulin resistance in normal dogs following alloxan-induced insulin deficiency. Diabetologia 13: 459-462
58. Revers RR, Fink R, Griffin J, Olefsky JM, Kolterman OG (1984) Influence of hyperglycemia on insulin's in vivo effects in type II diabetes. J Clin Invest 73: 664-672
59. Rossetti L, Papachristou D, Shulman G, Smith D, DeFronzo R (1986) Insulin resistance in partially pancreatectomized rats: reversal with phloridzin therapy. Diabetes 35: 38A
60. Saito K, Yaginuma N, Takahashi T (1979) Differential volumetry of A, B, and D Cells in the pancreatic islets of diabetic and non-diabetic subjects. Tohoku J Exp Med 129: 273-283
61. Scarlett JA, Gray RS, Griffin J, Olefsky JM, Kolterman OG (1982) Insulin treatment reverses the insulin resistance of type II diabetes mellitus. Diabetes Care 5: 353-363
62. Seltzer HS, Allen EW, Herron AL, Brennan MT (1967) Insulin secretion in response to gly-

cemic stimulus: relation of delayed initial release to carbohydrate intolerance in mild diabetes mellitus. J Clin Invest 46: 323-335
63. Shoelson S, Haneda M, Blix P, Nanjo A, Sanke T, Inouye K, Steiner D, Rubenstein A,Tager H (1983) Three mutant insulin in man. Nature 302: 540-543
64. Simonson D, Ferrannini E, Bevilacqua S, Smith D, Barrett E, Carlson R, DeFronzo RA (1984) Mechanism of improvement in glucose metabolism after chronic glyburide therapy. Diabetes 33: 838-845
65. Srikanta S, Ganda OP, Gleason RE, Jackson RA, Soeldner JS, Eisenbarth GS (1984) Pre-type I diabetes: linear loss of beta cell response to intravenous glucose. Diabetes 33: 717-720
66. Starke A, Grundy S, McGarry JD, Unger RH (1985) Correction of hyperglycemia with phloridzin restores the glucagon response to glucose in insulin-dependent dogs: implications for human diabetes. Proc Natl Acad Sci USA 82: 1544-1546
67. Stefan Y, Orci L, Malaisse-Lagae F, Perrelet A, Patel Y, Unger RH (1982) Quantitation of endocrine cell content in the pancreas of non-diabetic and diabetic humans. Diabetes 31: 694-700
68. Swenne I (1982) The role of glucose in the in vitro regulation of cell cycle kinetics and proliferation of fetal pancreatic B-cells. Diabetes 31: 754-760
69. Tager HS (1984) Abnormal products of the human insulin gene. Diabetes 33: 693-699
70. Tomita T, Lacy PE, Matschinsky FM, McDaniel ML (1974) Effect of alloxan on insulin secretion in isolated rat islets perifused in vitro. Diabetes 23: 517-524
71. Toreson WE (1951) Glycogen infiltration (so-called hydropic degeneration) in the pancreas of human and experimental diabetes mellitus. Am J Pathol 27: 327-347
72. Trent DF, Fletcher DJ, May JM, Bonner-Weir S, Weir GC (1984) Abnormal islet and adipocyte function in young B-cell-deficient rats with nearnormoglycemia. Diabetes 33: 170-175
73. Truglia JA, Livingston JN, Lockwood DH (1985) Insulin resistance: receptor and post-binding defects in human obesity and non-insulin-dependent diabetes mellitus. Am J Med 79 B): 13-22
74. Turner RC, McCarthy ST, Holman RR, Harris E (1976) Beta-cell function improved by supplementary basal insulin secretion in mild diabetes. Br Med J 1: 1252-1254
75. Unger RH, Grundy S (1985) Hyperglycemia as an inducer as well as a consequence of impaired islet function and insulin resistance: implications for the management of diabetes. Diabetologia 28: 119-121
76. Vague P, Moulin JP (1982) The defective glucose sensitivity of the B-cell in non-insulin-dependent diabetes: improvement after 24 hours of normoglycemia. Metabolism 31: 139-142
77. Volk BW, Wellman KF (1977) Hormonal diabetes. In: Volk BW, Wellman KF (eds) The diabetic pancreas. Plenum, New York, pp 271-290
78. Ward WK, Beard JC, Halter JB, Pfeiffer MA, Porte Jr (1984) Pathophysiology of insulin secretion in non-insulin-dependent diabetes mellitus. Diabetes Care 7: 491-502
79. Ward WK, Taborsky GJ, Beard JC (1986) Reduced maximal potentiation of the insulin response to arginine: a sensitive indicator of B-cell damage. Diabetes 35: 98 A
80. Weibel ER (1963) Principles and methods for the morphometric studies of the lung and other organs. Lab Invest 12: 131-155
81. Weir GC, Clore ET, Zmachinski CJ, Bonner-Weir S (1981) Islet secretion in a new experimental model for non-insulin-dependent diabetes. Diabetes 30: 590-595
82. Weir GC (1982) Non-insulin-dependent diabetes mellitus: interplay between B-cell inadequacy and insulin resistance. Am J Med 13: 461-464
83. Weir GC, Leahy JL, Bonner-Weir S (1986) Experimental reduction of B-cell mass: implications for the pathogenesis of diabetes. Diabetes Metab Rev 2: 125-161
84. Westermark P, Wilander E (1978) The influence of amyloid deposits on the islet volume in maturity onset diabetes mellitus. Diabetologia 15: 417-421
85. Yamamoto H, Uchigata Y, Okamoto (1981) Streptozotocin and alloxan induce DNA strand breaks and poly (ADP-ribose) synthetase in pancreatic islets. Nature 294: 284-286

Perspectives of Islet Cell Transplantation in Diabetes

P. E. Lacy

Introduction

Basic investigations on a particular problem may lead to unexpected findings with the resultant initiation of research in a new field. This is a recurrent theme in science, and the history of the development of islet transplantation provides another example.

In the mid-1950s the only tool available for morphologic studies of hormonal secretion of the islets was light microscopy. This approach had many limitations and could provide only qualitative assessments of hormonal storage and release. Fortunately a new morphologic tool, electron microscopy, was under development at that time, providing hope that more definitive information might be obtained about the secretory process of islet cells. Our laboratory was the first to apply electron microscopy to the study of the islets of LANGERHANS and to define ultrastructural criteria for the identification of the different types of islet cells in different species of animals. Ultrastructural studies on B-cells from animals under different experimental conditions demonstrated that B-granules were released from the cells by the fusion of the membrane surrounding the granules with the plasma membrane and the subsequent dissolution of the granule in the extracellular space. We called this process "emiocytosis."

These morphologic studies on the B-cells provided new information; however, there were still limitations with this approach. What was needed was a method to separate the islets from the exocrine pancreas and therefore permit in vitro studies on insulin secretion so that a direct correlation of the structure and functional status of the cells could be accomplished. MOSKALEWSKI [1] described a technique using collagenase for the separation of guinea pig islets. Our laboratory modified this approach and developed a method for the mass isolation of intact islets from the rat pancreas [2, 3]. The development of this technique made it possible to commence studies on the hormonal secretion of islets in vitro and to begin to describe the biochemical, metabolic, and morphologic events associated with the secretory process. Using these approaches, we demonstrated that the microtubule-microfilament system of the B-cell was responsible for the intracellular translocation of B-granules to the cell membrane prior to their release by emiocytosis. The biochemical events involved in this intracellular trafficking of B-granules have still not been resolved. In vitro studies with isolated islets have been performed in many laboratories in an attempt to determine how glucose initiates the secretory process in the B-cell. The debate still continues as to whether glucose stimulates insulin release by activation of a specific receptor, or by glucose metabolism, or by a combination of these two mechanisms. It is extremely important that this basic problem be resolved, since this information may be helpful in understanding and demonstrating possible defects that may exist in the B-cells of certain forms of type 2 diabetes.

Since intact, functional islets could be isolated from the rat pancreas, the next obvious question was to determine whether transplants of normal islets into rats with experimentally induced diabetes would revert the diabetic state to normal. Inbred strains of rats were used for these studies to avoid the problem of rejection, and we demonstrated that transplants of normal islets in the diabetic animals were quite effective [4, 5]. Subsequently, many laboratories demonstrated that both adult isolated islets and the fetal rat pancreas could be used to produce normoglycemia in the recipients [6-8]. Many laboratories also demonstrated that these transplants reversed the early complications of diabetes in experimental animals [9-14].

These studies, demonstrating the effectiveness of islet transplants in rats, almost immediately led to the concept that islet transplantation might be used as a therapeutic approach to human diabetes. Some laboratories immediately attempted the transplantation of human islets into diabetic patients, but we believed this approach was premature, for the following reason: If islet transplantation was to be used as a therapeutic approach to human diabetes, then it would be necessary to maintain the transplants in the patients without the need for continuous immunosuppressive therapy of the recipient. Thus, our approach was to return to the experimental animal and attempt to develop methods to prevent the rejection of islet allografts without the continuous use of immunosuppressive drugs. This has been achieved and the methods developed for preventing rejection will be described later in this chapter.

The finding that rejection of islet transplants in experimental animals could be prevented without the use of immunosuppressive drugs created two fascinating areas of research that needed to be pursued. The first of these concerned the attempt to translate the animal studies on islet transplantation to human application. This would require the development of methods for mass isolation of human islets and then determine whether the procedures that worked effectively in animals to prevent rejection would also work in human diabetes.

The second area of research relates to basic investigations on the immunologic mechanism involved in the prevention of rejection and the use of this information to obtain further insight into the possible etiology and pathogenesis of type 1 diabetes. As described in other chapters, there is increasing evidence that type 1 diabetes is an autoimmune type of disease. In simplistic terms, autoimmunity means that the B-cells for the type 1 diabetic are recognized as being "foreign" and are destroyed by the immune system of that individual. The opposite situation exists in the animals with islet transplants that have been established by procedures which do not utilize immunosuppression of the recipients immune system. The islet transplants in these animals are still obviously "foreign"; however, the procedures that have been developed to prevent rejection have led to the lack of recognition of these cells as being "foreign" by the immune system of the recipient. Thus, basic investigations in this transplant model on how the immune system was altered to prevent recognition of the "foreign" islet cells should provide information that may be applicable to the treatment of patients identified prior to the development of overt diabetes or immediately after the onset of clinical diabetes.

The purpose of this chapter is to review the experimental approaches that have been developed for the prevention of rejection of islet transplants in animals without the use of immunosuppressive drugs, the present state of knowledge concerning the immune mechanisms involved in these procedures, and the present and future status of islet transplantation as a therapeutic approach to human diabetes.

Animal Islet Transplants

Prevention of Rejection of Islet Allografts

In 1957, SNELL [15] suggested that passenger leukocytes carried along with transplanted organs might be responsible for initiation of immune rejection, whereas the parenchymal cells of the organ would not initiate rejection. This suggestion lay fallow for many years. In 1974, JACOBS [16] reported that in vitro culture of the ovary for several days would prolong the survival of ovarian grafts transplanted across major histocompatibility barriers. Subsequently, LAFFERTY [17] prevented rejection of thyroid allografts in mice by culturing the donor thyroid in the presence of 95% O_2 for 3 weeks prior to transplantation. Lafferty suggested that the high oxygen tension might be destroying passenger lymphoid cells in the donor tissue, thus preventing rejection.

At the time of LAFFERTY's report, we were attempting to prevent rejection of islet grafts by perifusion of the islets in vitro for several weeks. This was a difficult procedure; thus, we immediately tried culturing individual rat islets in the presence of 95% O_2. We found that the islets would survive in this environment for only 3-4 days. Many other approaches were tested during the next 2 years without significant success, and finally we tried low-temperature culture of the donor islets as a means of altering the putative passenger lymphoid cells within these structures. The reason for using low-temperature culture was that OPELZ and TERASAKI [18] had reported that human lymphocytes maintained at 22 °C would survive, but lost their ability to stimulate a mixed leukocyte reaction in vitro. Using this approach, we found that culturing the donor rat islets at 24 °C for 7 days and giving a single injection of rat antilymphocyte serum to the recipient at the time of transplantation would completely prevent rejection of islet allografts transplanted across major histocompatibility barriers [19]. Neither low-temperature culture alone nor the single injection of antilymphocyte serum alone would prevent rejection, but the use of both modalities together prevented rejection.

The next question was whether one could induce rejection of the islet allografts established by low-temperature culture by injecting donor lympoid cells into the recipients bearing the transplants. We found that injection of donor peritoneal exudate cells would induce rejection of the established grafts, and that T-lymphocytes and macrophages from the donor would induce rejection whereas B-lymphocytes would not induce rejection [20, 21]. These findings clearly indicated that the return of donor lymphoid, antigen-presenting cells to the recipients would induce rejection and that the animals were dependent upon the islet grafts for the maintenance of normoglycemia.

The subsequent task was to determine whether the lack of ability of the individual islet cells in the islets cultured at low temperature to initiate rejection was due to a complete lack of histocompatibility antigens on their surface or the absence of one or more specific histocompatibility antigens. PARR et al. [22] had reported that mouse islet cells did not express any histocompatibility antigens using an electron-microscopic, immunohistochemical technique for their demonstration. Our laboratory used a more sensitive immunologic technique for demonstration of the histocompatibility antigens and found that mouse islet cells do express class I antigens but do not express class II histocompatibility antigens [23]. This finding has been confirmed in other species [24]. Since class II antigen (I a) expression is required for a lymphoid antigen-presenting cell to initiate an immune reaction, the lack of this histocompatibility antigen may explain the inability of the islet cells alone to initiate the immune rejection process. I shall return to this question later in this chapter. The presence of class I antigens on the islet grafts would explain how the foreign islet cells were recognized once the rejection process was initiated in the recipient following the injection of donor lymphoid, antigen-presenting cells.

Since mouse islet cells did not express Ia histocompatibility antigens, we could now determine whether treatment of donor mouse islets with specific Ia antisera and complement would destroy Ia^+ lymphoid, antigen-presenting cells in the islets and thereby prevent rejection. We found that such treatment completely prevented rejection of islets transplanted across a major histocompatibility barrier in mice [25].

The next problem was to determine whether the Ia^+ lymphoid cells were present within the islets and to establish their identity. Using immunofluorescence, we were able to demonstrate Ia^+ lymphoid cells within individual mouse islets [26]. Two types of lymphoid cells were present: one type resembled small lymphocytes and the other resembled macrophages with elongated processes.

A special type of lymphoid, antigen-presenting cell had been isolated and characteried by STEINMAN from lymph nodes and spleens of mice [27]. These special types of cells were called dendritic cells and were characterized by being Ia^+, having elongated, dendritic-like processes, lacking phagocytic activity, and being extremely potent in stimulating a mixed leukocyte reaction. Steinman's group [28] isolated mouse dendritic cells and produced a specific monoclonal antibody to these cells. In collaboration with STEINMAN, our laboratory used this monoclonal antibody and complement for treatment of the donor islets to determine whether elimination of dendritic cells would prevent rejection of mouse islet allografts. We found that this procedure did indeed prevent such rejection [26]. Rejection of established grafts could be initiated by injecting a small number of partially purified donor dendritic cells. These findings indicated that at least in the mouse, the intraislet, Ia^+ dendritic cells play a major role in the initiation of rejection of islet allografts.

Other methods have also been developed for the alteration or destruction of passenger leukocytes in the donor islets and prevention of islet allograft rejection. As indicated earlier, we had found that exposure of individual rat islets to 95% O_2

destroyed the islets after 3–4 days culture. LAFFERTY and his associates [29] overcame this problem by demonstrating that aggregates of mouse islets would withstand exposure to 95% O_2 for 1 week and that pretreatment of the donor mouse islets in this environment prevented rejection when the islets were transplanted across a major histocompatbility barrier. Ultraviolet irradiation has also been used to inactivate antigen-presenting cells in the islets and to prevent rejection of rat islets transplanted across a major histocompatibility barrier [30]. PIPELEERS et al. [31] have developed a method for isolating pure populations of B-cells and found that this procedure would apparently eliminate lymphoid antigen-presenting cells and allografts of the purified populations of islet cells would have a prolonged survival after transplantation [32]. Further studies have been accomplished with low-temperature culture of donor islets and TZE et al. [33] found that low-temperature culture alone would prevent rejection of islets transplanted into a recipient strain that had a relatively low immune responsiveness to the donor tissue. These different methods of altering and destroying passenger leukocytes and preventing rejection of the islets are summarized in Table 1.

Table 1. Methods for prevention of rejection of islet allografts in rodents

Animals	Pretreatment recipients	Pretreatment donor islets	Treatment recipients post-transplant	Site of islet implantation	Reference
Rats	None	Culture 24 °C, 7 days	One injection ALS	Liver via PV	19
Mice	None	Culture islet aggregates, 95% O_2, 7 days	None	Kidney capsule	29
Mice	None	Ia antibody + C′	None	Liver via PV	25
Mice	None	Antidendritic cell antibody + C′	None	Liver via PV	26
Rats	None	UV irradiation	Cyclosporin A, 30 mg/kg, 3 days	Liver via PV	30
Rats	None	Separation of pure islet cells	None	Liver via PV	32
Mice	None	None	L3T4 antibody 4 days	Liver via PV	74
Mice	Ia-depleted donor blood	None	None	Liver via PV	38
Rats	UV-irradiated donor blood	None	None	Liver via PV	39
Rats	None	None	Three injections ALS	Testes, intra-abdominal	55
Rats	None	None	None	Brain	54

ALS, antilymphocyte serum; PV, Portal Vein

Prevention of Rejection by Induction of Tolerance

Several key questions are raised by the finding that transplants of "foreign" islet cells can survive in the recipients and be undetected immunologically simply by removing or altering Ia^+, antigen-presenting cells in the donor islets prior to transplantation. Has a state of specific immune tolerance been induced in these recipients? If tolerance has been induced, what are the immunologic mechanisms involved in the maintenance of tolerance in the recipients? What are the mechanisms that lead to the development of tolerance in these recipients? These are important questions that are of significance not only to transplant immunology but also perhaps in understanding the etiology and pathogenesis of type 1 diabetes in human patients.

Some evidence has been obtained that a specific immune unresponsiveness or tolerance is induced in recipient animals bearing endocrine grafts established by removal or alteration of passenger leukocytes prior to transplantation. Mice with long-established thyroid allografts would immediately reject a second transplant of untreated thyroid from a third strain but would accept a second transplant of uncultured thyroid from the original donor strain [34]. Our laboratory obtained similar findings in rats in which the recipients with established islet allografts produced an acute rejection of transplants of untreated islets from a third strain, whereas transplants of untreated islets from the original donor strain were not rejected [35]. A relatively small number of donor lymphoid cells (10^3-10^4) would induce rejection of treated islets or thyroid grafts when injected immediately after transplantation, whereas a large number (10^6-10^7) of donor lymphoid cells were required to induce rejection of these grafts 6 months after transplantation [20, 36]. These findings indicate that a marked change has occurred in the immune system of the recipient requiring a massive number of donor antigen-presenting cells to induce rejection in the long-established endocrine grafts.

Repeated injections of specific anti-I-J serum were given to mice with established islet allografts in the hope of eliminating possible suppressor T-lymphocytes in the recipients and inducing rejection. This treatment alone did not induce rejection; however, only a small number of donor splenocytes (10^4) were required to induce rejection, whereas $>10^7$ donor splenocytes were needed to induce rejection of established islet allografts in mice that had not been treated with anti-I-J serum [37].

These findings indicate that a specific immune unresponsiveness or tolerance had been induced in recipient animals bearing established endocrine allografts. This lead to the development of another approach for preventing rejection of islet allografts in mice. The hypothesis was that since transplants of islets devoid of Ia^+ passenger lymphoid cells induced a tolerant status, then it should be possible to preimmunize recipients with Ia^- cells, induce a partial state of tolerance, and be able to transplant untreated donor islets. In the mouse, red blood cells are Ia^- but express H-2K and D antigens (class I), similar to mouse islet cells. Thus, we preimmunized recipient mice with Ia-depleted donor blood and transplanted untreated islet allografts into these animals. This regimen prevented rejection of the untreated islet allografts, whereas preimmunization with *untreated* donor blood caused an acceleration of rejection of the islets [38]. Recently, LAU et al. [39] have used ultraviolet light for irradiation and inactivation of antigen-presenting cells of donor rat blood and found that preimmunization of recipient rats with the treated blood would prevent rejection of rat islet allografts. These preimmunization methods are listed in Table 1.

Presumably, the maintenance of immune responsiveness in the recipients is due to suppressor T-lymphocytes. We have attempted to demonstrate suppressor T-lymphocytes in vitro from animals with established islet allografts, but have been unsuccessful so far. Thus, extremely important questions remain to be resolved in this area. Is the mechanism of maintenance of the grafts and prevention of recognition of the islet cells as being "foreign" due to suppressor T-lymphocytes? If suppressor T-lymphocytes are involved, what are the mechanisms that lead to their development following transplantation of the treated islets? Are cells expressing only class I antigens capable of initiating the tolerant status, or are a few Ia^{+} lymphoid antigen-presenting cells required to initiate this response? Do islet cells acquire Ia expression after transplantation due to certain lymphokines? If the islet cells do have induced Ia after transplantation, are these nonlymphoid cells with Ia expression responsible for initiating the production of suppressor T-lymphocytes or initiating another immunologic mechanism that may prevent rejection?

Prevention of Rejection of Islet Xenografts

If transplantation of human islets is shown to be successful as a therapeutic approach to human diabetes, then the demand for human islets will undoubtedly exceed the available supply. Thus, studies are needed to determine whether xenografts of islet tissue can be prevented from rejecting without the continuous use of immunosuppressive drugs, not only from the standpoint of providing a possible supply of islet tissue for human transplants but also to provide further basic information in transplantation immunology.

The first attempt to transplant animal tissue into human diabetics was by Dr. P. Watson Williams and his surgical colleague, Mr. Harsant, in 1893 [40]. Three pieces of freshly slaughtered sheep pancreas were transplanted into the subcutaneous tissue of a 15-year-old diabetic child. The transplant had no effect on the diabetic state. In 1927, Luisada [41] transplanted pieces of duct-ligated baboon pancreas beneath the tunica vaginalis of the testis in two diabetics, again with no effect on the diabetic state. No further attempts were made to use animal tissue for transplantation into diabetic patients.

In recent years, attempts have been made to transplant islets across a wide species barrier in animals by using fish islets for transplantation into diabetic rats [42]. If the recipient animals received total body irradiation, then function of the fish islets could be demonstrated for a period of 1-2 days. Eloy et al. [43] reported that intrahepatic transplants of 15-day-old chick embryo pancreases into diabetic rats improved the diabetic state of the recipients for as long as 18 months. In contrast, intrahepatic transplants of 18-day-old chick embryo pancreases were rapidly rejected. To my knowledge, these intriguing observations have never been confirmed in other laboratories.

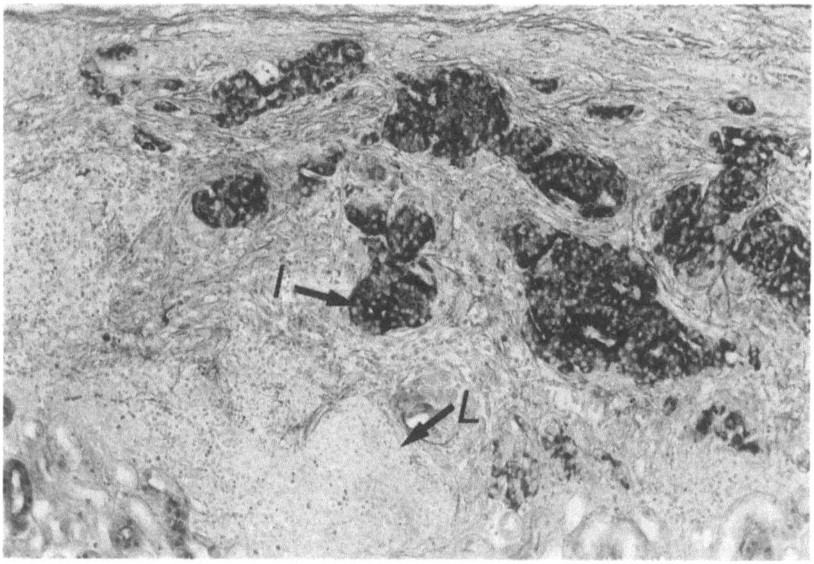

Fig. 1. Hamster islet graft *(I)* in the kidney capsule of a mouse 60 days after transplantation. The B-cells have a normal degree of granulation and the recipient was normoglycemic. The mouse became diabetic when the kidney bearing the islet graft was removed. Focal nodules of lymphocytes *(L)* are present adjacent to the islet grafts but not invading the islets. Aldehyde-fuchsin stain, ×600

Transplants of endocrine tissue across a closely related species barrier (rat to mouse) have been successful using procedures which destroy or alter passenger lymphoid cells in the donor grafts prior to transplantation. SOLLINGER et al. [44] prevented the rejection of thyroid xenografts by culturing rat thyroids in the presence of 95% O_2 prior to transplanting the grafts beneath the renal capsule of mice. Our laboratory demonstrated that the rejection of rat islets transplanted into diabetic mice could be prevented by the use of low-temperature culture in conjunction with either a single injection of antilymphocyte serum [45] or a short course (3 days) of cyclosporin A therapy after transplantation [46]. In vitro culture of aggregates of rat islets in the presence of 95% O_2 for 1 week prior to transplantation into diabetic mice also produced a marked prolongation of islet xenograft survival [47]. In recent studies, we have obtained a marked prolongation of survival of hamster islets transplanted beneath the renal capsule of diabetic mice by the use of low-temperature culture for a 1-week period prior to transplantation. The mean survival time of the cultured islets was $>43.3 \pm 4.7$ days, with 20% survival at 60 days after transplantation, whereas the uncultured, control hamster islets had a mean survival time 21.7 ± 4.9 days. Figure 1 illustrates a hamster islet graft at 60 days after transplantation beneath the renal capsule of a diabetic mouse. The animal was normoglycemic throughout this period of time and the B-cells in the graft have a normal degree of granulation. Removal of the kidney bearing the graft at 60 days resulted in immediate return to a diabetic state. The methods used for preventing rejection of islet xenografts are listed in Table 2.

Table 2. Methods for prevention of rejection of islet xenografts

Donor animal	Pretreatment of donor islets	Treatment of recipient mice post-transplant	Site of implantation	Reference
Rat	Culture 24 °C, 7 days	One injection mouse and rat ALS	Liver via PV	45
Rat	Culture 24 °C, 7 days	Cyclosporin A, 50 mg/kg, 3 days	Liver via PV	46
Rat	Culture islet aggregates, 95%, O_2, 7 days	One injection mouse and rat ALS	Kidney capsule	47
Hamster	Culture 24 °C, 7 days	None	Kidney capsule	
Rat	None	None	Testes	53

ALS, antilymphocyte serum; PV, Portal Vein

It is interesting that the hamster islet grafts maintained the blood glucose levels in the recipient mice at the same level present in normal hamsters. The nonfasting plasma glucose in normal hamsters is 66.2 ± 4.7 mg/dl and this level was maintained in the mice, whereas the normal nonfasting level in the mice was 128.4 ± 6.4 mg/dl.

Our laboratory has recently developed a method for the mass isolation of pig islets [48] and now studies can be initiated on attempting to prevent rejection of islet xenografts across an even wider species barrier by alteration of the passenger leukocytes in the donor tissue.

Insulitis in Established Islet Xenografts

As described in other chapters in this volume, an insulitis composed of mononuclear cells is one of the cardinal morphologic findings in the islets of type 1 diabetics following the onset of clinical diabetes. Histologic studies of islet allografts in rodents established by procedures which remove or alter passenger leukocytes in the islets prior to transplantation have shown that the islet grafts are free of any mononuclear cell infiltration or insulitis. In contrast, xenografts of either rat or hamster islets into mice always have a rim of mononuclear cells around the islets even though the grafts have become established and are not undergoing rejection. Figure 1 illustrates a focal accumulation of lymphocytes adjacent to an established hamster islet xenograft at 60 days after transplantation. These lymphoid cells have been isolated from renal subcapsular transplants of rat islets in mice and were shown to be T-lymphocytes that were predominantly Lyt-2^+ cells [49]. Lymphocytes that are Lyt-2^+ may be either cytotoxic T-lymphocytes or suppressor T-lymphocytes. Since the lymphocytes were not infiltrating the islets and the grafts were maintaining normoglycemia in the recipients and were not undergoing rejection, it is possible that the focal accumulation of Lyt-2^+ T-lymphocytes may represent focal accumulation of suppressor T-lymphocytes around the established islet xenografts.

Effect of Site of Transplantation

Islet grafts have been shown to be effective in reversing the diabetic state to normal when implanted in several different anatomic sites in the recipient animals. These effective sites include the liver by injecting the islets into the portal vein [5], the peritoneal cavity [4], a peritoneal-omental pouch [50], spleen [51], subcapsular space of the kidney [52], testis [53], and the brain [54].

The site of transplantation has a marked effect on the rate of rejection of untreated islet allografts and xenografts. The most rapid rate of rejection of freshly isolated islets is in the spleen [53]. Presumably this is due to the placement of the foreign grafts directly in contact with the lymphoid system of the recipient resulting in a rapid initiation of immune rejection. In contrast, a marked prolongation of survival is obtained if the islets are placed within the testis [53] or in the brain [54]. SELAWRY [55] has shown that allografts of rat islets transplanted into the testis of diabetic BioBreeding (BB) rats in conjunction with a short course of immunosuppressive therapy would survive and achieve normoglycemia in the recipients, whereas islets transplanted into the liver via the portal vein in these rats were rapidly rejected. It has been known for many years that these two sites are partially immunologically privileged sites for the implantation of allogeneic tissue. The subcapsular space of the kidney has also been shown to produce some degree of protection from rejection of the islet grafts: the survival time at this site was approximately twice that of similar grafts transplanted into the liver via the portal vein [52]. The mechanisms involved in delaying rejection in these semiprivileged sites are unknown.

The use of the renal subcapsular site for implantation may also provide a synergistic effect in preventing rejection of islets pretreated to destroy passenger leukocytes. In our recent studies on xenografts of hamster islets into mice, we have found that low-temperature culture produced a marked prolongation of hamster islet xenograft survival when the islets were transplanted beneath the kidney capsule of the recipients, whereas the same treatment had no effect in prolonging survival of islets transplanted into the liver via the portal vein.

These findings on the effect of the site of implantation may be of importance to human islet transplantation in the future, since it may be necessary to utilize the renal subcapsular site or the testis in conjunction with pretreatment of the donor islets in order to prevent rejection without the use of immunosuppressive drugs.

Role of Lymphokines in Islet Rejection

Prevention of rejection of islet allografts without the use of immunosuppressive drugs provides an experimental model which is opposite to the presumed rejection or destruction of B-cells that apparently occurs by an autoimmune mechanism in type 1 diabetes. Thus, the elucidation of the mechanisms involved in preventing rejection of islets in this experimental model should provide information that will be useful in understanding the etiology and pathogenesis of type 1 diabetes, as well as providing approaches that may be helpful in preventing the onset of this disease. These studies should also provide new and more specific approaches for the prevention of rejection of islet transplants without the need for immunosuppressive drugs.

Interaction of donor antigen-presenting cells with recipient T-lymphocytes and the resultant generation of cytotoxic T-lymphocytes involves the production of several lymphokines that are required for the establishment of this immune response. Gamma-interferon (gamma-IFN), interleukin-1 (IL-1), and interleukin-2 (IL-2) are three lymphokines that play critical roles in this process. IL-1 is released from activated antigen-presenting cells and not only induces T-lymphocytes proliferation but also has an effect on many other cell systems. It has been shown to stimulate acute-phase protein synthesis by the liver, proliferation of fibroblasts, and initiation of bone resorption [56-59]. Nerup and associates [60-62] reported recently that IL-1 has a cytotoxic effect on isolated rat islets. In vitro culture of rat islets in the presence of IL-1 for 6 days caused the islets to disintegrate into small clumps with an accompanying impairment of glucose-induced insulin secretion and loss of insulin and glucagon from the islet cells. Subsequently, our laboratory [63] found that incubation of isolated rat islets in the presence of IL-1 for 15 h would produce a 60%-80% inhibition of glucose-induced insulin release. This 15-h effect of IL-1 was reversible, since continued incubation of the islets in the absence of this lymphokine for an additional 3 days returned their responsiveness to glucose-induced insulin secretion to normal. Thus it is possible that this lymphokine may play an important role in the impairment of function of B-cells or lead to their destruction during rejection of islet transplants or in type 1 diabetes. Monoclonal antibodies are being prepared to IL-1 and it will be of great interest to determine the effect of these antibodies on the prevention of rejection of islet allografts.

Bottazzo [64] has suggested that in type 1 diabetes mellitus a viral infection involving B-cells may result in localized gamma-IFN production with resultant induction of Ia expression on B-cells, presentation of autoantigens by the B-cells, and induction of autoimmune T- and B-lymphocytes against the presumed islet B-cell autoantigens with destruction of these cells. Bottazzo [65] has reported the presence of rare Ia^+ B-cells in the pancreas of a 12 year-old diabetic girl soon after the onset of type 1 diabetes. Thus, the key critical questions are: Can Ia expression be induced on islet cells with gamma-IFN, and if this is possible, are the Ia^+ cells capable of antigen presentation?

Gamma-IFN has been shown to induce Ia antigens not only on macrophages but also on cells that normally do not express class I histocompatibility antigens, such as mast cells, endothelial cells, fibroblasts, and melanoma cells [66-70]. Our laboratory has shown recently that Ia expression can be induced on mouse islet cells from B10.BR and Balb/C mice by in vitro culture of isolated islets in the presence of gamma-IFN for 5-6 days [71]. Dual immunofluorescent staining for Ia antigens and insulin indicated that both B-cells and non-B-cells in the islets were induced to express Ia antigens. Approximately 20%-40% of the islet cells were induced to express Ia with this procedure.

The islet transplant model provides an opportunity to determine whether islet cells with induced Ia expression are capable of antigen presentation, by treating the donor islets with Ia antibody and complement to remove Ia^+ lymphoid cells and then inducing Ia expression on the islet cells with gamma-IFN prior to transplantation. Initial studies in our laboratory indicate that induction of Ia expression on the islet cells does not convey the capability of antigen presentation; however, many more detailed investigations are needed to confirm these preliminary findings. Antigen presentation by a cell requires not only the expression of Ia, but also the capability of synthesizing and releasing IL-1. Studies are in progress to determine whether islet cells, with or without induced expression of IA, are capable of releasing IL-1. If it is shown that islet cells are not capable of synthesizing IL-1 and presenting antigens, then the possibility is raised that the aberrant expression of Ia on these cells may play a role in the induction of tolerance. The islet transplant model provides a superb opportunity to investigate these basic and extremely important questions.

In an immune response, IL-1 and gamma-IFN are apparently released, initially resulting in activation of T-lymphocytes and the production of IL-2 with the resultant induction of IL-2 receptors on the activated lymphocytes and the formation of cytotoxic T-lymphocytes. The induction of IL-2 receptors on the activated T-lymphocytes provides a specific marker for the identification and elimination of these cells. KIRKMAN et al. [72] obtained a marked prolongation of cardiac allograft survival in mice following the administration of an anti-IL-2 receptor antibody to the recipient animals during a 10-day interval following transplantation of the cardiac grafts. Apparently the monoclonal antibody to IL-2 receptors caused specific destruction of these activated lymphocytes and prevented rejection of the grafts. Studies are needed to determine whether IL-2 receptor antibodies will affect the survival of islet allografts. Another activation marker on lymphocytes is L3T4, which is shown to be present on helper T-lymphocytes [73]. SHIZURU et al. [74] have prevented rejection of islet allografts in mice by repeated injections of a monoclonal antibody to L3T4 to the recipient animals. Thus the presence of specific activation markers on lymphocytes provides an opportunity for the production of monoclonal antibodies to these markers and to use these specific immunotherapeutic agents to prevent rejection of islet allografts and xenografts in conjunction with procedures to destroy or alter passenger leukocytes within the islets.

Fetal Pancreas Transplantation

An advantage of the fetal pancreas for transplantation is that islets in the fetus are capable of replication and comprise a higher proportion of the pancreas than in the adult. Isografts of fetal pancreas in rodents have been used successfully in reversing diabetic states to normal within inbred strains of rodents [8].

Prevention of rejection of allografts of the fetal pancreas by culture in vitro has not been as successful as that with allografts of isolated adult islets [75]. In vitro culture of donor fetal pancreas in the presence of 95% O_2 for 3 weeks produces only a slight to moderate reduction in immunogenicity of the fetal allografts. Low-temperature culture of the fetal pancreas or treatment of the preparation with Ia antibody and complement have not been successful in preventing rejection of fetal pancreatic allografts.

This difference between adult islets and the fetal pancreas is probably due to the large amount of immature lymphoid tissue present in the fetal pancreas. Large masses of lymphoid tissue have been observed in established isografts of fetal mouse pancreas [75]. Apparently neither in vitro culture nor treatment of the pancreas with Ia antisera and complement is able to decrease the immature lymphoid cells below the critical level that is required for the prevention of rejection.

LAFFERTY's group has developed a method for the isolation of proislets from the fetal mouse pancreas [76]. Proislets are composed of undifferentiated tissue elements that differentiate and form islets following transplantation as isografts. In vitro culture of fetal proislets for 10 days in 95% O_2 resulted in approximately 50% survival of the proislet allografts at 4 weeks after transplantation, whereas intact fetal pancreases cultured under the same conditions were rejected at this time interval [77]. The use of fetal proislets is one approach to the problem of rejection of fetal islet tissue; however, the yield of islet tissue by this isolation procedure is low. The prevention of rejection of fetal pancreas allografts is a very important area of investigation, particularly because the fetal pancreas may be usable as a source of islet tissue for human transplants.

Human Islet Transplantation

Isolation of Human Islets

After demonstrating that it was possible to prevent rejection of islet allografts in animals without the use of immunosuppressive drugs, attention was now focused on the mass isolation of human islets. Procedures were needed which would make it possible to isolate a sufficient quantity of islets from a single human pancreas to be used in transplantation. We found that the collagenase technique as used for rodent islet isolation was not effective when applied to the human pancreas. Earlier attempts had been made by others to transplant human islets isolated by the rat collagenase technique and these were unsuccessful. The lack of success was undoubtedly due to the methodology of isolating the islets. In recent years several procedures have been developed for the mass isolation of canine, bovine, and human islets [78-81]. Our laboratory developed a method which yielded approximately 100000-150000 islets per human pancreas, and the preparation contained approximately 20% islets and 80% acinar tissue [81]. The islets isolated by this procedure were functional in vitro, and since a large mass of islets could be obtained from a single pancreas, we decided to test this preparation, even though it was impure, by transplanting it into diabetic patients who were already receiving immunosuppressive drugs to maintain a kidney transplant. The site of transplantation was the spleen due to the impurity of the preparation. Six diabetic patients received the transplants, and in three of the recipients the islet graft functioned for 1-2 months after transplantation as indicated by elevated plasma C-peptide levels and a decrease in insulin requirements of 50%-90% during this time. A seventh patient received an autotransplant of islets isolated by this procedure. The patient had chronic pancreatitis and a total pancreatectomy was performed. The tail of the pancreas was removed first, and islets were isolated from this resected portion. The islet preparation was extremely pure since the acinar tissue had been destroyed, and approximately 70000 islets were obtained. Since the preparation was almost pure islet tissue, it was possible to reimplant the islets into this patient via the umbilical vein so that the islets would lodge in the liver. Function of this autotransplant of islets has been present for over 18 months as demonstrated by a low level of plasma C-peptide and a decrease in insulin requirements from 20 units/day after surgery to 4 units/day. These findings in both groups of patients were most encouraging, since they indicated that the islet isolation technique did provide viable islets and that these would function in the patients.

The next step in these investigations was to develop a method for the further purification of the islet preparation. Recently we have developed a procedure for purification of the human islets by centrifugation in a Ficoll gradient. The preparation contains approximately 80% islets and 20% acinar tissue. The development of this procedure will now make it possible to transplant the islets via the portal vein into the liver of diabetic recipients and to utilize procedures that have been effective in animals for destruction or alteration of passenger leukocytes in the islets preparation.

MINTZ and associates have developed a different method for human islet isolation and have transplanted islets into diabetic patients who are already receiving immunosuppressive drugs for a kidney transplant. The purity of the preparation made it possible to transplant these islets into the liver via the portal vein. Initial reports from these studies indicated that temporary function lasting one to several months occurred following transplantation of the human islets [82].

Human clinical trials have also been initiated using the fetal pancreas for transplantation into diabetic patients receiving immunosuppressive drugs to maintain a kidney transplant. At the present time the reports from these studies are fragmentary. No definite function has been demonstrated in these human fetal pancreas transplants; however, many months will be required to evaluate their status fully.

Future Perspective of Human Islet Transplantation

The passenger leukocyte concept has been established and validated for islet transplants in animals. Removal of alteration of passenger leukocytes in isolated, adult donor islets will prevent rejection of islet allografts without the continuous use of immunosuppressive therapy. As reviewed in this chapter, many procedures have been developed to accomplish this effect on the donor islets and methods have been devised to induce a specific tolerant status in recipient animals prior to transplantation of the islets. Thus the problems that remain for human islet transplantation are purely technical. These consist of having methods that will provide massive quantities of adult islets from the pancreas for transplantation and to adapt and modify these pretreatment procedures to the human islet preparations.

A key question in these investigations is whether the presumed autoimmune state in type 1 diabetes will cause destruction of the human islet transplants when immunosuppression is not utilized. SUTHERLAND et al. [83] reported that segmental pancreas transplants between nondiabetic and diabetic identical twins without the use of immunosuppressive drugs resulted in destruction of the B-cells in the grafts and a return to a diabetic state. This finding would appear to indicate that the human islet allografts would be destroyed unless immunosuppressive agents were given to the recipient. If the destruction of the B-cells is mediated by lymphoid cells, then recognition of the B-cells by cytotoxic T-lymphocytes would be linked to a close similarity of the histocompatibility antigens expressed on both the donor B-cells and the recipient lymphocytes. It is possible that this cellular-mediated reaction might be avoided if the donor islets expressed histocompatibility antigens different from the recipient. Recent studies by WOEHRLE et al. [84] provide evidence that this concept may be true for islet transplants in BB animals. Donor Wistar-Furth islets were incubated at 24 °C prior to transplantation and a single injection of antilymphocyte serum was given to the BB diabetic recipients. The BB rat has the same haplotype as Wistar-Furth rats and the islets were rejected after transplantation. In contrast, treatment of donor Lewis islets with this same procedure prevented rejection of the islet allografts. A major histocompatibility difference exists between Wistar-Furth and Lewis rats. If the BB rat model has similarities to type 1 diabetes in man, then these findings provide hope that such an approach might be helpful in human diabetes. Others have reported rejection of islet allografts in BB rats; however, these investigators utilized procedures which have not been established as being effective in preventing rejection of islet allografts in normal rats. When the human islet transplant trials are initiated again in our institution, we will mismatch the donor islet tissue with the recipient.

In summary, the future perspective of islet transplantation is extremely exciting. Within the next few years, it will be determined whether human islets can be transplanted into type 1 diabetic patients without the necessity of continuous immunosuppressive therapy. If such proves to be the case, this will provide a promising new therapeutic approach to the prevention of complications of diabetes. If the islet tissue is rejected by the autoimmune status of the recipient, then on the one hand these findings will provide insight into the pathogenesis of type 1 diabetes and on the other, islet transplantation will be attempted in diabetics in which autoimmunity does not play a role in rejection. From an experimental standpoint, the islet transplant model provides a superb opportunity both to delineate the events involved in normal rejection of tissue and to ascertain the immunologic mechanisms involved in the induction of tolerance. Basic investigations with this model should provide information of great importance in understanding the pathogenesis of autoimmune diseases and may lead to definitive immunologic, therapeutic approaches for the abrogation of autoimmunity.

References

1. Moskalewski S (1965) Isolation and culture of the islets of Langerhans of the guinea pig. Gen Comp Endocrinol 5: 342-353
2. Lacy PE, Kostianovsky M (1967) A method for the isolation of intact islets of Langerhans from the rat pancreas. Diabetes 16: 35
3. Lacy PE, Walker MM, Fink CJ (1972) Perifusion of isolated rat islets in vitro. The participation of the microtubular system in the biphasic release of insulin. Diabetes 21: 987
4. Ballinger WF, Lacy PE (1972) Transplantation of intact pancreatic islets in rats. Surgery 72: 175-186

5. Kemp CB, Knight MJ, Scharp DW, Lacy PE, Ballinger WF (1973) Transplantation of isolated pancreatic islets into the portal vein of diabetic rats. Nature 244: 447
6. Reckard CR, Barker CF (1973) Transplantation of isolated pancreatic islets across strong and weak histocompatibility barriers. Transplant Proc 5: 761-763
7. Leonard RJ, Lazarow A, Hegre OD (1973) Pancreatic islet transplantation in the rat. Diabetes 22: 413-428
8. Brown J, Molnar IG, Clark W, Mullen Y (1974) Control of experimental diabetes mellitus in rats by transplantation of fetal pancreases. Science 184: 1377-1379
9. Mauer SM, Sutherland DER, Steffes MW, Leonard RJ, Najarian JS, Michael AF, Brown DM (1974) Pancreatic islet transplantation. Effects on the glomerular lesions of experimental diabetes in the rat. Diabetes 23: 748-753
10. Steffes MW, Brown DM, Basgen JM, Mauer SM (1980) Amelioration of mesangial volume and surface alterations following islet transplantation in diabetic rats. Diabetes 29: 509-515
11. Federlin KF, Bretzel RG (1984) The effect of islet transplantation on complications in experimental diabetes of the rat. World J Surg 8: 169-178
12. Krupin T, Waltman SR, Scharp DW, Oestrich C, Feldman SD, Becker B, Ballinger WF, Lacy PE (1979) Ocular fluorophotometry in streptozotocin diabetes mellitus in the rat. The effect of pancreatic islet isografts. Invest Ophthal Vis Sci 18: 1185-1190
13. Silberberg R, Hirshberg GE, Lesker P (1977) Enzyme studies in the articular cartilage of diabetic rats and of rats bearing transplanted pancreatic islets. Diabetes 26: 732-735
14. Schmidt RE, Plurad SB, Olack BJ, Scharp DW (1983) The effect of pancreatic islet transplantation and insulin therapy on experimental diabetic autonomic neuropathy. Diabetes 32: 532-540
15. Snell GD (1957) The homograft reaction. Annu Rev Microbiol 2: 439-458
16. Jacobs BB (1974) Ovarian allograft survival. Prolongation after passage in vitro. Transplantation 18: 454-457
17. Lafferty KJ, Cooley MA, Woolnough J, Walker KZ (1975) Thyroid allograft immunogenicity is reduced after a period in organ culture. Science 188: 259-261
18. Opelz G, Terasaki PI (1974) Lymphocyte antigenicity loss with retention of responsiveness. Science 184: 464-466
19. Lacy PE, Davie JM, Finke EH (1979) Prolongation of islet allograft survival following in vitro culture (24 °C) and a single injection of ALS. Science 204: 312-313
20. Lacy PE, Davie JM, Finke EH (1979) Induction of rejection of successful allografts of rat islets by donor peritoneal exudate cells. Transplantation 28: 415-420
21. Zitron IM, Ono J, Lacy PE, Davie JM (1981) The cellular stimuli for the rejection of established islet allografts. Diabetes 30: 242-246
22. Parr EL (1979) The absence of H-2 antigens from mouse pancreatic B-cells demonstrated by immunoferritin labeling. J Exp Med 150: 1-9
23. Faustman D, Hauptfeld V, Davie JM, Lacy PE, Shreffler DC (1980) Murine pancreatic B-cells express H-2K and H-2D but not Ia antigens. J Exp Med 151: 1563-1568
24. Baekkeskov S, Kanatsuna T, Klareskog L, Nielsen DA, Peterson PA, Rubenstein AH, Steiner DF, Lernmark A (1981) Expression of major histocompatibility antigens on pancreatic islet cells. Proc Natl Acad Sci USA 78: 6456
25. Faustman D, Hauptfeld V, Lacy PE, Davie JM (1981) Prolongation of murine islet allograft survival by pretreatment of islets with antibody directed to Ia determinants. Proc Natl Acad Sci USA 78: 5156-5159
26. Faustman DL, Steinman RM, Gebel HM, Hauptfeld V, Davie JM, Lacy PE (1984) Prevention of rejection of murine islet allografts by pretreatment with anti-dendritic cell antibody. Proc Natl Acad Sci USA 81: 3864-3868
27. Steinman RM, Witmer MD (1978) Lymphoid dendritic cells are potent stimulators of the primary mixed leukocyte reaction in mice. Proc Natl Acad Sci USA 75: 5132-5136
28. Nussenzweig MC, Steinman RM, Witmer MD, Gutchinov B (1982) A monoclonal antibody specific for mouse dendritic cells. Proc Natl Acad Sci USA 79: 161-165
29. Bowen KM, Lafferty KJ (1980) Reversal of diabetes by allogeneic islet transplantation without immunosuppression. Aust J Exp Biol Med Sci 58: 441-447
30. Lau H, Reemtsma K, Hardy MA (1984) Prolongation of rat islet allograft survival by direct ultraviolett irradiation of the graft. Science 223: 607-608

31. Pipeleers D, Pipeleers-Marichal M (1981) A method for the purification of A, B or D cells and for the isolation of coupled cells from isolated rat islets. Diabetologia 20: 654-663
32. Pipeleers D, Pipeleers-Marichal M, Gepts W, Van De Winkel M (1986) Purified islet cell grafts are tolerated without immunosuppressive treatment in allotransplanted diabetic rats. (Abstract). Presented at the second Assisi international symposium on advanced models for the therapy of insulin-dependent diabetes. Assisi, Italy
33. Tze WJ, Tai J (1983) Prolongation of islet allograft and xenograft in nonimmunosuppressed rat recipients. Metabolism 32: 279-282
34. Donohoe JA, Andrus L, Bowen KM, Simeonovic C, Prowse SJ, Lafferty KJ (1983) Cultured thyroid allografts induce a state of partial tolerance in adult recipient mice. Transplantation 35: 62-67
35. Zitron IM, Ono J, Lacy PE, Davie JM (1981) Active suppression in the maintenance of pancreatic islet allografts. Transplantation 32: 156-158
36. Talmage DW, Dart G, Radovich J, Lafferty KJ (1976) Activation of transplant immunity: effect of donor leukocytes on thyroid allograft rejection. Science 191: 385-388
37. Faustman D, Hauptfeld V, Lacy PE, Davie JM (1982) Demonstration of active tolerance in maintenance of established islet of Langerhans allografts. Proc Natl Acad Sci USA 79: 4153-4155
38. Faustman D, Lacy PE, Davie JM, Hauptfeld V (1982) Prevention of allograft rejection by immunization with donor blood depleted of Ia-bearing cells. Science 217: 157-158
39. Lau H, Reemtsma K, Hardy MA (1983) Pancreatic islet allograft prolongation by donor-specific blood transfusions treated with ultraviolett irradiation. Science 221: 754-756
40. Williams PW (1894) Notes on diabetes treated with extract and by grafts of sheep's pancreas. Br Med J 2: 1303
41. Luisada (1927) Cited by Fichera G Implanti omoplastici feto-umani nei cancro e nel diabete. Tumori 14: 434
42. Weber C, Weil R, McIntosh R, Hogle H, Warden G, Reemtsma K (1975) Xenotransplantation of piscine islets into hyperglycemic rats. Surgery 77: 208-215
43. Eloy R, Haffen K, Kedinger M, Grenier JF (1979) Chick embryo pancreatic transplants reverse experimental diabetes of rats. J Clin Invest 64: 361-373
44. Sollinger HW, Burkholder PM, Rasmus WR, Bach FH (1977) Prolonged survival of xenografts after organ culture. Surgery 81: 74-94
45. Lacy PE, Davie JM, Finke EH (1980) Prolongation of islet xenograft survival without continuous immunosuppression. Science 209: 283-285
46. Terasaka R, Lacy PE, Bucy RP, Davie JM (1986) Effect of cyclosporine A and low temperature culture on prevention of rejection of islet xenografts (rat to mouse). Transplantation 41: 661-662
47. Lacy PE, Finke EH, Janney CG, Davie JM (1982) Prolongation of islet xenograft survival by in vitro culture of rat megaislets in 95% O_2. Transplantation 33: 588-592
48. Ricordi C, Finke E, Lacy PE (1986) A method for the mass isolation of islets from the adult pig pancreas. Diabetes 35: 649-653
49. Janney CG, Davie JM, Lacy PE, Finke EH (1982) Characterization of lymphocytes from rejected and nonrejected islet xenografts. Transplantation 33: 585-587
50. Yasunami Y, Lacy PE, Finke EH (1983) A new site for islet transplantation - a peritoneal-omental pouch. Transplantation 36: 181-182
51. Finch DRA, Wise PH, Morris PJ (1977) Successful intra-splenic transplantation of syngeneic and allogeneic isolated pancreatic islets. Diabetologia 13: 195-199
52. Reese-Smith H, DuToit DF, McShane P, Morris PJ (1981) Prolonged survival of pancreatic islet allografts transplanted beneath the renal capsule. Transplantation 3k: 305-306
53. Bobzien B, Yasunami Y, Majercik M, Lacy PE, Davie JM (1983) Intratesticular transplants of islet xenografts (rat to mouse). Diabetes 32: 213-216
54. Tze WJ, Tai J (1983) Successful intracerebral allotransplantation of purified pancreatic endocrine cells in diabetic rat. Diabetes 32: 1185-1187
55. Selawry H, Fajaco R, Whittington K (1985) Intratesticular islet allografts in the spontaneously diabetic BB/W rat. Diabetes 34: 1019-1024
56. Oppenheim JJ, Stadler BM, Siraganian RP, Mage M, Mathieson B (1982) Lymphokines: their role in lymphocytes responses. Properties of interleukin-1- Fed Proc 41: 257

57. Lachman LB (1983) Human interleukin-1: purification and properties. Fed Proc 42: 2639
58. Postlethwaite AE, Lachman LB, Kang AH (1984) Induction of fibroblast proliferation by interleukin-1 derived from human monocytic leukemia cells. Arthritis Rheum 27: 995
59. Canalis E (1986) Interleukin-1 has independent effects on deoxyribonucleic acid and collagen synthesis in cultures of rat calvariae. Endocrinology 118: 74
60. Mandrup-Poulsen T, Bendtzen K, Nielson JH, Bendixen G, Nerup J (1985) Cytokines cause functional and structural damage to isolated islets of Langerhans. Allergy 40: 424
61. Mandrup-Poulsen T, Bendtzen K, Nerup J, Dinarello CA, Svenson M, Nielson JH (1986) Affinity-purified human interleukin-1 is cytotoxic to isolated islets of Langerhans. Diabetologia 29: 63
62. Bendten K, Mandrup-Poulsen T, Nerup J, Nielsen JH, Dinarello CA, Svenson M (1986) Cytotoxicity of human pI 7 interleukin-1 for pancreatic islets of Langerhans. Science 232: 1545
63. Comens PG, Wolf BA, Sullivan FP, Unanue ER, McDaniel ML (1986) Effects of interleukin-1 on insulin secretion. Diabetes, 35, 46A
64. Bottazzo GF, Pujol-Borrell R, Hanafusa T, Feldman M (1983) Role of aberrant HLA-DR expression and antigen presentation in induction of endocrine autoimmunity. Lancet 2: 1115
65. Bottazo GF, Dean BM, McNally JM, MacKay EH, Swift PGF, Gamble DR (1985) In situ characterization of autoimmune phenomena and expression of HLA molecules in the pancreas in diabetic insulitis. N Engl J Med 313: 353
66. Wong GHW, Clark-Lewis I, McKimm-Breschkin JL, Schrader JW (1982) Interferon-γ-like molecule induces Ia antigens on cultured mast cell progenitors. PNAS 79: 6989
67. Pober JS, Gimbrone MA Jr, Cotran RS, Reiss CS, Burakoff SJ, Fiers W, Ault KA (1983) Ia expression by vascular endothelium is inducible by activated T cells and by human γ interferon. J Exp Med 157: 1339
68. Pober JS, Collins T, Gimbrone MA Jr, Cotran RS, Gitlin JD, Fiers W, Clayberger C, Krensky AM, Burakoff SJ, Reiss CS (1983) Lymphocytes recognize human vascular endothelial and dermal fibroblast Ia antigens induced by recombinant immune interferon. Nature 305: 726
69. Collins T, Korman AJ, Wake CT, Boss JM, Kappes DJ, Fiers W, Ault KA, Gimbrone MA Jr, Strominger JL, Pober JS (1984) Immune interferon activates multiple class II major histocompatibility complex genes and the associated invariant chain gene in human endothelial cells and dermal fibroblasts. PNAS 81: 4917
70. Fossati G, Taramelli D, Balsari A, Bogdanovich G, Andreola S, Parmiani G (1984) Primary but not metastatic human melanomas expressing DR antigens stimulate autologous lymphocytes. Int J Cancer 33: 591
71. Wright JR, Lacy PE, Unanue ER, Muszynski C, Hauptfeld V (1986) Induction of Ia antigens on isolated murine islet cells with interferon-γ. Diabetes, 35, 88A
72. Kirkman RL, Barrett LV, Gaulton N, Kelley VE, Ythier A, Strom TB (1985) Administration of an anti-interleukin-2 receptor monoclonal antibody prolongs cardiac allograft survival in mice. J Exp Med 162: 358
73. Dialynas DP, Quan ZS, Wall KA, Pierres A, Quintans J, Loken MR, Pierres M, Fitch FW (1983) Characterization of the murine T cell surface molecule, designated L3T4, identified by monoclonal antibody GK 1.5: similarity of L3T4 to the human Leu-3/T4 molecule. J Immunology 131: 2445-2451
74. Shizuri JA, Gregory AK, Chao CT, Fathman CG (1986) Anti-L3T4 mediated tolerance induction for allogeneic islet transplantation. Diabetes 35: 350
75. Simeonovic CJ, Bowen KM, Kitlarski I, Lafferty KJ (1980) Modulation of tissue immunogenicity by organ culture. Transplantation 30: 174
76. Simeonovic CJ, Lafferty KJ (1982) The isolation and transplantation of foetal mouse proislets. Aust J Exp Biol Med Sci 60: 383
77. Simeonovic CJ, Lafferty JH (1982) Immunogenicity of isolated foetal mouse proislets. Aust J Exp Biol Med Sci 60: 391
78. Horaguchi A, Merrell RC (1981) Preparation of viable islet cells from dogs by a new method. Diabetes 30: 455-458
79. Lacy PE, Lacy ET, Finke EH, Yasunami Y (1982) An improved method for the isolation of islets from the beef pancreas. Diabetes 31: 109-111
80. Harrison DE, Christie MR, Gray DWR (1985) Properties of isolated human islets of Langer-

hans: insulin secretion, glucose oxidation and protein phosphorylation. Diabetologia 28: 99-103
81. Scharp DW, Lacy PE (1985) Human islet isolation and transplantation. Diabetes, 34, 5 A
82. JDFI First World Conference on Diabetes Research. Held in Monaco, November, 1985. 125 pp. Copyright by JDFI, 1986
83. Sibley RK, Sutherland DER, Goetz F, Michael AF (1985) Recurrent diabetes mellitus in the pancreas isoand allograft. A light and electron microscopic immunohistochemical analysis of four cases. Lab Invest 53: 132-144
84. Woehrle M, Markmann JF, Silvers WK, Barker CF, Naji A (1986) Transplantation of cultured pancreatic islets to BB rats. Surgery 100: 334-341

Subject Index

a

b

C

h

i

j

k

l

p

r

s

t

u

v

w

y

z

MIX
Papier aus verantwortungsvollen Quellen
Paper from responsible sources
FSC® C105338

If you have any concerns about our products,
you can contact us on
ProductSafety@springernature.com

In case Publisher is established outside the EU,
the EU authorized representative is:
Springer Nature Customer Service Center GmbH
Europaplatz 3, 69115 Heidelberg, Germany

Printed by Libri Plureos GmbH
in Hamburg, Germany